Youth:
Choices *and* Change

Promoting Healthy Behaviors in Adolescents

SCIENTIFIC AND TECHNICAL PUBLICATION No. 594

Youth:
Choices *and* Change

Promoting Healthy Behaviors in Adolescents

Cecilia Breinbauer and Matilde Maddaleno

Produced with support from:

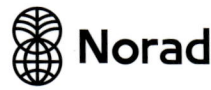

NORWEGIAN AGENCY FOR DEVELOPMENT COOPERATION

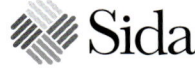

SWEDISH INTERNATIONAL DEVELOPMENT COOPERATION AGENCY

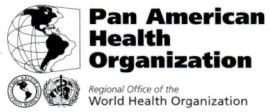

PAN AMERICAN HEALTH ORGANIZATION
Pan American Sanitary Bureau, Regional Office of the
WORLD HEALTH ORGANIZATION
525 Twenty-third Street, N.W.
Washington, D.C. 20037 U.S.A.

2005

PAHO HQ Library Cataloguing-in-Publication

Breinbauer, Cecilia
    Youth: Choices and Change. Promoting Healthy Behaviors in Adolescents
Washington, D.C.: PAHO, © 2005.
(Scientific and Technical Publication No. 594)

ISBN 92 75 11594 X

I. Title   II. Series
III. Maddaleno, Matilde

1. TEEN HEALTH
2. ADOLESCENT HEALTH SERVICES
3. ADOLESCENT PSYCHOLOGY — trends
4. ADOLESCENT BEHAVIOR

NLM WS460

The Pan American Health Organization welcomes requests for permission to reproduce or translate its publications, in part or in full. Applications and inquiries should be addressed to the Publications Area, Pan American Health Organization, Washington, D.C., U.S.A., which will be glad to provide the latest information on any changes made to the text, plans for new editions, and reprints and translations already available.

© Pan American Health Organization, 2005

Publications of the Pan American Health Organization enjoy copyright protection in accordance with the provisions of Protocol 2 of the Universal Copyright Convention. All rights are reserved.
The designations employed and the presentation of the material in this publication do not imply the expression of any opinion whatsoever on the part of the Secretariat of the Pan American Health Organization concerning the status of any country, territory, city, or area or of its authorities, or concerning the delimitation of its frontiers or boundaries.

The mention of specific companies or of certain manufacturers' products does not imply that they are endorsed or recommended by the Pan American Health Organization in preference to others of a similar nature that are not mentioned. Errors and omissions excepted, the names of proprietary products are distinguished by initial capital letters.

Cover design by Ultradesigns
Silver Spring, Maryland, U.S.A.

"Good habits formed at youth make all the difference."

–Aristotle (384–322 B.C.)
Greek philosopher

"In youth, we clothe ourselves with rainbows, and go as brave as the zodiac."

–Ralph Waldo Emerson (1803–1882)
U.S. philosopher, essayist, poet
"Fate" in The Conduct of Life, *1860*

"There is a period near the beginning of every man's life where he has little to cling to except his unmanageable dream, little to support him except good health, and nowhere to go but all over the place."

–E. B. White (1899–1985)
U.S. author and editor
"The Years of Wonder" Essays of E.B. White, *1977*

"The essence of our effort to see that every child has a chance must be to assure each an equal opportunity, not to be equal, but to become different—to realize whatever unique potential of body, mind, and spirit he or she possesses."

–John Fischer
Dean, Teachers College, Columbia University, 1973

Contents

Preface / xi

The Authors / xiii

Acknowledgments / xv

Foreword
Paving the Way from Adolescence to a Healthy Adulthood / *xvii*

Introduction
Healthy Choices and Changes / *xxi*

SECTION ONE

DEVELOPING EFFECTIVE HEALTH PROMOTION AND PREVENTION PROGRAMS FOR ADOLESCENTS / 1

Introduction / 2

Chapter One
Adolescent Lifestyles in Latin America and the Caribbean: The Challenges and Their Scope / *5*

Chapter Two
The Knowledge-Behavior Gap in Health Promotion / *13*

Chapter Three
The Importance of Behavior Theories to Successful Adolescent Health Programs / *16*

Chapter Four
Adolescents Living in a Complex Environment of Multiple Levels of Influence / *20*

Chapter Five
Listening to Adolescents' Needs and Wants: A Respectful Intervention / *29*

Chapter Six
The Crucial Link between Theories and Developmental Stages of Adolescence / *34*

Chapter Seven
The Youth: Choices and Change Model for Designing Effective Interventions for Adolescents / *37*

SECTION TWO

THEORIES AND MODELS FOR HEALTH PROMOTION AND BEHAVIOR CHANGE:
THEIR APPLICATION TO ADOLESCENTS / 45

Theories and Models that Promote Change at the Individual Level / 46

Chapter Eight
The Health Belief Model / 49

Chapter Nine
The Transtheoretical Model and Stages of Change / 55

Chapter Ten
The Theory of Reasoned Action / 71

Chapter Eleven
The Theory of Planned Behavior / 78

Chapter Twelve
The Goal-Setting Theory / 87

Chapter Thirteen
The Self-Regulation Theory / 94

Chapter Fourteen
The Sensation-Seeking Theory / 102

Chapter Fifteen
At a Glance: The Individual Level Theories and Models for Behavior Change / 111

Theories and Models that Promote Change at the Interpersonal Level / 118

Chapter Sixteen
The Social Cognitive Theory / 119

Chapter Seventeen
The Social Networks and Social Support Theories / 137

Chapter Eighteen
The Authoritative Parenting Model / 153

Chapter Nineteen
The Resiliency Theory / 168

Chapter Twenty
The Stress and Coping Theories / 176

Chapter Twenty-one
At a Glance: The Interpersonal Level Theories and Models for Behavior Change / 190

Theories and Models that Promote Change at the Community Level / 195

Chapter Twenty-two
The Community Organization Models / 196

Chapter Twenty-three
The Diffusion of Innovations Theory, Behavior Change Communication Models, and Social Marketing / *209*

Models that Promote Change at the Policy Level / *224*

Chapter Twenty-four
Models of Policy and Legislation Development / *226*

Chapter Twenty-five
At a Glance: The Community and Policy Level Theories and Models for Behavior Change / *244*

SECTION THREE

ADOLESCENT DEVELOPMENTAL CHANGES AND GOALS:
THE IMPORTANCE OF EARLY INTERVENTION / 253

Introduction / *254*

Chapter Twenty-six
A New Approach to Classifying Adolescent Developmental Stages / *257*

Chapter Twenty-seven
Gender Differences and Adolescent Behaviors / *269*

Chapter Twenty-eight
Early Intervention during Adolescence: The Preadolescent Period / *277*

Chapter Twenty-nine
Early Intervention during Adolescence: The Early Adolescent Period / *306*

SECTION FOUR

CONCLUSIONS AND RECOMMENDATIONS / 333

Introduction / *334*

Chapter Thirty
The Next Decade: Perspectives for Improving Adolescent Health and Development / *337*

Afterword / *347*

References / *349*

Selected List of Web Resources on Adolescence and Health Behaviors / *387*

Preface

The book you hold in your hands is quite unique in numerous respects. While the behavioral change theories and models presented in it have been utilized by social science researchers for several decades, the findings of their application, specifically to adolescents, have been systematically collected and are being reported here for the first time. This book also represents the first attempt to incorporate a developmental perspective in the conceptual analysis of these classical theoretical constructs when applied to various stages of adolescence. Such a perspective will enable planners and developers of health promotion interventions to identify and address differences in behavioral and socio-emotional capabilities between 13-year-olds and 18-year-olds, for example, and then design programs that effectively respond to the specific needs and wants of each developmental stage.

Cultural, ethnic, and gender differences are also given special consideration, as are the role of poverty and the ability of some adolescents to secure physical and emotional well-being despite circumstances of adversity. In addition, much of the information included in this book regarding critical developmental distinctions between the preadolescent and early adolescent stages, while gleaned by clinicians through years of experience working with these age groups, has been compiled and is being presented here for the first time, with a particular focus on its implications for public health interventions.

This book also breaks new ground in explaining why some health promotion interventions aimed at positive adolescent behavior change produce the desired results, while others fail. The thoroughness of the analysis extends to the diversity of geographical settings that provide a backdrop for the studies cited: from Africa to the United States, Canada to Jamaica, Brazil to the Netherlands, El Salvador to Japan, and India to Mexico, to name only a few. My specific desire is that the experiences of the global research community presented here will find fertile ground among a variety of publics throughout Latin America and the Caribbean. This audience would include local health promoters, designers of community health promotion programs, health professionals, the academic and research community, ministries of public health and of youth affairs, those who study and those who create mass media trends, parents and teachers, school counselors, and all others who play a significant role in adolescents' lives.

By working together across a variety of levels—interpersonal, community, and policy—these groups, and their counterparts in countries across the world, hold tremendous potential to encourage the adoption of health-promoting lifestyles among adolescents. One of this book's central lessons is that the cornerstone for success in instilling lifelong healthy behaviors is early intervention, beginning in the preadolescent years, before health-compromising behaviors have taken deep root. This lesson forms the underpinning of the Youth: Choices and Change Model created by PAHO and also being presented for the first time here. By following the steps proposed, developers of adolescent health programs can help young people master the developmental goals appropriate for their age group, strengthen their ability to make conscious decisions for health, and achieve their self-set goals for the future.

Young people, particularly those in the 15-to-24 age group, figure prominently in four of the Millennium Development Goals adopted by member countries of the United Nations in 2000. Nearly one in every three persons in Latin America and the Caribbean today is between 10 and 24 years of age. Therefore, actions for the empowerment of tomorrow's generation—such as ensuring universal education and gender equality, and improving HIV/AIDS prevention strategies and socioeconomic opportunities for youth as they commence their economically productive years—can play a pivotal role in the achievement of the umbrella goal of extreme poverty reduction by the year 2015.

Mirta Roses
Director

The Authors

Cecilia Breinbauer is a psychiatrist specializing in child and adolescent health. She received her medical degree from the University of Chile, followed by postgraduate training in child psychiatry. Since then, Breinbauer has dedicated her professional life to working with children, adolescents, and their families in the promotion of healthy development and parenting. She has enjoyed the close mentorship of Stanley Greenspan, Clinical Professor of Psychiatry, Behavioral Sciences, and Pediatrics at The George Washington University School of Medicine, who is internationally recognized for his research in the area of healthy childhood emotional development. Breinbauer is a member of the Interdisciplinary Council on Developmental and Learning Disorders Advisory Board, where she serves as chair of the public health committee, coordinator for the Latin America and Caribbean network, and president of the Chilean chapter. With the goal of adding a public health perspective to her extensive clinical experience, Breinbauer is currently pursuing a master's degree in public health at The George Washington University in Washington, D.C. Since 2001, she has also served in the Pan American Health Organization's Child and Adolescent Health Unit. Breinbauer is the proud mother of three early adolescents.

Matilde Maddaleno is a pediatrician specializing in adolescence. Following receipt of her medical degree from the University of Chile, she completed postgraduate training in pediatrics. She also holds a master's degree in public health from The George Washington University. From 1986 to 1995, Maddaleno directed the Adolescent and Youth Program in Peñalolen, Chile, and, until 1996, served as assistant professor in pediatrics at her alma mater, where she was also a member of the Curricula Development and Research Advisory Group. From 1992 to 1994, Maddaleno directed the W.K. Kellogg Foundation's Project to Promote Comprehensive Services for Children and Adolescents in the Eastern Metropolitan Area of Santiago, and from 1994 to 1996 was an advisor to the Chilean National Adolescent Health Program. From 1999 until April 2004, Maddaleno served as Adjunct Assistant Professor of Global Health at The George Washington University. Since 1996, she has served as Regional Advisor in Adolescent and Youth Health and Development for the Pan American Health Organization. In this role, she has overseen the provision of technical cooperation to Latin America and the Caribbean designed to enable governments to develop integrated national programs and services in adolescent health, including strengthening institutional capacity and increasing opportunities for professional training in adolescent public health. During her time at PAHO, Maddaleno has been an outspoken advocate for youth policy development within and outside the Organization, and she and the PAHO adolescent health team have successfully promoted fundraising and resource mobilization at the national and regional levels. In 2001, she was the recipient of an International Association for Adolescent Health Founders' Award for excellence in the field. Maddaleno is the proud mother of two late adolescents.

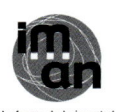

THE PAHO IMAN PROJECT
This book is part of the PAHO Child and Adolescent Health Unit's Integrated Management of Adolescent Needs (IMAN) Project, which focuses not only on the provision of health services, but additionally on health promotion and prevention measures, and seeks to offer priority countries in the Region of the Americas an integrated package of successful interventions in adolescent and youth health and development. IMAN consists of four components: information services, health services, human resources development, and family and community interventions.

Acknowledgments

The authors wish to express their appreciation for the input of numerous PAHO technical staff and consultants whose valuable expertise and insights helped to sharpen the focus and strengthen the messages presented in this book. These include Benjamin Berman, Paul Bloem, Jose Miguel Caldas, Gloria Coe, Lucimar Coser Cannon, Jane Ferguson, Rafael Flores, Francisca Infante, Enrique Jacobby, V. Chandra Mouli, Rafael Obregón, Armando Peruga, Marilyn Rice, Jessie Schutt-Aine, Heather Selin, Sylvia Singleton, and Alex Vega. Practical feedback was additionally provided by numerous professionals working in adolescent health promotion and prevention programs in Latin America and the Caribbean. The authors especially thank Gina Tambini, PAHO's Family and Community Health Area Manager, and Yehuda Benguigui, PAHO's Child and Adolescent Health Unit Chief, for their continuous support to our work. A special debt of gratitude is owed to Stanley Greenspan and Georgia DeGangi, who generously shared their time and clinical experiences, thereby providing important underpinnings for Section Three's focus on the preadolescent and early adolescent stages of development and on the importance of early intervention. Finally, the authors reserve a special mention for the leadership and talent of PAHO's Publications Area team, without whom this book could not have been possible.

The Pan American Health Organization extends its appreciation to the Norwegian Agency for Development Cooperation (Norad) and the Swedish International Development Cooperation Agency (Sida) for their collaboration on this project. The support of these organizations has been crucial to the formation of this book's developmental approach and focus on innovative ways to promote healthy lifestyles among youth.

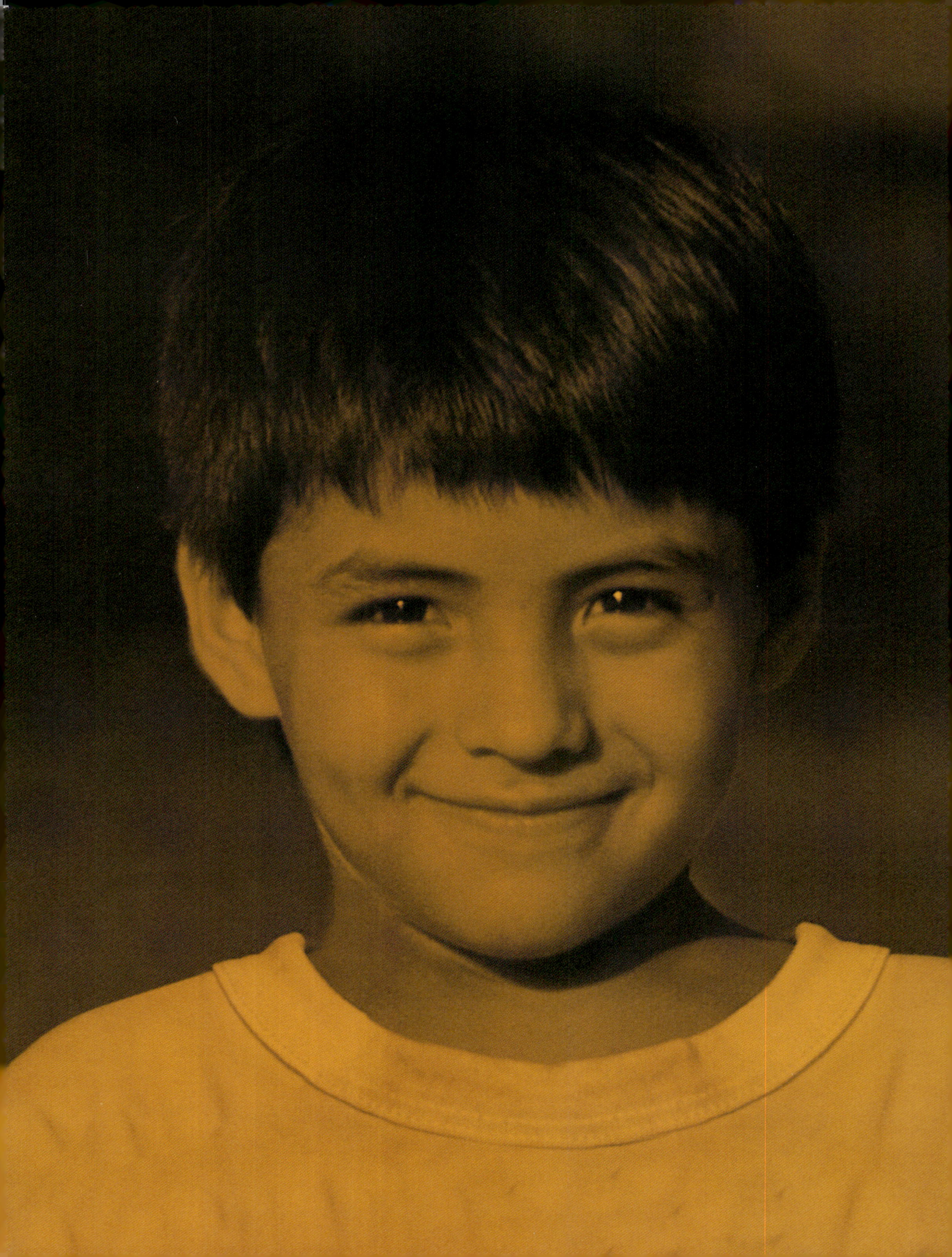

[Foreword]

Paving the Way from Adolescence to a Healthy Adulthood

"Oh youth, youth! You don't worry about anything; you seem to possess all the treasures of the universe. . . . And perhaps the whole secret of your charm lies not in your ability to do everything, but in your ability to think that you will do everything."
—Ivan Sergeevich Turgenev (1818–1883)
  Russian author

Adolescence is a time of unprecedented curiosity about life and the decoding of its inner workings. This curiosity is fueled by boundless energy and a nascent sense of independence and power as the prospects of becoming a full-fledged adult draw ever nearer. The possibilities for experimentation proliferate, opening unexpected doors leading to previously unimagined roads. The opportunities for accelerated sociopsychological growth and the consolidation of personal identity are counterbalanced by the equally potent dangers adolescents face as they navigate this vast uncharted territory called "coming of age."

All those who work to improve and protect the health and well-being of adolescents are, perhaps more than any other care-giving profession, faced with a series of unique challenges. In the physical sense, none is more robust and uncompromised by debilitating health conditions than this age group. At the same time, mental acuity is never sharper nor powers of information retention stronger.

Perhaps for these very reasons, traditional adolescent health programs and policies, whether local or national in scope, have tended to be narrow in focus and curative in nature in addressing such behavior-related issues as HIV/AIDS, pregnancy, gang violence, and abuse of tobacco, alcohol, and drugs. To the degree to which the services developed are oriented to specific problems, they have differed little from those of disease prevention and control programs in that they have often defined success by the absence or disappearance of the problem at hand.

Because these programs tend to be vertical in approach, they usually do not take into account the broad social context within which the problem first arose. Nor are the needs, concerns, and rights of the adolescents themselves fully recognized or incorporated into the design of interventions. The input of family, teachers, peers, and other significant others is often overlooked and/or underutilized, as are gender- and culture-related considerations and the changing developmental needs of young people at different ages.

Latin America and the Caribbean have been at the forefront of developing policies, programs, and services for adolescents in the Region of the Americas. But in these countries, as elsewhere around the world, many of these initiatives currently adhere to the traditional approaches described above. Yet over the past decades, awareness has grown of the need to move beyond a problem-oriented approach to adolescent health to a developmental approach based on the basic precepts of health promotion, as highlighted in the historic Ottawa Charter adopted by the countries of the Americas and others around the world at the International Conference on Health Promotion on 21 November 1986.

As stated in the Charter,

> Health promotion is the process of enabling people to increase control over, and to improve, their health. To reach a state of complete physical, mental, and social well-being, an individual or group must be able to identify and to realize aspirations, to satisfy needs, and to change or cope with the environment. . . . Good health is a major resource for social, economic, and personal development and an important dimension of quality of life. Political, economic, social, cultural, environmental, behavioral, and biological factors can all favor health or be harmful to it.

The cornerstones of the health promotion strategy—building healthy public policy, creating supportive environments, strengthening community actions, developing personal skills, and reorienting health services—are particularly relevant in addressing the challenges of improving and protecting the health and well-being of adolescents in that they widen the playing field of potential resources and indicate new variables to be considered by program planners and designers.

The central element of all successful health promotion and prevention programs is the underlying theoretical framework (DiClemente, Crosby, and Kegler 2002; Glanz, Rimer, and Lewis 2002) and determining why this particular framework is meaningful and effective in addressing local challenges. There has been a growing effort to identify, describe, analyze, and replicate those evidence-based intervention models which have produced the most positive results in enabling adolescents to adopt and maintain health-promoting lifestyles and/or change health-compromising lifestyles.

Of particular concern is the growing body of evidence that while public health interventions can successfully increase young people's knowledge about the health issues most affecting them—such as risky sexual practices and substance abuse—the mere provision of information is not enough to lead to positive and sustained behavior change. What is missing are interventions that successfully *motivate* adolescents to *use* the information and services available and *develop the skills* necessary to become *actors of their own change*.

Youth: Choices and Change is being produced by the Pan American Health Organization (PAHO) as a guide to help those who work with adolescents and youth[1] identify the most effective theoretical frameworks for health promotion and prevention programs that are tailored to the distinct developmental goals, needs, and wants of young people at different ages and that take into account gender and cultural background considerations. In addition, it provides tools that will enable program developers to design, implement, and evaluate interventions and services that are relevant and appropriate to local conditions and circumstances. It reviews literature containing the classical health promotion and behavior change theories and models most frequently utilized in health education today and includes a critical analysis of their application and effectiveness.

The systematic compilation of these theories and models in one source—combined with a comprehensive conceptual analysis of each, as applied specifically to adolescent behavior and incorporating a developmental perspective—make this publication a unique contribution to the study of adolescent health. PAHO's Child and Adolescent Health Unit, as part of the Family and Community Health Area, is pleased to present this book with the desire that it find resonance among a variety of audiences: policymakers, program designers at the local and national levels, health professionals, university professors and students, researchers, and all others interested in the fields of health promotion and adolescent health.

---

[1] PAHO and the World Health Organization define adolescence as the period between 10 and 19 years of age and youth as the period between 15 and 24 years; the term "young people" is used to indicate both groups.

[Introduction]

Healthy Choices and Changes

"Perfection of means and confusion of goals seem, in my opinion, to characterize our age."
—Albert Einstein
  Out of My Later Years, 1950

Einstein's observation was made over a half century ago, yet it still holds true today: the search for precision and "excellence" in the means often causes us to lose sight of the ultimate goal. The resulting confusion can claim its toll on public health initiatives, no matter how well intentioned. In the case of adolescent health, program developers must remember that while different behavior change models might represent effective *means* to the adoption of health-promoting lifestyles, the ultimate goal is *positive, sustainable behavioral change which enables young people to become actors of their own change and achieve their self-set goals.* As expressed in the Ottawa Charter, health promotion is a means to increase the control people have over the determinants of their own health by increasing self-care capacities, which are the decisions and actions individuals take regarding their health.

Youth: Choices and Change provides a variety of theoretical frameworks within which health professionals and others dedicated to improving the health of adolescents and youth may design mechanisms to stimulate the development of healthy lifestyle choices. By strengthening youths' decision-making capacity and encouraging them to take advantage of enhanced social support systems within the community, the impetus for behavioral change receives both immediate and ongoing positive reinforcement.

From a broad health promotion perspective, encouraging adolescents to adopt and maintain healthy lifestyles and behaviors is crucial to reducing the burden of chronic diseases in Latin America and the Caribbean countries, given that many of the unhealthy habits that later produce morbidity and mortality in adults are acquired during the period of adolescence (PAHO 1998). At the same time, as we will see in Chapter One, young people in this region of the world represent a growing segment of the overall population, and therefore their health and development will be a key element for the region's socioeconomic and political progress now and in the coming years (PAHO 2000a).

In today's world of sophisticated targeting of young people by the fast food, tobacco, and alcohol industries; nearly universal access to television; the glamorization of sexual experimentation; and peer pressure; youth are inundated with messages that both subtly and blatantly push health-compromising activities. The social pressure to adopt the risky lifestyles depicted in commercial advertising is enormous. In this sense, promoting the importance of healthy lifestyles and environments must compete with other messages that young people often find more attractive. At the same time, evidence shows that while public health interventions can successfully increase adolescent and youths' knowledge about health risks, this awareness is not, in and of itself, always enough to change unhealthy behaviors.

This means that while young people may have access to information and may even know that certain behaviors and practices are unsafe, this is not sufficient to persuade them to change their actions. Instead, youth must be motivated to develop the skills and assets necessary to prepare for the coming years of change through a sense of positive empowerment and the personal conviction that they have the capacity to make conscious choices about their lives, including the desirability of moving away from negative influences and situations as a means of self-preservation and enrichment.

Youth: Choices and Change has four sections. In the first, an overview is provided of adolescent lifestyles in Latin America and the Caribbean, indicating the scope of the challenge for health promotion programs and policymakers. The need to bridge the knowledge-behavior change gap is highlighted, followed by a discussion of the importance of adopting a suitable theoretical framework as the basic foundation for achieving successful and respectful interventions. The book's first section also underscores the crucial link between the different stages of adolescent development and the use of behavior change and health promotion theories and models specifically tailored to these stages, including appropriate gender and cultural background considerations. In Section One's final chapter, the authors describe the Youth: Choices and Change Model and explain why the Pan American Health Organization recommends it as an effective tool for the design of health interventions for adolescents.

The book's second section analyzes the most prominent theories and models on behavior change and health promotion in use with a developmental perspective, noting that program developers should not only consider theories and models focusing on individual change but also those which promote change at the interpersonal, community, and policy levels. The reader will find an extensive literature review of the applications of the different theories and models when encouraging the adoption and maintenance of health-promoting behaviors and the cessation of health-compromising behaviors in adolescents.

Section Three underscores the importance of understanding the different developmental processes through which adolescents will pass and how this progression must serve as the context within which any given theoretical framework will be applied. The authors note that while many of the classical behavior change and health promotion theories and models described in the previous section hold great promise, they can only achieve the desired results if program designers understand the changing needs and wants of adolescents at different stages of development and tailor interventions and goals accordingly. PAHO considers the preadolescent and early adolescent age groups[1] to be the most overlooked by adolescent health programs and emphasizes the importance of promoting the adoption and maintenance of healthy behaviors beginning with preadolescence, instead of waiting until later, when health-compromising behaviors have already begun and may be well entrenched, thus becoming more difficult to change. In this section's closing chapters, PAHO presents a series of developmentally appropriate goals to be considered when planning health promotion and prevention programs for these two age groups.

The fourth and final section synthesizes the contents of the previous three sections and highlights the unique contributions of this book, particularly its emphasis on early intervention during the preadolescent and early adolescent years and on the incorporation of a growth and developmental perspective in the creation of adolescent health promotion programs. It also offers insight into the current socioeconomic challenges and advantages facing youth in Latin America and the Caribbean and presents a review of international commitments undertaken by the member countries of the United Nations designed to strengthen the health and development of young people in the Region of the Americas. The section concludes with a series of recommendations for improving health and development opportunities for this group over the next decade.

PAHO's Child and Adolescent Health Unit presents this book in the hope that it will stimulate and further refine dialogue—in the academic and public health communities, on national political agendas, and beyond—about the need to promote and protect the health and well-being of young people everywhere, as today's precious resource and a solid investment in tomorrow's sustained socioeconomic development.

---

[1] Preadolescence refers to girls ages 9–12 and boys ages 10–13; early adolescence refers to ages 12–14 and 13–15, respectively.

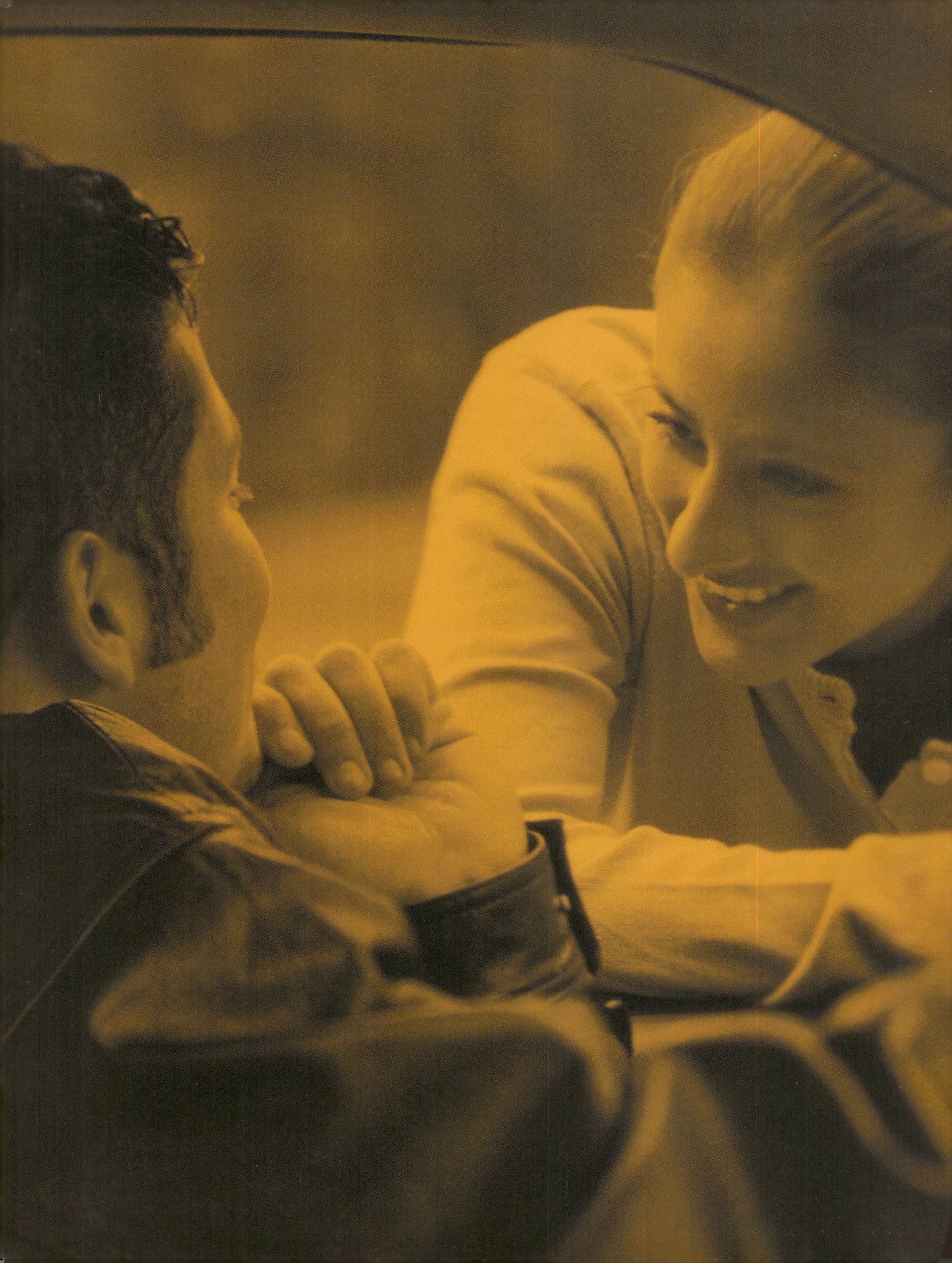

[Section One]

Developing Effective Health Promotion and Prevention Programs for Adolescents

Introduction

The first section of *Youth: Choices and Change* opens with an overview of the status of adolescent health in Latin America and the Caribbean, the principal focus of technical cooperation activities of the Pan American Health Organization (PAHO). The four areas of adolescent lifestyle behavior introduced in Chapter One—sexual activity; violence; alcohol, tobacco, and drug abuse; and nutrition and physical activity—will continue to be those of interest in subsequent analyses throughout the remainder of the book. Chapter Two will discuss why increasing access to health information and enabling adolescents to become more knowledgeable about health issues in general are oftentimes not enough to convince them to adopt healthier behaviors and lifestyles. Chapter Three highlights the importance of designing health promotion programs and interventions that are guided by the appropriate health behavior theory or theories. Too often, though, health promotion and prevention programs are based primarily on precedent, tradition, intuition, or general principles, without a full understanding of the theoretical frameworks that lead to interventions that achieve actual behavior change (Glanz, Rimer, and Lewis 2002). It is PAHO's hope that publication of this book will contribute to measurable improvements in the near future of this current situation.

Chapter Four identifies the multiple levels of influence found in the adolescent's world and stresses the need for behavior change interventions to incorporate both individual and environmental approaches, as well as to apply multiple strategies in multiple settings and include various levels of assessment (e.g., social, epidemiological, behavioral, environmental, educational, ecological, administrative, policy) and of evaluation (e.g., process, impact, outcome). This chapter concludes with a guide proposed by PAHO that builds on the factors that *predispose*, *enable*, and *reinforce* the choice of individual lifestyles and/or shape environmental conditions, as found in the classical PRECEDE-PROCEED model for health promotion planning and evaluation, by linking these three forces to the framework of theories and models to be presented in Section Two of this book.

The importance of listening to and understanding adolescent *needs* and *wants*—and integrating a response to these into the intervention design—is the subject of Chapter Five, whereas Chapter Six presents another crucial step that is also often overlooked, as well: assessing adolescents within their current developmental stage and tailoring interventions specifically for the abilities and interests of that particular age group.

The basic elements presented in Chapters One through Six provide a complete framework within which health promoters may develop a series of interventions to enable adolescents to achieve and maintain healthy behaviors and lifestyles. The Youth: Choices and Change Model, developed by PAHO and presented in Chapter Seven, is an embodiment of this framework and allows designers to build programs using a step-by-step approach.

[Chapter One]

Adolescent Lifestyles in Latin America and the Caribbean: The Challenges and Their Scope

Young people in the Region of the Americas represent a growing and increasingly important socioeconomic segment of the population. In Latin America and the Caribbean countries, young people between the ages of 10 and 24 make up 30% of the population, with adolescents aged 10–19 representing 20% of the population and 80% of them living in urban areas (Comisión Económica para América Latina y el Caribe 2000). Of the 155 million young people living in the Americas, the highest percentage is concentrated in the Region's poorer countries and communities (Pan American Health Organization 2002b, 2000b). Many youths are indigenous and are subsequently marginalized from mainstream culture. According to census data, there are close to a million indigenous youths living in Bolivia (1992) and Guatemala (1994), and 2.7 million in Peru (1992) (Comisión Económica para América Latina y el Caribe 2001).

Sexual Activity

Approximately one-half of all adolescents in the Region under the age of 17 are sexually active. The average age of first sexual intercourse in many Latin American countries is approximately 15–16 years for girls and 14–15 years for boys (Pan American Health Organization 2002b). Adolescent boys in certain Caribbean countries initiate sexual activity as early as 10–12 years of age (Pan American Health Organization 2002b), and by age 15, 90% have had sex (Pan American Health Organization 2002c). Of the sexually active, between 48% and 53% never use contraceptives, and among those who do, approximately 40% do not use any protection on a regular basis (Pan American Health Organization 2002c). In the Dominican Republic, 44% of girls have had sex before 15 years of age, and 78% of this group have been pregnant (Calderón 2002). A high rate of Peruvian women (62%) who had initiated sexual activity before age 15 reported a coercive sexual initiation (Cáceres et al. 2000). Data from Guatemala indicate that although 69% of adolescents between the ages of 15 and 19 report knowledge of at least one family planning method, only 4% of sexually active adolescents report using one regularly (Pan American Health Organization 2002c). Surveys in the Caribbean suggest that 40% of girls and 50% of boys had no access to contraceptives during their first sexual intercourse.

Around half of all new HIV infections are in individuals aged 15–24, the range during which most people start their sexual lives (Joint United Nations Programme on HIV/AIDS 1998). Youths in Brazil, Haiti, Honduras, Panama, and various English-speaking Caribbean countries are particularly affected by the epidemic. It is estimated that 4.9% of males between the ages of 15 and 24 are infected in Haiti, and 1.7% of adolescent girls and 1.4% of adolescent boys in Honduras. In Brazil, 0.7% of adolescent boys are estimated to be infected but, given the country's large population size, the actual number of adolescents with HIV is reason for concern because it greatly increases the potential to spread the virus (United Nations Children's Fund 2000). The Bahamas reports a 25% increase in the incidence of HIV/AIDS in adolescents from 1999 to 2000 (Pan American Health Organization 2002c).

Program designers are confronted with an urgent but sensitive challenge. It is urgent because of the growing AIDS epidemic, and it is sensitive because the systems of values and beliefs regarding adolescent sex vary widely from community to community. The resulting situation has revived the traditional debate about whether it is best to promote condom use or abstinence in a social culture where enormous gender differences continue to prevail: a "macho" culture that promotes early sexual initiation among boys and abstinence among girls. The challenge is how to help adolescents become more mindful about their sexual lifestyle choices and see the value of avoiding early sex, even when this age group is flooded with conflicting social messages and pressures (media, older and more experienced peers) that encourage adolescents, particularly boys, to engage in sexual activity.

Other kinds of social messages tend to encourage ignorance and shame when dealing with sexual situations, especially when targeted to girls. For this reason, being able to decide when to have sex and how to protect themselves from early pregnancy, HIV, sexually transmitted infections, and sexual coercion is crucial to a girl's sense of being in control. Evidence shows that education on sexual health and/or HIV does not encourage increased sexual activity among adolescents (World Health Organization 2002a). The challenge is to go beyond traditional sexuality education programs that only increase information (Eggleston et al. 2000) and instead seek to strengthen adolescents' skills to adopt and maintain safer sex practices, either through a delay in sexual initiation or contraceptive and/or condom use. To achieve this, interventions need to target not only individual adolescents but also their parents and the community, by allowing access to condoms and contraceptives when needed and pushing for changes in social norms that encourage early sex.

Violence

In Latin America and the Caribbean countries, violence surrounds adolescents, especially poor, urban youths. The pervasiveness of violence is clearly recognized as one of the most urgent threats to adolescent health and development throughout the Americas. The leading causes of death among those ages 10–19 years are external and include violence and homicide. Twenty-nine percent of all homicides in the Americas occur in this age group. Violence in adolescence is not limited to physical or sexual trauma but also includes emotional and verbal abuse, threats, and other types of psychological abuse (Pan American Health Organization 2002b, World Health Organization 2002d).

Sexual abuse and domestic violence have also increased their profile: in the Caribbean Adolescent Health Survey (CAHS), conducted in 2000 among youths from nine English-speaking Caribbean countries, 17% of adolescent males and 15% of adolescent females reported having been physically abused. Nearly one in three of those surveyed expressed concern about the level of violence in their community. To the extent that violence is seen as a socially accepted method of anger expression and conflict resolution, these young people said they grow up in fear of being either the victim of violence or a witness to it before reaching adulthood.

The CAHS also found that owning or shooting a gun is viewed as a symbol of manhood in several countries. Seventeen percent of males reported having been in a fight where weapons were used, 20% said they had carried a weapon to school in the past 30 days, 31% had carried a weapon at times other than during school hours in the last 30 days, and 22% admitted that they have belonged to a gang at one point or another in their lives. In the same survey, 39% of 13–15-year-olds reported sometimes thinking about hurting or killing someone, while 5% reported always thinking about it (Pan American Health Organization 2000a).

Program designers are confronted with the challenge of how to address the multi-level determinants of youth violence, involving individual characteristics (e.g., difficult temperament and impulsiveness), family variables (e.g., economic stress, poor parenting, family abuse, parental substance abuse), and societal factors (e.g., access to weapons, media violence, inequitable educational and occupational opportunities, political violence) that contribute to this epidemic (World Health Organization 2002b, Weist and

Cooley-Quille 2001, Webber 1997, Ollendick 1996).

Gender violence also plays a key role in youth violence and development in Latin America and the Caribbean, where the culture of machismo accepts violence as a way to solve conflicts as part of the social norm. Masculinity development is embedded in this culture where the traditional path to becoming a man involves being verbally and physically aggressive, solving conflicts through fights, and exercising power and control over women (Aguirre and Güell 2002). In the design of programs, early intervention and prevention are key: programs targeted to younger children should be coordinated with those directed toward preadolescents and adolescents, with a view toward developing nonviolent capabilities for anger expression and conflict resolution across the life cycle, focusing on new alternative paths to masculinity development, and addressing gender inequities at the different environmental levels (family, school, community at large).

Alcohol, Tobacco, and Drug Use

The use of tobacco, alcohol, and other drugs poses a special threat to young people because of the short- and long-term consequences of substance abuse. Alcohol is the most commonly used substance by adolescents in the Caribbean countries. The CAHS showed that 40% of females and 54% of males (ages 12–18) drink alcohol. Beer, spirits, and marijuana are not only easily available but have become part of everyday life for most adolescents in Belize, where their early use is considered a rite of passage for young males (Pan American Health Organization/Belize 2002). One in ten 16- to 18-year-olds reports consuming four or more drinks at one time.

Because their growth and development process is far from complete, preadolescents should not drink alcohol. Nevertheless, this is a frequent reality in Latin America and the Caribbean. When living under conditions of extreme poverty, age of initiation and likelihood of frequent consumption may be greater. Forster and colleagues found that 25% of children between ages 6 and 18 in Brazil who spent all day in the streets and slept there, drank alcohol on a regular, nearly daily basis (Forster, Tannhauser, and Barros 1996). Pechansky and Barros published the results of a household survey of 950 adolescents between the ages of 10 and 18 in the urban area of Porto Alegre, Brazil, which showed a mean age of onset to be 10.1 years, with no gender differences (World Health Organization 2001, Pechansky and Barros 1995). In another Brazilian study, approximately 50% of young people between the ages of 10 and 12 reported having used alcohol, compared to 74% of those between the ages of 10 and 18. Thirty percent of those ages 10–18 had used alcohol to the point of intoxication, and 19.3% reported heavy use (six or more times within the past 30 days) (Galduroz et al. 1997). Studies point to an increase in drinking in Brazil, Chile, Costa Rica, and

Mexico, especially among young women (World Health Organization 2001, Carlini-Cotrim 1999, Medina-Mora 1999, Consejo Nacional para el Control de Estupefacientes (Chile) 1996, Urzúa 1993). Data from a Costa Rican survey support the proposition that an earlier age of initiation may predict a greater likelihood of alcohol problems later in life (Bejarano, Carvajal, and San Lee 1996). Heavy drinking by adolescents has been positively correlated with adolescents' perception that their parents were drinking too much (Pechansky and Barros 1995).

Since the consumption of alcohol enjoys generalized cultural acceptance, setting the goal of alcohol abstinence among adolescents might not be a realistic one for health promotion program planners. Alcohol's relationship to harm is mediated by two factors: per capita consumption (how much the general population drinks) and consumption patterns (Jernigan 2002). Adult per capita consumption has been related to liver cirrhosis. Patterns of consumption have been linked, among other factors, to motor vehicle accidents, suicides, and sexual and physical violence. The challenge, therefore, for program designers is how to promote a delay in the starting age for alcohol exploration, how to encourage the adoption of reasonable and responsible drinking behaviors among youth, and how to reduce per capita consumption among young people, all the while taking into account this group's vulnerability to subliminal media images and their desire to emulate adult role models who encourage drinking as a rite of passage or a way to cope with problems.

The challenge also requires establishing a clearer delineation of the boundaries of "reasonable and responsible drinking" as an accepted social norm. The definition should be generally agreed upon by the community, should protect the population from the unhealthy effects of alcohol, and should establish social and legal limits (e.g., legal minimum age for purchase and consumption, media advertising) and responsibilities based on what would be considered "unreasonable and irresponsible" among the adult population. Adolescents need clear messages from their parents and the community to counteract the glamorous packaging of alcohol consumption by the media in an increasingly impersonal and globalized world.

Youth are not only targeted by the alcohol industry but by the tobacco companies, as well. Exposure of middle adolescents (ages 14–17) to tobacco advertising in Latin American and Caribbean countries is extremely high, reaching over 90% in Argentina, Bolivia, Costa Rica, Mexico, and Uruguay (The Global Youth Tobacco Survey Collaborative Group 2002). In Uruguay, 35% of students between the ages of 11 and 15 reported having tried their first cigarette (Pan American Health Organization 2002c), and 21.6% of adolescents were offered free cigarettes by a tobacco company between 1999–2001 (The Global Youth Tobacco Survey Collaborative Group 2002). In Argentina, 35% of adolescents 12 to 15 years of age reported tobacco use within the last 30 days (Pan American Health Organization 2002c). Argentina is the country with the highest percentage in the world of adolescents exposed to secondhand smoke in public spaces (86.7%). Ironically, 70.4% of Argentine adolescents think smoking should be banned from public places, a percentage that closely corresponds to the number of nonsmoking adolescents in this country (The Global Youth Tobacco Survey Collaborative Group 2002).

The overwhelming evidence of the negative health consequences produced by direct and indirect exposure to tobacco smoke demands a strong effort to encourage adolescents to stay tobacco-free. Urging changes in community social norms requires a comprehensive and multifaceted approach comprised of policy and program interventions that take place at schools and other places frequented by adolescents, and are reinforced by public service campaigns and advocacy in the media, as well as by legislative and fiscal measures. Unfortunately, changing social norms becomes more complicated when there is a significant percentage of adults (e.g., parents, teachers, community leaders, government officials, lawmakers) who are themselves struggling with the addictive effects of nicotine. These individuals might possibly resist (or, at least, not actively support) policies to ban smoking in public spaces, despite the findings of a recent study of 106,071 adolescents ages 13–15 in 24 Latin American and Caribbean countries, which revealed that 79.1% think smoking should be banned in public areas (The Global Youth Tobacco Survey Collaborative Group 2002). The challenge of empowering adolescents to stay free of tobacco consumption, therefore, includes promoting their right to secure smoke-free zones in the neighborhoods where they live, work, and play.

The use of illegal drugs among youth poses a double threat, not only through the mental health consequences of addiction but also because of the increased risk for HIV/AIDS infection. It is estimated that 46% of Argentine adolescent males and 32% of Argentine adolescent females acquired the infection through the use of intravenous drugs (Pan American Health Organization 2002c). Marijuana is readily available in most of the countries of the Americas, and it has been widely recognized in scientific literature as a gateway drug for the use of cocaine and other more powerful substances (Morral, McCaffrey, and Paddock 2002, Wagner and Anthony 2002). A series of surveys conducted among high school students by the Inter-American Observatory on Drugs found that more than 60% of students feel it is easy or very easy to access illicit drugs. The amount of cannabis seized in Latin America and the Caribbean increased from 2,088,834 kg in 1996 to 3,545,643 kg in 2001. The amount of cocaine and heroin seized in these countries also increased significantly between 1996 and 2001 (Inter-American Observatory on Drugs 2002). Although marijuana is the illegal drug most frequently consumed by adolescents in several of the countries, inhalants have become the second-most used illegal drug over the past few years. The rate of marijuana dependence among Brazilian adolescents has reached 6.9%, while the rate for inhalant dependence is 5.8% (Observatorio Brasileiro de Informaciones sobre Drogas 2002; Consejo Nacional para el Control de Estupefacientes 2001, 1999).

Nutrition and Physical Activity

Another worldwide health concern—obesity—is also on the rise among adolescents in the Region of the Americas, with preliminary findings of prevalence ranging from 8% to 22% (Pan American Health Organization 2002d; Atalah et al. 2001; McArthur, Peña, and Holbert 2001). Fifty percent of obese adolescents become obese adults, and the greatest relative risk is among 10- to 15-year-old obese adolescents (Dietz 1998). Although the relationship between obesity and health consequences has been widely proclaimed, the future negative outcomes of obesity are of little immediate interest to Latin American adolescents. The majority—regardless of socioeconomic status—is interested, instead, in keeping a healthy weight and positive body image in the present, by learning about fat and calorie content of foods and beverages, weight loss methods, and energy expenditure (McArthur, Peña, and Holbert 2001). Anorexia nervosa among young people, particularly adolescent girls, is a growing health concern. Contemporary research indicates that eating disorders and body dissatisfaction have been reported among poor, as well as affluent, teenagers and among black and Hispanic, as well as Asian and Caucasian, teens (Steinberg 1999).

Obesity, eating disorders, and the importance of healthy nutrition and regular physical activity are all topics that are not adequately addressed (if at all) either at school or in the family setting. At the same time, many Latin American and Caribbean countries do not have regulations requiring nutritional labeling of locally produced food, which would increase the awareness of both parents and adolescents and enable them to make better informed choices in the purchase, preparation, and consumption of food.

As they progress through the adolescent years, physical activity among both girls and boys tends to decline steadily, coinciding with an increase in academic and/or work demands and a focus on other areas of interest. The increase in the prevalence of overweight among children and adolescents is not only related to their eating habits but also to their levels of physical activity. Data from the Youth Media Campaign Longitudinal Survey, conducted in 2002 in the United States by the Centers for Disease Control and Prevention, revealed that 61.5% of children aged 9–13 years do not participate in any organized physical activity during their nonschool hours and that 22.6% do not engage in any free time physical activity (U.S. Department of Health and Human Services

2003a). Decreases in physical activity and in the number of physical education programs in schools is also an alarming trend worldwide. Schools have unique opportunities to provide adequate physical activity for all young people through official compulsory physical education programs as well as through school sports programs and after-school leisure-time physical activity initiatives (World Health Organization 2004b). The Statistics Canada series of reports, *How Healthy Are Canadians?*, analyzed factors that help overweight preadolescents to become more active. The series concludes that for overweight/obese preadolescents, a relatively high number of hours in physical education class were predictive of becoming physically active, and overweight/obese preadolescents who were frequent television viewers had low odds of adopting and maintaining an active lifestyle (Statistics Canada 2003).

The challenges to the successful promotion of healthy nutrition and adequate physical exercise are found, as in other areas, at multiple levels: how to introduce healthy eating habits and regular physical activity into family and school routines; how to encourage adolescents to adopt and maintain adequate eating habits and physical activity in a world governed by frequent fast food consumption, prolonged hours of television viewing, and sedentary learning and/or job activities; and how to support communities to invest in environments for youth that encourage healthy nutritional and exercise choices, including the development of policies to increase the nutritional value of foods targeted to adolescent consumption, as well as their availability and proper nutritional labeling, and the provision of community venues designed for sports and other types of physical activity.

[Chapter Two]

The Knowledge-Behavior Gap in Health Promotion

There is ample evidence that while public health interventions can successfully increase adolescent and youths' knowledge about health issues (Eggleston et al. 2000, Cunha et al. 1998), cognitive knowledge is not enough for a sustained change in behaviors (Merson, Dayton, and O'Reilly 2000; Leyva et al. 1995). Providing factual information about risky health behaviors and thereby enhancing knowledge may be necessary to the extent that they can lead to subsequent behavioral modification, but the literature suggests that the link between knowledge and behavior is only moderate, at best (Rimal 2000). Therefore, translating knowledge about health issues into healthy behaviors remains a challenging and difficult task in health promotion (Mandu et al. 2000; Merson, Dayton, and O'Reilly 2000). This can be especially true in the case of adolescents, when the immediate consequences of an unhealthy behavior are nonetheless pleasurable, and when the health threat posed by the behavior is perceived as distant and far-removed. Such is the case for smoking, overeating, drinking, drug use, and unprotected sex (Kelly 2000).

The *information deficit model*, utilized by the early tobacco prevention programs of the 1960s and 1970s, assumed that adolescents would refrain from cigarette smoking if they were provided with adequate information demonstrating that this habit causes serious harm to the body. Many programs based solely on this objective did increase knowledge among children and adolescents, as intended, but the programs were consistently found to be ineffective in the long term in dissuading young people from smoking.

The limitations of this approach led to efforts in the 1970s to identify a more complex set of personal factors possibly linked to cigarette smoking by young people. Utilizing the *affective education model*, efforts were oriented to help young people develop stronger intrapersonal resources (building self-esteem) and general social competence (decision-making, communication, and assertiveness). However, evaluations of these programs demonstrated that they were almost as ineffective in reducing cigarette smoking among young people as programs based on the information deficit model. On a positive note, the affective education strategy did mark the beginning of promising trends in the design of education programs to prevent smoking. For the first time, many programs began to directly incorporate research regarding factors that influence smoking initiation, and they began to include more powerful theoretical models of behavior change.

The concept of "behavior change" describes not only the shift from health-compromising behaviors to health-promoting behaviors, but also explains the *process of change* in adopting and maintaining new behaviors. For example, early adolescents are less likely to engage in sexual activity, but as they begin to explore their sexuality, it is important for them to adopt safe sex practices once they decide to initiate sexual activity. Another example is the process of adopting and maintaining responsible and reasonable drinking habits as young people increase the frequency of their participation in social events with their peers.

The failure of various kinds of programs targeting adolescents to reduce health-compromising behavior and to enable the adoption of health-promoting behaviors has led to two questions: "What are the factors influencing health behaviors in adolescence?" and "How does behavior change occur in adolescents?"

The factors that influence the likelihood of engaging in health-compromising behaviors during adolescence can be quite complex. They include, but are not limited to, the following:

- *individual factors*, such as an impulsive or sensation-seeking temperament, the influence of hormones on aggression and sexual behavior, and high levels of anxiety and mood regulation difficulties;
- *interactive patterns*, such as an opposition-defiant, aggressive, or extremely self-absorbed personality type;
- *relationship factors*, such as negative emotional experiences and climate within the family, with peers, and with others in the community, and caregivers with poor parenting skills; and
- *social influences* in the immediate environment, as well as those drawn from the wider community and culture, which promote health-compromising lifestyles (e.g., mass media messages, industry marketing targeting youth, harmful adult role models, economic hardship and inequity, and violence).

Having identified these factors, it is important to clarify that the display of one or two in isolation does not determine the likelihood that adolescents will engage in health-compromising lifestyles. Risky behavior, instead, results from the buildup of many factors. Behavior change theories describe how these factors and other determinants of behaviors (e.g., beliefs, values, self-efficacy) can be changed, reinforced, or introduced to achieve a desired behavioral change.

Seeking to answer the second question—how behavior change can occur in adolescents—experts developing programs to promote healthy eating, physical activity, nonsmoking, delay in sexual initiation and adoption of safer sex practices, and other similar ones have focused over the last decade on introducing concepts of behavior change and health promotion theories into their interventions. Several school and community-based programs, and some behavior change communication interventions, are examples of this approach. Longitudinal research increasingly supports a wide-ranging, but well-coordinated and integrated approach incorporating interventions at several levels simultaneously—interpersonal, community, and policy, for example—rather than concentrating solely on changing individual behaviors. The U.S. Surgeon General, in a recent report on reducing tobacco use (U.S. Department of Health and Human Services 2000), and the International Consultation on Tobacco and Youth, in its final conference report, *What in the World Works?* (World Health Organization 1999), contributed an assessment of the value and efficacy of the major approaches that have been implemented to reduce tobacco use. According to the WHO report, "no single policy or program measure will be effective. Rather, a broad mix of initiatives is required, with the interventions varying according to the circumstances of each country" (World Health Organization 1999). These conclusions are supported in the 2000 U.S. tobacco reduction report, in which Dr. David Satcher, then U.S. Surgeon General, noted unequivocally: "Our lack of greater progress in tobacco control is more the result of failure to implement proven strategies than it is the lack of knowledge about what to do."

[Chapter Three]

The Importance of Behavior Theories to Successful Adolescent Health Programs

In *Health Behavior and Education: Theory, Research, and Practice*, the authors observe that:

> "Programs to influence health behavior, including health promotion and education programs and interventions, are most likely to benefit participants and communities when the program or intervention is guided by a theory of health behavior. Theories of health behavior identify the targets for change and the methods for accomplishing changes. Theories also inform the evaluation of change efforts by helping to identify the outcomes to be measured, as well as the timing and methods of study to be used."
> (Glanz, Rimer, and Lewis 2002)

The importance of theories to successful adolescent programs has been described by different authors (Kirby 2001, Jemmot and Jemmot 2000). In a review of more than 250 effective sex education programs designed for young people, Kirby found 10 common characteristics. One is that the programs were "based on theoretical approaches that have been demonstrated to influence other health-related behavior and identify specific important sexual antecedents to be targeted."

During the last decade, attention has focused on the fact that too often in public health practice, interventions are adopted and applied although no real evidence exists of their effectiveness. It follows that all countries and communities—but especially those with scarce economic resources—pay a high opportunity cost if the interventions chosen do not yield the highest possible health return on the investment made. In this light, it is imperative that decision-makers carefully investigate what the research literature has identified as the best interventions, taking this knowledge as the departure point for the design of locally appropriate programs.

In today's environment of "accountability" and the need to demonstrate impact, promotion and prevention programs must produce tangible results. Governments and private donors are interested in funding programs with measurable outcomes. The new emphasis on performance means that promotion and prevention practitioners must show that the programs they propose will achieve the results predicted. Using scientifically defensible principles will help practitioners respond to demands for accountability and will simultaneously ensure that program participants receive the most effective services available (U.S. Department of Health and Human Services 2001c).

There are increasing efforts to identify programs that meet various sets of criteria that define what is science- or evidence-based. In general, a program designated as *evidence-based* has been reviewed by a panel of experts who determine that the program meets a set of predetermined standards of empirical research; for example, if a program is theory-based, if it has sound research methodology, and if it can show results that are clearly linked to the intervention itself and not to extraneous factors (Education Development Center 2001).

The effort to identify "best practices" for adolescent health promotion and prevention programs is the result of a new era of "evidence-based medicine," in contrast to earlier programs designed according to tradition, intuition, or general principles. The use of a strong and effective theoretical framework allows program developers to evaluate interventions and obtain the necessary evidence of effectiveness.

Theories help in the stages of planning, implementing, and evaluating an intervention. They help to identify *what* the program designer needs to know before developing and implementing an intervention program. They can provide insight into *how* to choose program strategies to reach and impact adolescents within their environment. Theories also help to pinpoint *what* should be monitored, measured, or compared in a program evaluation (Glanz, Lewis, and Rimer 2002; Glanz and Rimer 1995). The theoretical framework is the basic foundation upon which evidence-based interventions are built in order to achieve successful programs or "best practices" for adolescents.

Nevertheless, not all theoretical frameworks are equally helpful in designing, implementing, and achieving successful interventions for young people. This book intends to guide program designers in the selection of health promotion and behavior change theories that have shown to provide useful, practical concepts and constructs that have been successfully tested and applied to interventions with adolescents.

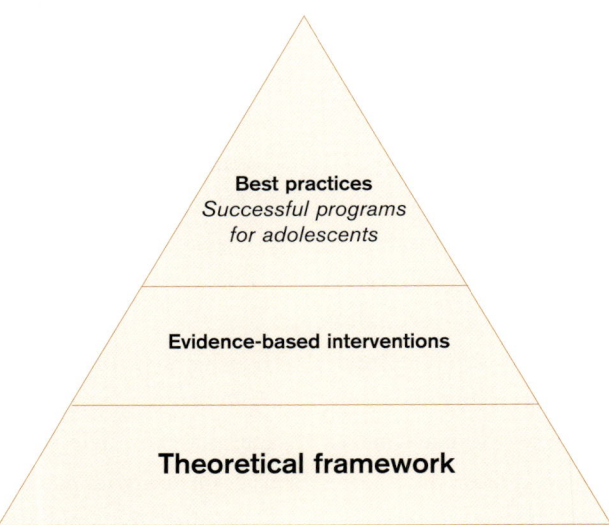

Figure 3-1. **The Theoretical Framework as the Basic Foundation for Successful Adolescent Health Programs**

Kok, Schaalma, De Vries, Parcel, and Paulussen, for example, have had significant experience in the study of tobacco and AIDS prevention programs for adolescents. These authors emphasize the importance of using "problem-driven applied social psychology," versus "theory-driven applied social psychology," when selecting a theoretical framework. In other words, Kok and colleagues insist on the need to select not one single theory, but a theoretical framework that includes a series of theories which lead to a better understanding of the specific problem to be addressed and of how best to solve it. They warn against using theory-driven applied psychology, whose end goal is to test the theory itself, thereby considering practical problems from a single theoretical perspective, instead of allowing oneself the flexibility to choose from among a variety of theoretical constructs that can best address the problem. This dichotomy harks back to Einstein's words of caution regarding perfection of means and confusion of goals. It is important to not lose sight of the final goal, which is to enable the adoption and maintenance of healthy behaviors, through the development of effective health promotion and prevention programs for adolescents, in which theories serve as a navigator or roadmap along the continuum to behavior change.

Problem-driven psychology requires a thorough analysis of the practical problem in question and involves the consideration of multiple theoretical perspectives to find answers to the problem. Before potential theoretical frameworks are selected, program designers need to answer such questions as: What is the problem? Why is it a problem? Whose problem is it? What are the possible causes? A narrow focus on only one theory, or a restrictive sampling of only a few theories, can lead to hypotheses that may not contribute to a reduction or solution of a practical problem (Kok et al. 1996). Nor should the selection of a given framework be guided solely by prior familiarity with it or because it currently happens to be in vogue (Glanz, Rimer, and Lewis 2002), but instead by its proven ability to respond adequately to the problem and achieve the established goal (Sussman and Sussman 2001).

[Chapter Four]

Adolescents Living in a Complex Environment of Multiple Levels of Influence

The U.S. Center for Substance Abuse Prevention, in a review of evidence-based programs for adolescents, states that successful programs in substance abuse prevention possess three key characteristics: they are guided by "theories that blend both individual and environmental approaches," apply "multiple strategies in multiple settings," and follow "a logical design that includes assessment and evaluation" (U.S. Department of Health and Human Services 2002a).

Bartholomew, Parcel, Kok, and Gottlieb, in their book *Intervention Mapping: Designing Theory- and Evidence-Based Health Promotion Programs*, propose using a *social ecological approach*. Through this approach, health is viewed as a function of individuals and the environments in which the individuals are *embedded*, including the family, social networks, organizations, communities, and society as a whole (Bartholomew et al. 2001, Stokols 1996). Since adolescent behavior is influenced by determinants at these various levels, Bartholomew and colleagues encourage program developers to see these various levels as *embedded systems*, in which higher-order systems (e.g., society) set constraints and pro-

---

Box 4-1. **Three Key Aspects in the Development of Successful Adolescent Health Programs**
- They are guided by theories that blend both individual and environmental approaches.
- They apply multiple strategies in multiple settings.
- They follow a logical design that includes assessment and evaluation.

U.S. Center for Substance Abuse Prevention, 2002

vide input to lower-order systems (e.g., individuals), and the lower-order systems in turn provide input back to systems at a higher level.

In view of new knowledge and ongoing research, Lawrence Green and Marshall Kreuter (1999) have had to revise the subtitle of each subsequent edition of their groundbreaking work *Health Promotion Planning*, first published in 1980. The three editions taken together reflect a shift over the past quarter century from a health education approach (1st edition) into one that incorporates a more comprehensive environmental approach (2nd edition, 1991), and finally a more multi-sectoral and multilevel, or ecological, approach (3rd edition, 1999). In addition, in the work's most recent edition, the authors further refine the so-called *magic bullet approach* by importing from the medical field the concept of *evidence-based practice* and then applying it to the health promotion arena, noting that "Human biology is relatively uniform across the human species; however, human behavior, culture, and social change processes are not uniform enough to permit a single set of best practices to suffice the way medical best practices might" (Green and Kreuter 1999).

Within this redefined framework, then, it is important to select theories that help to achieve change at different *ecological levels* in a complex environment. The levels of influence for health-related behaviors and conditions that have been identified are as follows (McLeroy et al. 1988):

(1) individual factors;
(2) interpersonal factors;
(3) institutional, or organizational, factors;
(4) community factors; and
(5) public policy factors.

Table 4-1. presents a list of behavior and social change theories and models as presented in three major health promotion works, selecting those that are particularly relevant to the development of healthy adolescent behaviors. (The majority of these theoretical constructs will be discussed in greater detail in Section Two of this book.)

An important contribution of Green and Kreuter's work has been the development of the PRECEDE-PROCEED model for health promotion planning and evaluation, which highlights the three characteristics presented in Box 4-1., i.e., the application of theory-based approaches and multiple strategies in a logical design allowing for adequate assessment and evaluation. The PRECEDE component of the model includes assessment at five different levels: social, epidemiological, behavioral and environmental, educational and ecological, and administrative and policy, while the PROCEED component focuses on developing the implementation and evaluating its process, impact, and outcome.

Figure 4-1. illustrates the structure of Green and Kreuter's model, including the five levels, or phases, of the PRECEDE

Table 4-1. **Categorization of Selected Theories by Level of Influence and Reference Source**[1]

Level of Influence and Changes	**Health Behavior and Health Education: Theory, Research, and Practice** (Glanz, Rimer, and Lewis 2002, 1997)	**Intervention Mapping: Designing Theory- and Evidence-Based Health Promotion Programs** (Bartholomew et al. 2001)	**Emerging Theories in Health Promotion Practice and Research: Strategies for Improving Public Health** (DiClemente, Crosby, and Kegler 2002)
Individual	- The Health Belief Model - The Theory of Reasoned Action and the Theory of Planned Behavior - The Transtheoretical Model and Stages of Change	- The Health Belief Model - The Theory of Reasoned Action and the Theory of Planned Behavior - The Transtheoretical Model and Stages of Change - The Goal-Setting Theory - The Self-Regulation Theory	- The Authoritative Parenting Model - The Theory of Gender and Power
Interpersonal	- The Social Cognitive Theory - The Social Networks and Social Support Theories - The Stress and Coping Theories	- The Social Cognitive Theory - The Social Networks and Social Support Theories - The Diffusion of Innovations Theory	
Community	- The Community Organization and Community-Building Models - The Diffusion of Innovations Theory - The Organizational Change Theories	- The Community Organization and Community-Building Models - The Organizational Change Theories	
Policy		- The Agenda-Building Theory - The Policy Windows Theory - The Policy Development Model	

[1] Note: Of the three publications, the first two group the various theories according to different levels of influence, while the third one does not. Also, while these works provide examples of the theories' application in youth health promotion and prevention programs, this is not their exclusive focus, nor do they include a detailed analysis of the various stages of adolescent development and this group's changing needs and wants.

component and the four corresponding to the PROCEED component.

Green and Kreuter (1999) emphasize the importance of identifying the pertinent *determinants of health* as the first step in the design development of any health promotion intervention. Green and Kreuter refer to health determinants as a broad group of forces or factors that *predispose*,

Box 4-2. **Acronyms for the PRECEDE-PROCEED Model**

P-R-E-C-E-D-E	P-R-O-C-E-E-D
Predisposing	Policy
Reinforcing	Regulatory
Enabling	Organizational
Constructs	Constructs
Educational/Ecological	Educational
Diagnosis	Environmental
Evaluation	Development

Figure 4-1. **The PRECEDE-PROCEED Model for Health Promotion Planning**

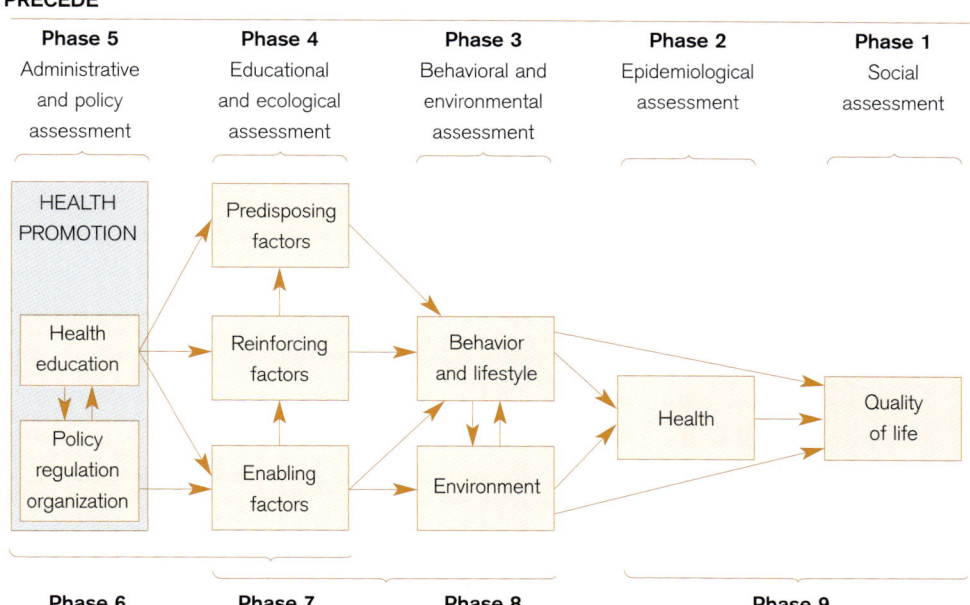

Source: *Health Promotion Planning: An Educational and Ecological Approach, 3rd Edition*, by L. W. Green and M. W. Kreuter © 1999. Reproduced with permission of The McGraw-Hill Companies.

enable, and *reinforce* individual lifestyles and/or shape environmental living conditions in ways that affect the health of populations, with aggregated effects, even though each of them individually might only explain a small amount of variance in health outcomes. Based on this definition, Green and Kreuter suggest that program designers identify the particular determinants of health to be targeted in the intervention by classifying them into the following three categories:

- *predisposing factors*: According to Green and Kreuter, these are "antecedents to behaviors that provide the rationale or *motivation* for the behavior" and would include socio-demographic factors (e.g., socioeconomic status, age, gender, ethnic group, family size and history) that may be used to identify a target population, even though many of these factors cannot be "changed" by health promotion programs. Also included are "changeable" factors, such as knowledge, attitudes, beliefs, values, and confidence, or self-efficacy. Green and Kreuter also include in this group several constructs described within the Health Belief Model (to be discussed in Chapter Eight of this book) and the Theory of Planned Behavior (Chapter Eleven), both at the individual level of influence and change, as well as the Social Cognitive Theory (Chapter Sixteen) at the interpersonal level of influence and change and its *self-efficacy* construct (which was also later incorporated by the Health Belief Model). Regarding *values* as predisposing factors, the authors establish an important ethical distinction that sometimes gets lost in the efforts to achieve behavioral change: "We do not set out in short-term health education or health promotion programs to *change* values. We seek instead to help people recognize inconsistencies between their values and their behavior or environment" (Green and Kreuter 1999).

- *enabling factors*: The authors define these as the "factors that *facilitate* the performance of an action by individuals or organizations." These factors include the availability, accessibility, and affordability of health care; community resources; and health-compromising consumer products (e.g., cigarette machines, laborsaving devices, the majority of "fast foods"); community and government commitment to good health through policies and legislation; as well as barriers to adopt a healthy behavior (e.g., lack of smoke-free school zones, playgrounds and other recreational areas, legal drinking age laws), including health-related skills to carry out a behavioral or environmental change. Most of these enabling factors have been addressed by community and policy level interventions based on theories and models that help to promote change at this level (e.g., community organization, organizational change, diffusion of innovations, development of policies and legislation models) which will be discussed later on in the community and policy level sections of this book.

- *reinforcing factors*: According to Green and Kreuter, "reinforcing factors are those consequences of actions that determine whether the actor receives positive (or negative) feedback and is supported socially afterward." These factors include feedback and pressure, as well as the kinds of social support provided by family members, peers, teachers, employers, health providers, community leaders, and decision-makers. Furthermore, Green and Kreuter highlight, in the case of adolescents, the characteristics of the distinct developmental stages will need to be taken into account when identifying reinforcing factors (e.g., preadolescents will more likely first seek social support from parents, while middle adolescents tend to seek out friends).

Figure 4-2. presents a more detailed rendering of the fourth phase of the PRECEDE-PROCEED model shown in Figure 4-1. In this configuration, the predisposing, enabling, and reinforcing factors that determine behavior form the fourth phase of the PRECEDE-PROCEED model, educational and ecological assessment.

Although Green and Kreuter's three categories can be extremely helpful in identifying health determinants at different levels of influence, they nonetheless rely on the most traditional concepts in behavior and social change, without a particular focus on young people and without addressing additional important theories that incorporate other factors that predispose, enable,

Figure 4-2. **The Predisposing, Enabling, and Reinforcing Factors of the PRECEDE-PROCEED Model (Phase 4: Educational and Ecological Assessment)**

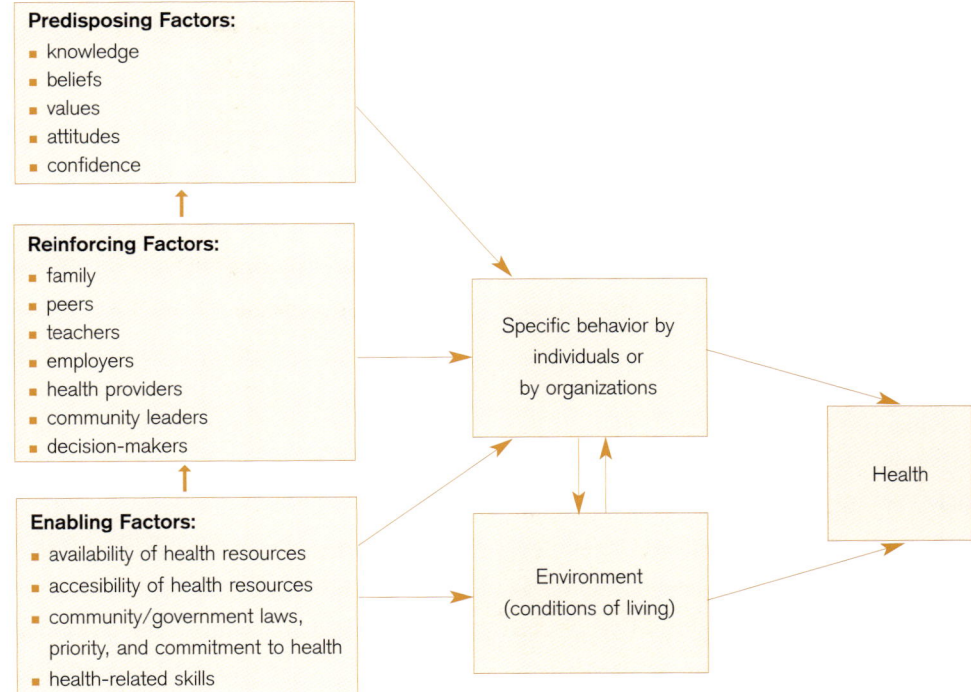

Source: *Health Promotion Planning: An Educational and Ecological Approach, 3rd Edition*, by L.W. Green and M.W. Kreuter © 1999. Adapted and reproduced with permission of The McGraw-Hill Companies.

and/or reinforce specific behaviors among adolescents and youth. Furthermore, the distinction between predisposing, enabling, and reinforcing factors is perhaps merely didactic in purpose, but it also can inadvertently lead to confusion. As the authors themselves admit, sometimes the same factor may play different roles simultaneously (e.g., learning enabling skills about how to use condoms can also become a predisposing factor for adolescents to actually use them, and gaining improved nutritional knowledge can predispose individuals to make healthier food choices as well as enable them to plan individualized diets to meet any specific goals they have set). A final observation regarding the PRECEDE-PROCEED model is that even though the use of theories to help identify health determinants and to develop theory-based interventions is present in this model, the lack of sufficient explicitness regarding the sequence of steps and actions that need to be taken may increase the temptation of program developers to devote insufficient time to theoretical framework choices and overall intervention structure and to move too prematurely into actual practice.

Having said this, PRECEDE-PROCEED is an excellent model for health promotion planning and program development addressing multiple levels of influence. *Youth: Choices and Change* will attempt to serve as a complement to Green and Kreuter's latest iteration of *Health Promotion Planning* by providing a review of theories pertinent to the promoting, predisposing, enabling, and reinforcing of healthy adolescent behaviors, while also incorporating a developmental (and, whenever possible, gender) perspective. This publication will also strive to complement other worthy publications that emphasize the need to follow a logical model for project assessment, design, and evaluation to address behavioral change at multiple levels, but which perhaps do not expand in sufficient depth in their coverage of the underlying theories and models that are helpful in guiding intervention design, particularly as regards adolescents and youth. One of the most recent contributions is *Behavior Change Interventions for Sexual Health Promotion: A Manual* published by the Caribbean Epidemiology Center (2003), which urges its readers to "refer to the research literature, experts in the field, [and] common sense and knowledge of behavior or learning theories/models" to select the appropriate intervention approach.

Figure 4-3. is a guide proposed by the authors of this book that builds on the three factors described by Green and Kreuter as determining individual lifestyles and shaping environmental living conditions. The figure is intended to facilitate a closer look by program designers at the underlying theories and models that help to identify, promote, or change predisposing, enabling, and reinforcing factors for adolescent health behaviors. The principal concepts of each are enclosed in parentheses and will be discussed within the framework of the corresponding theory or model

Figure 4-3. **Developing Interventions for Health-Promoting Behaviors in Adolescents: Theories that Contribute to the PRECEDE-PROCEED Model's Educational and Ecological Assessment (Phase 4)**

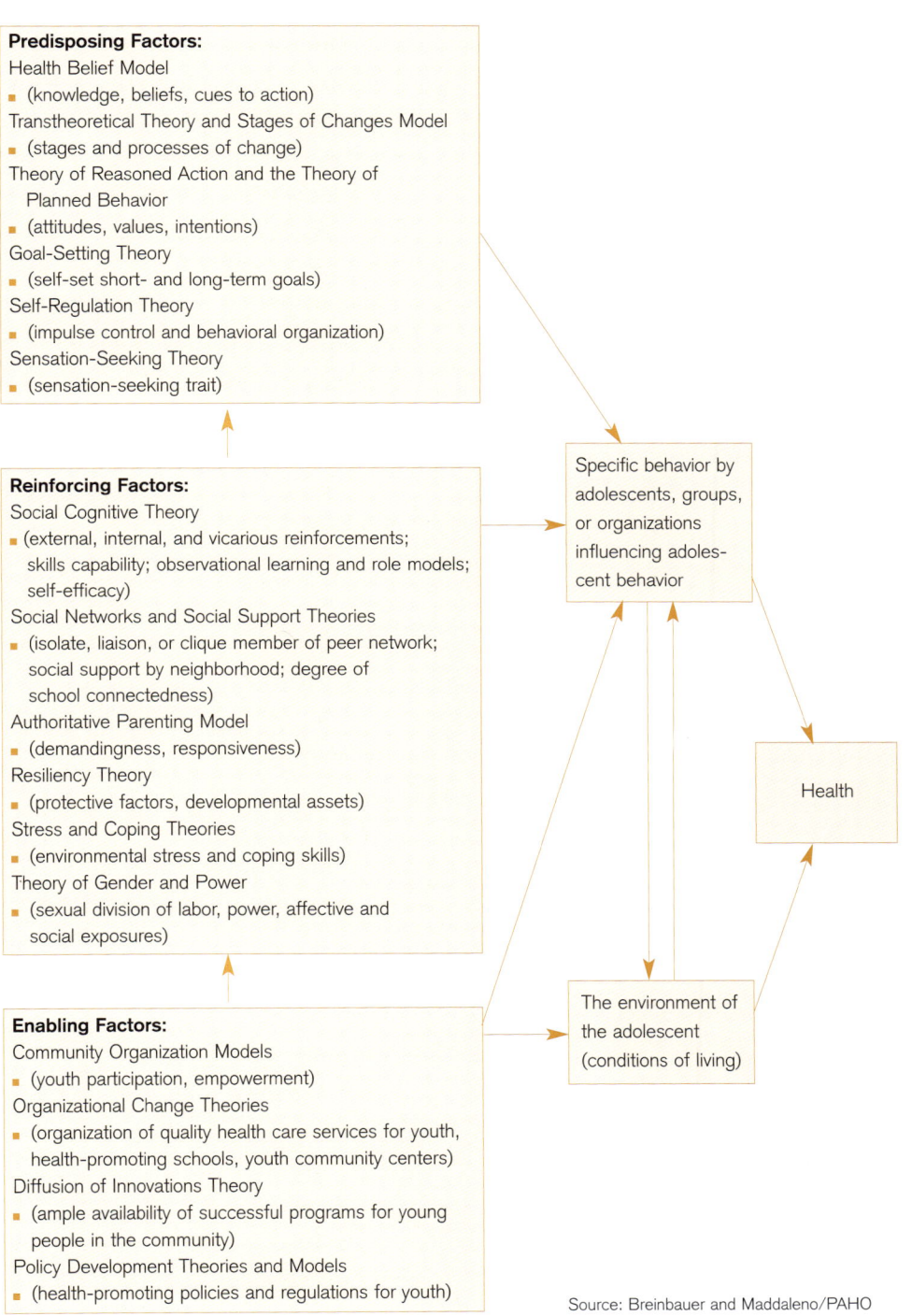

Source: Breinbauer and Maddaleno/PAHO

in Section Two of this book. In presenting this proposal, the authors of *Youth: Choices and Change* wish to note that they share in Green and Kreuter's preference to think of predisposing, enabling, and reinforcing factors as human capacities to be strengthened, rather than deficits or problems to be overcome.

The theories and models presented in Figure 4-3. are a selection of those the authors of this book consider particularly important to keep in mind when designing health promotion and prevention programs for adolescents and youth. This selection is based on a body of evidence found in the literature regarding theoretical frameworks whose constructs predict youth health behavior and/or support effective interventions for young people. The authors recognize that, since *Youth: Choices and Change* represents the first attempt to present a compilation of theories and models and the corresponding empirical evidence regarding their usefulness as regards adolescent behavior change, some inadvertent omissions might have occurred. At the same time, in future editions, it will be important to include any relevant emerging theories and corresponding evidence, for which insufficient information was available at the time of this book's printing.

[Chapter Five]

Listening to Adolescents' Needs and Wants: A Respectful Intervention

Different authors (Buchanan 2000, Kipnis 1994) have criticized the use of behavior change theories and strategies in vertical programs designed by government agencies, international organizations, or other "outside" entities, which do not include community participation and which attempt to manipulate and/or coerce individuals and groups to change their lifestyles without according due consideration to basic issues related to human dignity, integrity, and autonomy.

The Pan American Health Organization (PAHO) and the authors of this book share these criticisms and consider adolescent and community participation in the planning of health promotion interventions and programs to be fundamental. The use of behavior change theories and strategies is merely part of understanding successful interventions. While many of these theories show great promise, they are empty without an understanding of adolescent development processes, their social context, and how adolescent needs and wants change as adolescents mature. A special concern is that changing beliefs and attitudes and teaching skills to adolescents might not be enough to improve their health and well-being. Adolescents must be *motivated* to utilize the information they are provided, practice the skills they are taught, and take advantage of the services that are targeted to them.

Youth culture has, perhaps always throughout history, been misunderstood and misrepresented by older generations, resulting in an unfortunate situation of victimization, discrimination, stereotyping, and mass generalization. Researchers have focused on identifying behavioral determinants of health utilizing a problem-based approach that has tended to place blame on individuals rather than searching farther beyond for environmental explanations. Adolescents have been transformed into "cases" and labeled as different categories of problems ("youth at risk for substance abuse," "youth at risk of early sexual initiation," "youth at risk for HIV infection," etc.). Yet, as young people see when they observe their parents and others around them who are older, risk-taking in and of itself is not necessarily an undesirable trait. In some instances, such as when making certain career-related decisions, risk-taking is viewed as a very positive quality, conducive to personal growth and maturity. So when should adolescents be encouraged and allowed to take risks, and how do they develop the ability to distinguish between good choices and bad ones, given that so many mixed messages and double standards exist in the environment they share with others?

The opportunities for risk-taking and the need to make choices are nowhere more plentiful and powerful than for youth living in poor communities. These youth, too, bear the brunt of significant discrimination and exclusion by a larger society that often engages in "blaming the victim" when patterns emerge that many in this group are engaging in early unprotected sexual relations, defending themselves on the streets using violence, and warding off loneliness with alcohol and/or drugs.

Adolescence is a transitional period in which gradually increasing autonomy co-exists with the more traditional relationships of dependency upon parents, teachers, and other figures of authority. Adolescents need more freedom and trust in making their own choices within the limits that family and society provide. Families, communities, and society as a whole also need to define their beliefs, attitudes, and limits regarding different behaviors, in order to protect young people from harming themselves or others. Some behaviors already have a clear limit, with clear legal consequences set by society which are accepted by the majority of the population (e.g., rape, drug possession). Other compromising behaviors lack a clear consensus among individuals in certain communities (e.g., coercive use of sex, tobacco use) and usually lack legal consequences as well. The United Nations' Convention on the Rights of the Child provides a global framework for protecting adolescents from these types of behaviors, but as long as key members of society (parents, teachers, community authorities) don't clarify their beliefs and attitudes toward these behaviors, they will have no moral authority to pursue changes and limits among adolescents.

The challenge for those who work and interact with adolescents is how to best support them as they learn how to improve their own capacity for practical autonomy, to become more mindful about their choices (e.g., the value of not having early sex and of using contraceptives when needed), and to act accordingly, as these choices become part of their internal set of standards and sense of personal identity. An accumulating body of research suggests that taking a positive approach by promoting skills and assets instead of preventing deficits seems more likely to engage adolescents, helping them to realize their potential and avoid negative influences (Child Trends 2002). This approach also takes into account the needs and wants of adolescents, thereby helping to set the stage for a *respectful intervention*. As we have seen in the Ottawa Charter, the final goal of health promotion is to increase people's control over the determinants of their health by increasing their self-care capacities, which are the decisions and actions individuals take in the interest of their own health.

In order to help adolescents take an active interest in optimizing their own health, it is necessary to understand their *needs* and *wants*. For the purposes of this book, *needs* are defined as *the requirements to promote adolescent health and development* and *wants* as *the interests, desires, and wishes that motivate the adoption of different behaviors*.

According to UNICEF (1997), adolescents have *basic requirements* (rights) that governments and society must ensure are satisfied: nutrition, exercise, recreation, and access to services. Several authors (Brazelton and Greenspan 2000, Reich 1991, Wilson 1987) and institutions (United Nations Children's Fund 1997, Takanishi and Hamburg 1996, World Health Organization 1989) have produced a list of basic conditions, or "needs," for the healthy development of adolescents and youth:

(1) to have had a healthy childhood, in a safe setting, characterized by positive and nurturing emotional experiences and interactions;

(2) to live in a safe environment that provides the basic necessities of food, rest, and protection from violent surroundings and traumatic experiences;

(3) to maintain positive affective relationships and interactions with peers and adults who offer support and opportunities, as well as set limits and realistic expectations and provide structure;

(4) to have access to information and opportunities that are appropriate for adolescents' level of development

---

Box 5-1. **The Definition of Needs and Wants**

Needs
Needs are the requirements to promote adolescent health and development.
Wants
Wants are the personal interests, desires, wishes, and goals that motivate the adoption of different behaviors.

and individual differences and allow them to develop a wide range of practical, vocational, and life skills;

(5) to have equal access to a wide range of services, such as those related to education, employment, health, justice, recreation, and mental and emotional well-being;

(6) to live in a supportive environment molded by policies and legislation, social values, positive role models, and behavioral norms, with positive reinforcement of these by the mass media;

(7) to live in supportive, stable communities that provide cultural continuity;

(8) to have a sense of belonging and the opportunity to participate and be active, contributing members of their societies as parents, workers, and citizens;

(9) to believe in a promising future that offers real social and economic opportunities, in awareness that without the hope of achieving a modicum of socioeconomic stability, youth have little incentive to invest in their own education and to avoid unhealthy habits;

(10) to develop technical and analytical skills that allow adolescents to compete in the technologically savvy world economy; and

(11) to develop a motivation for continuous learning, the preparation for living with uncertainty and change, and the values needed to grow up in communities with different ethnic, religious, and cultural groups.

While satisfying these basic requirements or "needs" will support adolescent health and development, it might not be enough to motivate young people to adopt healthy behaviors when confronted with new choices. According to Acuff and Reiher (1997), a deep understanding of the adolescent consumer provides a "winning formula" for the development of products and programs that succeed with young people. In their book *What Kids Buy and Why*, the editors describe a series of "wants" of adolescents regarding media interests and recreation. Yet as child and adolescent psychiatrist and developmental theorist Stanley Greenspan notes, "it is affect (feelings) that gives rise and organizes thinking" (Greenspan 1993). He also states that the ability *to be intentional* is the ability to create and direct *desire*, which in its very nature is experienced as an *affective or emotional sense of purpose* (Greenspan 1997a). Adolescents want to explore novel challenges and experiences, partake in "grown-up" activities, be part of a social group, have money and access to buy things of interest to them, listen to music, watch TV, play video games and sports, and, overall, have fun in life. Table 5-1. compares common needs and wants of adolescents.

In order to develop effective health promotion and prevention programs for adolescents, it is crucial to understand the "needs and wants" of each gender as adolescents progress through different stages and begin identifying the choices that they can safely make on their own, the limits

Table 5-1. **Comparison of Common Needs and Wants of Adolescents**

NEEDS	WANTS
Love, ongoing nurturing relationship	Autonomy
Acceptance	Social interaction
Developmentally appropriate experiences and success	"Grown-up" experiences
Opportunities and guidance	Novelty
Expectations, limits, and values	Humor and fun
Safe and supportive environments at home and school and in neighborhoods	Music, television shows and movies, video and computer games, magazines and books, hang out with friends at social places, parties
Structures that provide healthy nutrition, physical activity, and proper sleep	Fast foods, sports, stay up late

Source: Breinbauer and Maddaleno/PAHO

that they still need, and the healthy but enjoyable and challenging activities they can participate in. Behavior change theories can provide effective behavior change strategies that will help adolescents achieve their self-set goals. Theories can also contribute strategies that strengthen adolescents' capabilities to organize among themselves and make positive changes in their social group and the community to support new healthy lifestyle choices. The challenge facing designers of programs and interventions is how to achieve an adequate balance of response to both adolescent needs and their wants, while providing opportunities, protecting, and motivating young people to adopt and maintain healthy behaviors.

[Chapter Six]

The Crucial Link between Theories and Developmental Stages of Adolescence

The importance of acknowledging the developmental processes of adolescents when planning health promotion and prevention programs has been emphasized previously in the literature. Linda Juszczak and Lois Sadler (1999), in their article "Adolescent Development: Setting the Stage for Influencing Health Behaviors," underscore the importance of assessing individuals within the stage of adolescence they are currently undergoing, and tailoring interventions specifically for the abilities and interests of that age group. Joy Dryfoos (1998), in her book *Safe Passage (Making It through Adolescence in a Risky Society: What Parents, Schools, and Communities Can Do)*, also emphasizes the importance of developmentally appropriate programs to achieve effectiveness. She notes that the most effective programs relate to teenagers according to where the young people "are" developmentally speaking, instead of where health and other types of professionals think they ought to be, based on their body size, appearance, and/or chronological age.

One of the key concepts of social marketing, increasingly used in the field of public health and social communications projects, is audience segmentation, or differentiation of large groups of people into smaller, more homogeneous subgroups. Acuff (1997) divides the period from 8 to 19 years of age into 4 different stages (preadolescence, and early, middle, and late adolescence). In 2001, the National Youth Anti-Drug Media Campaign in the United States adjusted its campaign targets from the original group of 9–17-year-olds to those ages 11 to 14 (U.S. Office of National Drug Control Policy 2002b).

PAHO and the World Health Organization define "adolescence" as the period between 10 and 19 years of age and "youth" as the period between 15 and 24 years of age. This distinction has been made to highlight the growing consensus that effective interventions can no longer pretend to target "adolescence" and "youth" as a unified homogeneous group, since strategies and the goals of the interventions developed will vary for different adolescent stages and by gender. With this in mind, Section Three of this book is devoted to a thorough discussion of the various stages of adolescent development, with particular emphasis on preadolescence and early adolescence, the needs and wants specific to these age groups, and how they are further differentiated by gender.

At this juncture, it should also be noted that PAHO considers that the single-most important of all these groups to be targeted by health promotion and prevention programs is the preadolescence period. Until recently, the great majority of interventions promoting safer sex practices, for example, have been directed to middle and late adolescents (e.g., increasing condom use and developing other necessary negotiation skills to ensure safe sexual practices). Yet preadolescence marks the advent of increased sexuality and intimacy development, which will continue through early, middle, and late adolescence. In this sense, *Youth: Choices and Change* is intended to serve as a practical guide for program designers to plan developmentally appropriate goals for interventions, with an emphasis on promoting the adoption and maintenance of health behaviors beginning with preadolescence, instead of later on, when health-compromising behaviors have already begun and may be well engrained, thus making them more difficult to change.

Section Three of this book will stress the overarching importance of integrating behavior change theories with developmental goals to improve adolescent health, a strategy that PAHO believes has, for too long, been overlooked and underutilized in the design of adolescent health programs. Other authors (Mummery, Spence, and Hudec 2000; Bush 1996; Sturges and Rogers 1996; Petosa and Jackson 1991) have also noted the paucity of efforts to analyze the concepts and constructs of behavior change theories with a developmental perspective.

Part of the explanation for this situation lies in the fact that traditional behavior change theories are often referred to in the literature as "learning theories." Learning theorists stress the context within which behavior takes place and are not especially developmental in their approach. For learning theorists, the basic processes of human behavior are the same during adolescence as they are during other periods of the life span. The introduction of behavior change theories to increase effectiveness of health education and health promotion interventions was first used to address adult behaviors (e.g., the Health Belief Model, discussed in Chapter Eight of this book) and then extrapolated to target adolescent lifestyles.

The shortcomings and gaps of a "theories-only" approach, within the context of adolescent health, are quite clear, since this age group is in a state of constant change and rapid development. As Mary Pipher, author of *Reviving Ophelia* (1994), writes: "Adolescence is a fascinating time of marked internal development and massive cultural indoctrination." The benefit of tailoring the application of behavior change theories, concepts, and constructs to the developmental stage and by gender enables the resulting interventions to better guide adolescents through the complex and ever-changing web of socio-environmental factors that make up their lives.

An integrated approach allows programs to be developed that analyze adolescent behavior with the framework of social environment and developmental stage and enables program designers to orient interventions by considering the following questions:

- Do determinants of adolescent health behaviors described by different theories (e.g., subjective norm, perceived behavioral control) change through different developmental stages? If so, in what ways?
- Are there adolescent gender-specific behavior determinants for tobacco, alcohol, and drug use; nutrition and physical activity; sexual activity and contraceptive use; and violence? If so, how and why must interventions for girls and boys be structured differently?
- Are there any other preadolescent behaviors that have not been sufficiently addressed that should be promoted to help adolescents adopt health-enhancing behaviors?

The answers to these and other similar types of questions will vary from community to community, culture to culture, and age group to age group in response to local realities. Therefore, the mix of program design elements will be unique as well, requiring health promoters to approach program design with a clear understanding of the target audience, the behavior change theories which may applied, and why (or why not) they might be appropriate.

[Chapter Seven]

The Youth: Choices and Change Model for Designing Effective Interventions for Adolescents

As we saw in Chapter Two of this book, longitudinal research is increasingly pointing to the efficacy of adopting broad-based, multilevel approaches to behavior change rather than concentrating on changing individual behavior in isolation. Chapter Four presents three ecological levels—interpersonal, community, and public policy—at which, optimally, change also needs to occur in order to support and reinforce change at the individual ecological level. Chapter Six discusses the importance of identifying the target group by stage of development (preadolescence; early, middle, or late adolescence), while Chapter Five shows why adolescent needs and wants need to be taken into account when developing respectful health-promoting interventions. Chapters Two and Three illustrate how behavioral change theories may be used to close the gap between the knowledge young people possess about how to lead healthy lives and actual positive changes they decide to make on their own to initiate these healthy lifestyles.

The basic elements highlighted in the first six chapters of this book provide a complete framework within which program designers may develop a series of interventions to support adolescents and youth in achieving and maintaining healthy behaviors and lifestyles. In this chapter, the Youth: Choices and Change Model is presented to enable designers to better visualize what their fully constructed program might look like. The model, developed by PAHO, provides a grid interlinking the components described above (Figure 7-1.) and allows designers to build programs utilizing a step-by-step approach. The model's key conceptual components are further defined and/or reviewed in Box 7-1.

Figure 7-1. **The Youth: Choices and Change Model**

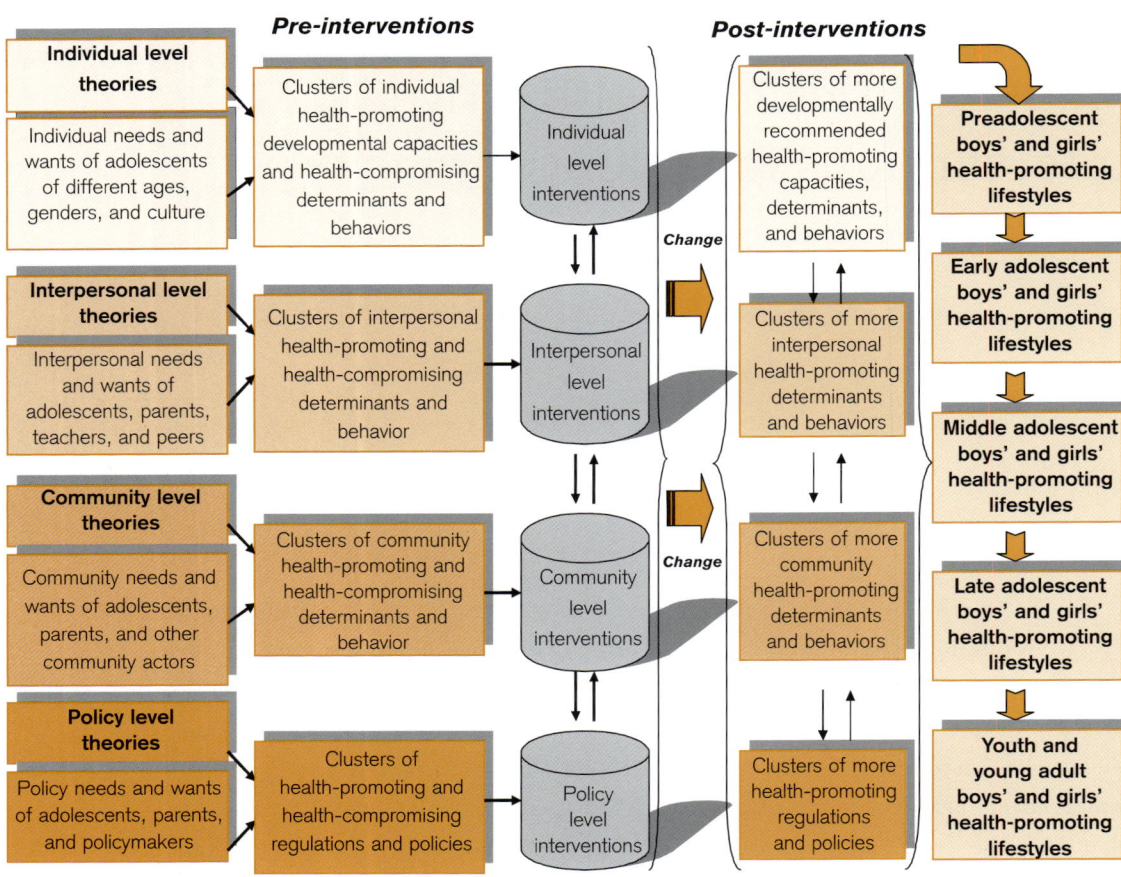

Source: Breinbauer and Maddaleno/PAHO

During the design of adolescent health programs, it is important to distinguish between *health behavior determinants*, as described in most of the health education textbooks (Box 7-1.), and *health determinants*, as described by the *population health approach* (Health Canada 2003, Frankish et al. 1996), which aims to improve the health of the entire population and to reduce health inequities among population groups. The population health approach describes a broad range of factors and conditions that have a strong influence on our health, which are described as *health determinants*, and are identified as the following:

- income and social status
- social support networks
- education and literacy
- employment/working conditions

> Box 7-1. **Definition of Terms Used in the Youth: Choices and Change Model**
>
> **Health behavior determinants** are the conditions and circumstances that influence behaviors which, in turn, affect health. Within the framework of behavior change theories, they consist of a series of theoretical constructs that predict behavior (e.g., attitudes, perceived benefits, intentions, subjective norms). These conditions or behavior determinants can be identified at all four ecological levels: the individual (e.g., attitudes), interpersonal (e.g., role models), community (e.g., youth empowerment), and policy (e.g., public policies). Determinants may be expressed as variables, may be measured and changed, and may serve as indicators of progress towards behavior change.
>
> **Health-promoting determinants** are those determinants, at different levels of intervention, which facilitate the adoption of healthy behaviors (e.g., positive attitudes towards condom use, positive role models, youth participation in HIV prevention campaigns, effective policies for condom availability). Protective factors, described by the Resiliency Theory (see Chapter Nineteen), as well as developmental assets, are health-promoting determinants.
>
> **Health-compromising determinants** are those determinants which facilitate the adoption of unhealthy behaviors (e.g., negative attitudes towards condom use, role models favoring early unprotected sex, lack of social support and networks, policies restricting condom distribution). Risk factors are health-compromising determinants.
>
> **Health-promoting developmental capacities** are those age-appropriate developmental capacities which facilitate the adoption of healthy behaviors (e.g., to have developed a personal conviction against early sexual relationships during preadolescence, to be able to set limits in sexuality exploration and negotiate alternative behaviors to intercourse for channeling sexual arousal during early adolescence).
>
> **Needs** are the requirements, by different actors at different levels (e.g., adolescents, parents, teachers, community leaders, policymakers), to promote adolescent health and development.
>
> **Wants** are the personal interests, desires, wishes, and goals of different actors (e.g., adolescents, parents, teachers, community leaders, policymakers) at different levels that motivate the adoption of various types of behaviors.
>
> **Heath-promoting lifestyles** refer to a cluster of behaviors that can help to preserve adolescent health, including sexual behaviors, and those related to violence; alcohol, tobacco, and drug use; and nutritional habits and physical activity.
>
> In identifying developmental stages:
> **preadolescent** refers to girls who are ages 9–12 and boys who are ages 10–13;
> **early adolescent** refers to girls ages 12–14 and boys ages 13–15;
> **middle adolescent** refers to girls ages 14–16 and boys ages 15–17;
> **late adolescent** refers to girls ages 16–18 and boys ages 17–18;
> **youth** refers to boys and girls ages 18-21; and
> **young adult** refers to boys and girls ages 21-24.

- social environment
- physical environment
- personal health practices and coping skills
- healthy/unhealthy child development
- biological and genetic makeup
- availability and quality of health services
- gender
- cultural background

Within the definition of health determinants utilized by the population health approach, *health behavior determinants* would be one of those listed above; specifically, the "personal health practices and coping skills" determinant. This differentiation particularly applies when the concept of health behavior determinants is used to describe those determinants that affect individual behaviors at the individual level, without considering the other levels of influence. Nevertheless, experts working in the health education and health behavior fields have also incorporated more and more this broader notion of health determinants, defining health behavior as "the actions of individuals, groups, and organizations as well as their determinants, correlates, and consequences, including social change, policy development and implementation, improved coping skills, and enhanced quality of life" (Glanz, Rimer, and Lewis 2002; Parkerson et al. 1993). However, for the health behavior approach, efforts to improve environmental factors, policies, and the above-listed broader health determinants should in the end be evaluated for their effects on measurable changes in health behavior or health outcomes. Glanz and colleagues (2002) caution that a policy change that does not lead to measurable changes in behavior may be either too weak or too short-lived, or be only a limited determinant of behavior.

Putting It All Together—The Youth: Choices and Change Model

The following steps will help developers of adolescent health programs to approach program planning systematically, allowing reflection about each of the components to be included in the design of interventions and facilitating the decision-making process:

(1) *Identify the target group: adolescent stage and gender.* In applying the Youth: Choices and Change Model, PAHO recommends that program designers begin by identifying the specific adolescent stage(s) and gender(s) they are going to target, given the stated needs and goals of the different actors involved. It is worthwhile noting that, historically, the needs frequently stated as being urgent are those related to changing middle and late adolescent behaviors, without due consideration being given to the value of focusing instead on building the strengths and positive behaviors of these age groups. As pointed out in Chapter Five, recent research shows that taking a positive approach by promoting skills and assets instead of preventing deficits has a better chance of engaging the interest and participation of adolescents, helping them to achieve their potential and avoid negative influences (Child Trends 2002). For these reasons, PAHO advises that program designers make special efforts to intervene early and to also target pre- and early adolescents, even when community members in these age groups might not yet show overt signs of health-compromising behaviors.

(2) *Identify adolescent needs and wants.* As we will see in much greater detail in Section Three of this book, adolescent

needs and wants will vary according to gender and the various different stages of development. Nevertheless, an awareness and understanding of the needs and wants of girls and boys at different ages, within the cultural context of the community itself, is crucial to the development of successful health interventions. Since cultural and social values will vary from community to community, learning the specific needs and wants of the local adolescent population usually occurs by organizing small focus groups among the target population.

(3) *Identify level of intervention.* As we saw in Chapter Four, adolescents live in a complex environment in which they are subject to multiple levels of influence for health-related behaviors: individual, interpersonal, institutional and/or organizational, community, and public policy. Given that the body of research continues to grow indicating that successful behavior change is best achieved if multilevel inputs are provided to support and reinforce this change synergistically, PAHO recommends that interventions calling for positive change be incorporated at each ecological level rather than focusing exclusively on changing individual behavior.

(4) *Identify other actors' needs and wants.* In a multilevel approach, the needs and wants of the other actors involved in promoting healthy adolescent lifestyles—parents, other family members, caregivers, teachers, peers, community leaders, and others—will need to be taken into account in order to secure this group's active support of and participation in the interventions and programs created. Since the members of this diverse group relate to adolescents in different ways, each will bring unique perspectives to the design process, enhancing the possibility of designing and implementing respectful interventions that are meaningful and age-appropriate for the recipients, thereby stimulating greater interest and commitment on the latter's part.

(5) *Identify the theories that will support the design of the intervention.* The Youth: Choices and Change Model proposes that *at least one theory be selected at each ecological level* to guide the design of interventions. Table 4-1. shows the various theories that may be applied at each level, and Section Two of this book explores each of the theories within its ecological context. But before theoretical frameworks are selected, ideally composed of theories chosen from the different ecological levels, program designers will need to utilize a problem-driven psychological approach (see Chapter Three) to answer the questions that will lead to a better understanding of the specific problem at hand and what needs to be done to achieve change.

(6) *Translating theory into practice.* The selection of meaningful theories to address a specific adolescent behavior or challenge (e.g., adopting responsible and reasonable drinking habits, reducing overall alcohol drinking among adolescents) will help to identify clusters of health-promoting and

health-compromising determinants (e.g., attitudes, subjective norms, choice of role models, coping strategies, poverty, local alcohol regulations for youth) and behaviors (e.g., adolescent drinking behaviors, parental drinking habits, school connectedness, ease of access to alcohol products) at each ecological level. The challenge is to translate those theoretical constructs into measurable variables *before* the intervention, so that changes may be measured *after* the intervention. In this way, the interventions will follow a logical design that includes assessment and evaluation, one of the key elements in the development of successful adolescent health interventions and programs (U.S. Department of Health and Human Services 2002a), as we saw in Chapter Four.

The selected theories will also help to design the interventions at each ecological level in order to decrease the amount of health-compromising determinants and behaviors and increase the amount of health-promoting determinants and behaviors after the intervention takes place. Although adopting and maintaining health-promoting behaviors among adolescents and changing health-compromising behaviors at each level is the ultimate goal, the *process* of achieving this might require targeting determinants of behaviors first (e.g., attitudes), which can then serve as measurable *process indicators* before changes in *outcome indicators* (final behavior) are ultimately obtained.

The Youth: Choices and Change Model also proposes targeting not only adolescent-specific determinants and behaviors (e.g., attitudes toward alcohol, resistance skills when offered alcohol) but also promoting the strengthening of developmental capacities appropriately gauged for pre- and early adolescent boys and girls through the interventions, which will, in turn, strengthen their abilities to make conscious healthy decisions (e.g., to improve mood regulation, control expression of emotions, critically analyze role models that involve excessive or irresponsible drinking habits). These developmental capacities will be more fully discussed in Section Three of this book.

* * *

Throughout the world, there is a growing number of successful adolescent health initiatives that incorporate the elements discussed so far in this book. Many of these were presented at an international conference sponsored by the World Health Organization in Stockholm, Sweden, in 2001 (Foxcroft et al. 2001). One of these is "Strengthening Families," a highly effective alcohol and drug prevention program developed in the United States by Iowa State University and consisting of seven 2-hour sessions and four booster sessions during which parents work to improve their parenting skills and adolescents strive to achieve more effective communication with their parents (Iowa State University 1997). The program has been scientifically evaluated and shown to be effective and is recognized by four U.S. federal agencies: the National Institute on Drug Abuse and the Departments of Education, Justice, and Health and Human Services. Youth attending the program had significantly lower rates of alcohol, tobacco, and marijuana consumption, as well as school conduct problems, compared to their control group counterparts. Furthermore, the differences between program and control youth were shown to increase over time, indicating that the skills learned and the strengthening of parent-child relationships continued to manifest their influence as these youth progressed through their adolescent years.

Perhaps the proven effectiveness of the "Strengthening Families" program lies in two key ingredients: first, that it promotes simultaneous changes at the individual, interpersonal, and community levels; and secondly, that it targets pre- and early adolescents (in this case, ages 10 to 14), which, as we have already seen, is a critical age group to be targeted by any and all adolescent health promotion initiatives. Important, also, is the fact that the program takes into account the needs of other actors—from family members and caregivers to community leaders—and that it is based on theories that facilitate the design of integrated interventions occurring across the lines of the different ecological levels.

In Section Two, we will review a variety of behavior change theories at different levels of intervention that are considered particularly relevant in the design of adolescent health promotion and prevention programs. Like the components of the theoretical framework of "Strengthening Families," the theories presented have demonstrated their ability to achieve positive results. The participants themselves have reported that they find the interventions to be innovative and appealing, perhaps because adolescents are granted the opportunity for greater autonomy and challenged to make conscious choices that place them firmly in charge of their own growth and maturation process.

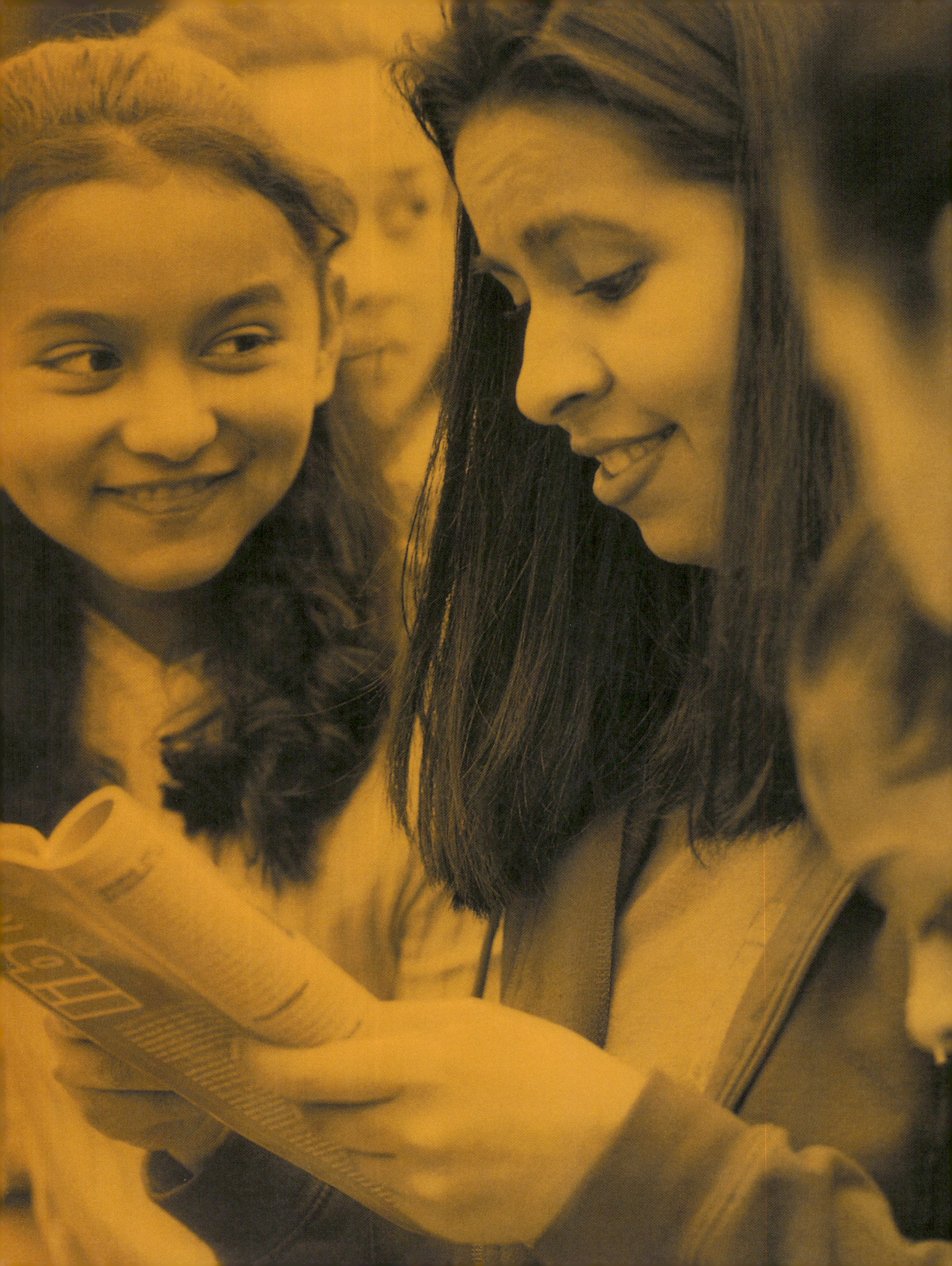

[Section Two]

Theories and Models for Health Promotion and Behavior Change: Their Application to Adolescents

Theories and Models that Promote Change at the Individual Level

As we saw in Chapter Four, behavior, when viewed from an ecological perspective, is affected by—and has an effect on—multiple levels of influence. The levels of influence for health-related behaviors and conditions that have been identified are the following (McLeroy et al. 1988):
   (1) individual factors;
   (2) interpersonal factors;
   (3) community and organizational factors; and
   (4) public policy factors

From this ecological perspective, behavior both influences and is influenced by the social environment. This multilevel, interactive perspective clearly shows the advantages of multilevel interventions, such as those that combine developmental, behavioral, and environmental components. For example, adolescents are less likely to take up smoking if they reach early adolescence with a strong internal sense of what is "right" and what is "wrong," and believe that smoking is unpopular, even if this feeling disagrees with that of other peers (individual level). Similarly, if their best friends also disapprove of the habit, their role models do not smoke, and they have developed healthy coping mechanisms to deal with the daily pressures of their personal lives, they will be less inclined to begin smoking (interpersonal level). Adolescents will also be less likely to adopt this behavior if they live and study in a smoke-free environment and listen to mass media advertising with attractively designed messages that encourage health-promoting lifestyles (community level). And finally, adolescents will also be more inclined to refrain from tobacco use if product prices are high and laws that prohibit tobacco sales to minors are strictly enforced (public policy level).

Theories on health behavior attempt to *explain* health behaviors ("explanatory theories or theories of the problem") and propose ways to reach *behavior change* ("theories of action that guide the development of interventions"). Oftentimes, one theory seems to be insufficient to explain the complexities of health behavior, leading to the development of *models* of health behavior. Models draw on a number of theories and empirical findings to help people understand a specific problem within a particular setting or context (Glanz, Rimer, and Lewis 2002). Theories also form the basis for evaluation, ensuring that the evaluator will set realistic and achievable expected results before the intervention begins and that these results can be measured following the intervention.

Chapters Eight through Fifteen of Section Two will deal with the first level, that of changing individual behavior. Individuals constitute the basic units of groups, families, organizations, schools, communities, and governments. Individual behavior shapes dimensions of collective health behavior and vice versa, including the complex interaction between the two. In the above-mentioned chapters, the following theories and models of individual health behavior will be reviewed in the context of working with adolescents:

- the Health Belief Model
- the Transtheoretical Model and Stages of Change
- the Theory of Reasoned Action
- the Theory of Planned Behavior
- the Goal-Setting Theory
- the Self-Regulation Theory
- the Sensation-Seeking Theory

As in the subsequent chapters in Section Two, which deal with the remaining three ecological levels of influence, a description of relevant theories and models will be presented, followed by a discussion of how these constructs may be applied to specific adolescent behaviors, such as reproductive health and sexual activity; violence; tobacco, alcohol, and drug use; and nutrition and physical activity. Each theory or model will be analyzed from a developmental perspective and include observations on its application as it relates to the different stages of adolescence. At the same time, gender differences for behavior determinants will be highlighted.

Recommended Bibliography for Section Two

For further reading on topics related to health education, health behavior, and health promotion, the following works may be of interest:

- *Theory at a Glance: Guide for Health Promotion Practice* (Glanz and Rimer 1995)
- *Health Behavior and Health Education: Theory, Research, and Practice* (Glanz, Rimer, and Lewis 2002, 1997)
- *Intervention Mapping: Designing Theory- and Evidence-Based Health Promotion Programs* (Bartholomew et al. 2001)
- *Emerging Theories in Health Promotion Practice and Research: Strategies for Improving Public Health* (DiClemente, Crosby, and Kegler 2002)
- *An Ethic for Health Promotion: Rethinking the Sources of Human Well-Being* (Buchanan 2000).

[Chapter Eight]

The Health Belief Model

The Health Belief Model was one of the first models to adapt theory from the behavioral sciences to health problems, and it remains today one of the most widely recognized conceptual frameworks of health behavior. It was originally introduced in the 1950s by psychologists Hochbaum, Kegels, Levanthal, and Rosenstock of the U.S. Department of Health and Human Services (Hochbaum 1958). This model predicts that individuals will take action to ward off, screen for, or control illness if they:

- regard themselves as susceptible to the condition (*perceived susceptibility*)
- believe the condition to have potentially serious consequences (*perceived severity*)
- believe that a course of action available to them would be beneficial in reducing either their susceptibility to the condition or the severity thereof (*perceived benefits*)
- believe that the anticipated barriers to (or costs of) taking action are outweighed by its benefits (*perceived barriers*)

An additional concept, *cues to action*, would activate the "readiness to act" in the model. These cues may be bodily events (symptoms) and/or environmental events (the use of reminders, how-to information, media publicity, and activities promoting increased awareness), which serve to instigate action. Another concept, *self-efficacy*, was added later by Rosenstock and others in 1988 to the model. Self-efficacy is defined as "the conviction that one can successfully execute the behavior required to produce the outcomes"

(Bandura 1977). This concept was added in recognition of the challenges presented in modifying lifestyles and behaviors in the long term, since the problems involved in modifying such habits as eating, drinking, exercising, smoking, and sexual practices require a good deal of confidence that one can, in fact, alter such lifestyles before successful change is possible.

In summary, in the Health Belief Model, for behavioral change to succeed, people *must feel threatened* by their current behavioral patterns, and they must believe that change of a specific kind will be beneficial by resulting in a valued outcome at an acceptable cost. At the same time, they must believe that they have the ability to overcome any and all perceived barriers to taking action.

Research and Evidence of Practical Applications of the Health Belief Model to Adolescent Lifestyles

The Health Belief Model can be a very useful one when working with adults, but it should be used with caution with adolescents. Because of the assumption that the person must feel threatened by their current behavior, the model may be used for certain adolescent concerns (e.g., body image and fat consumption for girls) but not necessarily for all risk behaviors, especially if the individual does not feel threatened. Younger children (i.e., 8–10 years) have reported higher levels of fear intensity than older children and adolescents (i.e., 10–16 years), although the latter group tends to report more fears relating to illness, disease, and school (Gullone 2000).

There is some evidence that sensation-seeking traits, which represent the optimistic tendency to approach novel stimuli and explore the environment, accompanied by increased risk behaviors, rise between 9 and 14 years of age and begin to decline in late adolescence (Zuckerman 1994). During adolescence, increases in risk behaviors can be accompanied by a greater perception of prevalence of the behaviors in the surrounding environment, along with decreases in perceptions of vulnerability and of the influence of health and safety concerns on behaviors. Al-

---

Box 8-1. The Health Belief Model: Key Theoretical Concepts in the Adoption of Healthy Behaviors

- **perceived susceptibility:** Individuals consider themselves at risk.
- **perceived severity:** Individuals consider the risk to have serious consequences.
- **perceived benefits:** Individuals consider that taking actions will be beneficial.
- **perceived barriers:** Individuals consider that the costs are less than the benefits.
- **cues to action:** reminders (e.g., symptoms, media publicity) that instigate action to adopt a health-promoting behavior
- **self-efficacy:** the conviction that one can successfully execute the health-promoting behavior required to produce outcomes

though adolescents can become more aware of risks, they can also modify their thinking in ways that enable their continued participation in risky situations (Gerrard et al. 1996). For the adolescent, risk-taking may have fewer perceived costs and more benefits, because of immature cognition; the need for novelty, esteem, and confidence; and a relative lack of life experiences.

Sturges and Rogers (1996) applied theories of health psychology, such as the Health Belief Model, to 10-year-old preadolescents ($n = 112$) who had not reached the stage of formal operational thought, 15-year-olds ($n = 67$), and 20-year-olds ($n = 93$). The authors found that among adolescents and young adults, the threat appeals worked only if people believed they could cope effectively with the danger; if they believed they could not cope, higher levels of the threat resulted in decreased intentions to refrain from tobacco use. Although preadolescents understood the information about threat severity and personal vulnerability, the fragility and malleability of the preadolescent's beliefs in self-efficacy demonstrated the importance of adding a developmental perspective to theories of preventive health psychology.

One promising future use of the Health Belief Model with adolescents and tobacco concerns their attitudes towards secondhand smoke, as seen in one recent study (Glantz and Jamieson 2000). The study found that the only statistically significant predictor of planning to stop or having actually stopped smoking among adolescents was believing that secondhand smoke harmed nonsmokers, which more than doubled the chances of planning to stop smoking or actually doing so. The same study found that nonsmoking teens were twice as likely to consider secondhand smoke dangerous as smokers. This suggests that educating young people about the dangers of secondhand smoke and, at the same time, empowering nonsmokers to speak out, should be strong elements of any tobacco control program. These findings are consistent with the results of two econometric studies. The first showed that the presence of an indoor clean air law was associated with lower teen smoking (Wasserman et al. 1991). The second indicated that secondhand smoke is a highly effective message for reaching young people through focus group studies of anti-tobacco advertising for teens (Goldman and Glantz 1998).

These findings also may be explained by understanding adolescent development. Although adolescents might not feel personally threatened by their current or future smoking behavior because of their sense of invulnerability and their need to explore risky situations, they might indeed feel threatened, concerned, or responsible for the possibility of harming others, especially those perceived as being more vulnerable than they are. During adolescence, standing up against unfair situations and the fear of contributing to these injustices might be a powerful motivation for change.

Another promising future use of the Health Belief Model in adolescents could be the use of short-term instead of long-term consequences as something adolescents would fear. This could be the case for discouraging driving while drinking alcohol. Although most adolescents know that this is a potentially harmful behavior, many of them still make the decision to do so. Reaching the legal age to obtain a driver's license is a universal dream among adolescents. A recent U.S. study, using the Health Belief Model (Gotthoffer 1999), revealed that the consequence youth fear most is being charged with driving under the influence (DUI), yet current anti-drinking and driving public service announcements rarely portray this as a possible negative consequence. This study provides information to effectively target youth with media campaigns oriented toward reducing drinking and driving by addressing the fear of receiving a DUI and the negative consequences this can bring.

The use of the model to promote regular physical activity among youths has been less successful. Messages that focus on the benefits of avoiding future chronic diseases are not effective in motivating youth. Nor do beliefs about the health benefits of physical activity correspond to actual activity levels among adolescents (Strauss et al. 2001). Yet, in another study, the perceived *immediate* benefits and barriers, two other key concepts in the Health Belief Model, have been shown to exert some influence on the physical activity of adolescents (Sallis et al. 1992). *Perceived barriers* in particular can be a very useful theoretical construct to apply when planning health promotion interventions. The design of the intervention can include youth participation when helping them identify the barriers they feel are interfering with adopting a new behavior. The intervention can include a change in those identified barriers; behaviors can be measured with and without the barriers. In a recent study of Hispanic and African-American middle adolescent girls, the perceived barriers to physical activity identified included negative experiences in physical education classes, concerns about personal appearance after the activity, and lack of opportunity and accessibility (Taylor et al. 1999).

The application of the Health Belief Model when promoting safer sex practices and reducing the risk of contracting HIV has also been challenging. Greater perceived chance for contracting HIV and lower concern about HIV infection have been associated with high-risk behaviors in runaway and homeless adolescents. Nevertheless, among Asian-American students (Yep 1993), the belief that the anticipated barriers to taking action are outweighed by its benefits, and awareness of the disease's graveness—more than fear of contracting the virus itself—have proven to be significant predictors of the adoption of HIV-preventive behaviors. Partner preference for condoms was a strong predictor of consistent condom use in another study (Larraque et al. 1997). The self-efficacy component of this model seems to play a crucial role in adolescents' confidence in their ability to discuss and insist on condom use with a partner (Mahoney, Thombs, and Ford 1995).

The Health Belief Model has also been used to explain parents' participation in at-home sexuality education activities for adolescents. Perceived self-efficacy and perceived barriers were the most significant factors differentiating parents involved in these activities from those not involved. Compared with highly involved parents, noninvolved parents were: (1) less confident that their children (ninth grade students) wanted to participate in the activities with them; (2) less sure of their children's desire to talk with them about sex-related issues; and (3) less certain that their own knowledge of AIDS-related issues was current. Parents highly involved in these activities reported becoming more comfortable talking with their adolescents about sexually transmitted infections (STIs) and felt that their children talked a little more openly with them about AIDS and STIs after participating in the activities. In contrast, uninvolved parents reported no changes relative to communicating with their children about sexuality (Brock and Beazley 1995).

This book's authors found only one article analyzing the Health Belief Model with a developmental perspective (Petosa and Jackson 1991). The purpose of this study was to use the model concepts to predict safer sex intentions among adolescents of different ages (seventh, ninth, and eleventh grade students). A predictive model was constructed of the Health Belief Model variables. The model was able to predict better safer sex intentions among younger students, accounting for 43% of the variance in safer sex intentions among seventh graders, and only 27% of the variance for ninth graders and 17% of the variance for eleventh graders. The results of this study suggest that the Health Belief Model variables can be useful in guiding the design of educational programs to promote safer sex intentions in younger students, but their effectiveness decreases as they get older.

Although the model has been widely used among the general population, its specific use with the adolescent population has not yet been analyzed. Research for this publication included an extensive MEDLINE search that retrieved all published articles using the Health Belief Model to address different adolescent lifestyles and behaviors. This review indicated that the majority of research using the model was in the area of sexual health in an attempt to reduce teen pregnancy, HIV/AIDS, and STIs, and to increase the use of safer sexual practices. Unfortunately, most of the reviewed articles using the model variables to promote safer sex practices targeted mainly middle and late adolescents and youth. It is not surprising to continue to find several safer sex educational programs based on Health Belief Model variables that target these instead of younger age groups. Table 8-1. shows the number of articles dedicated to each of the adolescent lifestyle areas of concern.

Table 8-1. **Most Commonly Researched Adolescent Behaviors Using the Health Belief Model (HBM)**

ADOLESCENT BEHAVIORS	NUMBER OF ARTICLES USING THE HBM	NUMBER OF ARTICLES BY KEYWORDS	
Sexual and Reproductive Health	37	Teen Pregnancy	12
		HIV/AIDS	17
		STIs	7
		Condom Use	21
Tobacco, Alcohol, and Drug Use	18	Tobacco	11
		Alcohol	10
		Drugs	7
Physical Activity and Nutrition	9	Obesity	5
		Physical Activity	4
		Nutrition	2
Violence	2		
TOTAL	**66**		

Box 8-2. **Summary of the Health Belief Model and Adolescent Lifestyles**

- The model has demonstrated its usefulness in guiding the design of educational programs to promote safer sex intentions in younger students, but its effectiveness decreases as they get older.
- The threat appeals work only if adolescents believe they can cope effectively with the danger.
- Believing that secondhand smoke harms nonsmokers is a significant predictor among adolescents of nonsmoking, planning to stop, or stopping smoking.
- Short-term, versus long-term, consequences for reducing drinking and driving are more effective, particularly if the consequence is the suspension of the adolescent's driver's license.
- Messages that focus on the benefits of avoiding future diseases are not effective in motivating youth to adopt and maintain physical activity.
- Perceived immediate benefits and barriers are helpful in promoting physical activity among adolescents.
- Perceived severity of HIV is a better predictor of the adoption of safer sex practices among adolescents than fear of contracting the disease.
- Self-efficacy plays a crucial role in adolescents' confidence in their ability to discuss and insist on condom use with a partner.
- Perceived self-efficacy and perceived barriers are significant factors differentiating parents involved in at-home sexuality education activities from those who are not involved.

[Chapter Nine]

The Transtheoretical Model and Stages of Change

This model emerged from a comparative analysis of leading psychotherapy and behavioral change theories. The comparative analysis identified 10 processes of change among these theories, such as consciousness-raising from the Freudian tradition, contingency management from the Skinnerian tradition, and helping relationships from the Rogerian tradition. The Transtheoretical Model uses stages of change to integrate processes and principles of change from across major theories of intervention, hence the name *trans*theoretical (DiClemente and Prochaska 1982, Prochaska 1979).

The model conceives behavioral change as a *process* and not an event, which involves a progression through six different *stages*:

- ***Pre-contemplation*** is the stage in which people have no intention of taking action to change their behavior in the foreseeable future, usually measured as the next six months. According to DiClemente and Prochaska, people may be in this stage because they are uninformed or insufficiently informed about the consequences of their behavior, or they may have tried to change a number of times in the past and have become demoralized about their inability to do so.

    The authors of this book think that there may be other reasons, as well, why adolescents do not move out of the pre-contemplation stage. It is particularly important in the case of young people to also explore the underlying emotional reasons that inhibit them from taking action to move into the next stage of change. For example, they might be afraid to adopt a new behavior (e.g., physical activity) because by changing a securely set habit or routine, they will be exposing themselves to a new, unknown reality (e.g., competition and potential failure). Not wanting to change a current health-compromising behavior (e.g., fast food consumption, drug use) could also result from a lack of motivation due to the potential loss of pleasure if they abandon a daily routine they look forward to and particularly enjoy (eating hamburgers, smoking marijuana). Adolescents may fail to recognize or even unconsciously deny they have a problem because of these last two reasons.

- ■ ***Contemplation*** is the stage in which people intend to change within the next six months. They are now aware of the advantages of changing but are also more acutely aware of the disadvantages. This balance between the costs and benefits of changing can produce profound ambivalence that can keep people "stuck" in this stage for long periods of time.

Adolescents may linger in this contemplation stage because a conscious weighing of the pros and cons provides insufficient motivation for them to take action; they may be overcome by an emotional awareness accompanied by intense feelings of anxiety, fear, or insecurity about how to take the next step. They might also feel a lack of self-efficacy in preparing a plan for action. This is a developmental skill that is not easily acquired by many adolescents, especially younger ones, who may therefore need external support.

- ■ ***Preparation*** is the stage in which people intend to take action in the immediate future, usually measured as the next month. They typically have already taken some significant steps within the past year. These individuals have a plan of action.

- ■ ***Action*** is the stage in which people have made specific overt modifications in their lifestyles within the past six months.

- ■ ***Maintenance*** is the stage in which people work to prevent relapses. They are less tempted to relapse and increasingly more confident that they can take on further changes. It is estimated that this stage lasts from six months to about five years.

- ■ ***Termination*** is a sixth stage that applies to some behaviors, especially those related to addictions. This is the stage in which individuals experience no temptations and enjoy complete self-efficacy.

Studies have shown that individuals go through these same stages when using self-help or self-management methods, or when they seek professional help or go to organized programs. It is important to note

> **Box 9-1. Key Stages of Behavior Change**
> - **Pre-contemplation:** no intentions of taking action in the next six months
> - **Contemplation:** intention to change within the next six months
> - **Preparation:** intention to take action in the next month
> - **Action:** engaging in new behavior within the past six months
> - **Maintenance:** continuing to implement new behavior and prevent relapse (six months to five years)

that this is a circular or spiral—and not a linear—model (Prochaska, DiClemente, and Norcross 1992). In other words, people do not go through the stages and "graduate;" instead they are thought to progress through these stages at varying rates, often moving back and forth along the continuum a number of times before attaining the goal of maintenance. According to this theory, tailoring interventions to match a person's readiness or stage of change is essential. For example, for people who are not yet contemplating becoming more active, encouraging a step-by-step movement along the continuum of change may be more effective than encouraging them to move directly into action. This is particularly true for pre- and early adolescents, who still need significant guidance on the sequencing and planning of new experiences (e.g., eating more fruits and vegetables or taking part in new sports).

This model states that people use different *processes of change* as they move from one stage of change to another. Efficient self-change thus depends on doing the right thing (*processes*) at the right time (*stages*). Processes of change provide important guides for intervention programs, because the processes are like independent variables that people need to apply to move from stage to stage. Below is a list of processes that have received the most empirical support to date:

From pre-contemplation to contemplation:

- *Raising consciousness* involves increased awareness about the causes that relate to a particular problem behavior, its consequences and cures. Interventions that can increase awareness include feedback, confrontations, interpretations of symbolic or somatic behaviors, and media campaigns.

In moving from pre-contemplation to contemplation, it is important to bring to a conscious level not only the current behavior and its consequences, but also the emotions that might be triggering the current behavior or lack of action towards a healthier behavior.

- *Dramatic relief* involves experiencing the negative emotions (fear, anxiety, worry) that go along with the unhealthy behavioral risks and their consequences. Psychodrama, role-playing, grieving, personal testimonies, and media campaigns are examples of techniques that facilitate acknowledgement of the emotions' existence and a greater awareness of why they are unpleasant and/or painful.

The use of dramatic relief strategies to elicit these types of negative emotions in adolescents needs to be accompanied by the modeling of healthy coping skills to deal with those intense emotions. Young people, especially early adolescent girls, are particularly vulnerable to stress during this period, and many of them have not yet fully developed healthy coping mechanisms. The exposure to dramatic relief strategies without the skills to cope with strong emotions might only increase anxiety and denial of the behavior. Having said this, one of the most effective dramatic relief techniques among young people tends to be personal testimonies, in which the adolescent shares with others the healthy coping mechanisms he or she has utilized to deal with the problematic behavior.

- *Environmental reevaluation* combines both emotional and cognitive assessments of how the presence or absence of a personal habit affects one's social environment, such as an assessment of the effect of smoking on others. It can also include the awareness that one can serve as a positive or negative role model for others. Empathy training, documentaries, and family interventions can lead to such assessments. This strategy might be more useful for middle or late adolescents, since it requires cognitive

Box 9-2. **Processes of Change: Pre-contemplation to Contemplation**
- Raising consciousness
- Dramatic relief
- Environmental reevaluation

and reflective empathy skills, which most pre- and early adolescents are still developing.

- **From contemplation to preparation for action:**
  - *Self-reevaluation* combines both affective and cognitive assessments of one's self-image with and without the presence of a particular unhealthy habit. Clarifying values, having healthy role models, and using mental imagery are techniques that can move people forward to the next stage. This strategy is particularly appropriate for use with pre- and early adolescents, since it helps to strengthen their identity development and self-regulation abilities, which do not become fully developed until late adolescence.

Other authors have suggested additional processes for moving ahead between these 2 stages (Bartholomew et al. 2001) when working with adolescents:

- *Self-efficacy and social support* (De Vries and Backbier 1994)
  This process can involve skills training in coping with the emotional dis-

advantages of change and provide guidance on how to prepare a plan of action. Mobilizing social support might be crucial for adolescents during this stage.

PAHO believes that this process of change is crucial in helping adolescents to move ahead, since preparing a plan of action requires developmental skills (sometimes called "executive functions," or self-directed actions the individual employs for self-regulation purposes) that are underdeveloped until late adolescence (especially in males). Adolescents also need social support to better regulate the intense emotions that accompany change and uncertainty (especially girls).

- *Decision-making perspective* (Holtgrave, Tinsley, and Kay 1995)
  This requires certain cognitive abilities that adolescents are strengthening during pre-, early, and middle adolescence, which include the ability to decompose problem-solving into small steps, visualize different consequences for different decisions, and overcome being overwhelmed by anxiety when confronted with several possible consequences.

- *Tailoring on time horizon* (Holtgrave, Tinsley, and Kay 1995)
  This can involve skills training in time management for adolescents, incorporating realistic, personal time horizons into their lives and taking into account their various interests. Helping adolescents with this process of change is particularly important. Good time management also requires the development of executive functions, which are related to the maturation of the prefrontal lobes, the last cerebral structures to reach full development.

- *Focus on important factors* (Holtgrave, Tinsley, and Kay 1995)
  This process refers to incorporating factors of high importance to adolescents that will likely motivate them to prepare for action. Generally, adolescents still need guidance on how to prioritize their activities. Motivation is a key aspect of deciding to change. Linking factors that highly motivate adolescents to embrace a plan of action for adopting a new behavior or changing a health-compromising behavior might be crucial to success. The Goal-Setting Theory (Chapter Twelve) expands on this aspect. It is important to remember that motivation in adolescents and adults often differs, even if the new behavior is the same. For example, adolescents might not be interested in increasing their level of physical activity for health reasons, but they might be motivated to participate in a new sport or pastime because of its novelty, high sensation level, ability to produce pleasure, or because they can enjoy it together with their friends

> **Box 9-3. Processes of Change: Contemplation to Preparation for Action**
> - Self-reevaluation
> - Self-efficacy and social support
> - Decision-making perspective
> - Tailoring on time horizon
> - Focus on important factors
> - Trying out new behavior
> - Persuasion of positive outcomes
> - Modeling

(e.g., rollerblading, mountain biking, rock climbing).

- *Trying out new behavior* (Maibach and Cotton 1995)
  This process involves changing something about oneself and gaining experience from that behavior. Although adolescents might be eager to try out new behaviors when they are motivated, they might also be afraid of the uncertainty of whether the new behavior is going to be a pleasurable experience. It is crucial to support adolescents by showing empathy for negative feelings of fear and uncertainty when they are trying out a new behavior.

- *Persuasion of positive outcomes* (Maibach and Cotton 1995)
  This involves promoting new positive outcome expectations and reinforcing already-achieved positive outcomes or progress to encourage adolescents to try out new behaviors. Adolescents are particularly in need of positive reinforcement while in the process of deciding to try new behaviors that are not popular among peers (e.g., eating healthier foods).

- *Modeling* (Maibach and Cotton 1995)
  This involves the illustration of models that effectively overcome barriers and/or provide how-to guides for behavior change. Adolescents need constant modeling of new behaviors, not only by observing positive role models but also by being explicitly coached by these positive role models on how to adopt new behaviors.

- **From preparation to action:**
  - *Self-liberation* is both the belief that one can change and the commitment and recommitment to act on that belief. New Year's resolutions and public testimonies are examples of mechanisms that can enhance the willpower necessary to follow through with actions signaling a new behavior.

  Maibach and Cotton (1995) suggested the following processes to move from the preparation stage to the action stage. They are particularly relevant within the context of adolescence because of the support and guidance that this age group needs from a developmental perspective:

  - *goal-setting*: helping set specific and incremental goals

- *skill improvement*: restructuring surroundings to contain important, obvious, socially-supported cues for the new behavior
- *coping with barriers*: identifying barriers and planning solutions to any obstacles to the desired behavior change
- *modeling*: perceiving the positive social reinforcement that peers or adults (positive role models) receive when demonstrating healthy behaviors

In addition to the above, PAHO would like to add an additional process of change relevant to the preparation-to-action juncture:

- *pleasing loved ones:* Very often, individuals, and particularly adolescents, make decisions to change in order to please an important person in their lives (e.g., girl- or boyfriend, parent, teacher). The Theory of Reasoned Action described in Chapter Ten captures this concept under the construct of "motivation to comply."

Box 9-4. **Processes of Change: Preparation to Action**
- Self-liberation
- Goal-setting
- Skill improvement
- Coping with barriers
- Modeling
- Pleasing loved ones

From action to maintenance:

- *Helping relationships* combine caring, trust, openness, and acceptance as well as support for the healthy behavior change. Rapport-building, a trusting relationship with a therapist or counselor, counselor calls, and buddy systems can be sources of social support. The existence of supportive relationships is perhaps the single-most important element in facilitating behavior change among adolescents.

- *Counter-conditioning* requires the learning of healthy behaviors that can effectively substitute for problem behaviors. Relaxation, assertion, desensitization, nicotine replacement therapy, and positive self-statements are strategies for discovering healthier, safer substitutes.

It is crucial to help adolescents identify healthy behaviors that can replace problematic behaviors. Young people will adopt new, healthier behaviors if they satisfy the need which the health-compromising behavior was formerly fulfilling (e.g., need for novelty, pleasure, high sensation-seeking; regulation of positive and negative affections or moods; belonging to a social group). Sometimes a health-compromising behavior might be serving as a strategy to achieve a highly motivating goal for adolescents (e.g., smoking to control weight among girls, being accepted by a particular social group). The challenge is to help adolescents identify effective health-promoting substitutes that can also satisfy these basic needs.

- *Contingency management* provides consequences for taking steps in a particular direction. Although contingency management can include the use of punishments, the literature asserts that individuals who want to make significant changes in their lives rely much more on rewards than on punishments. Therefore, reinforcements are emphasized, since the philosophy of the stages of behavioral change model is to work in harmony with a person's natural disposition towards change. Contingency contracts, overt and covert reinforcements, and group recognition are procedures for increasing rewards as well as the probability that healthier responses will be maintained. Adolescents need constant positive reinforcements and rewards when adopting a new behavior or changing a health-compromising behavior. They also need clear limits. Parents and adolescents should define in advance the consequences of overstepping those limits as a mechanism to reinforce recognition by adolescents that they will be held accountable for their actions.

- *Stimulus control* involves removing reminders or cues to engage in the unhealthy behavior and replacing them with cues or reminders to engage in the healthy behavior. Avoidance, environmental reengineering, and self-help groups can provide stimuli that support change and reduce risks for relapse. The ability to effectively apply stimulus control is directly related to the two key components of self-efficacy: *confidence* and *temptation*.
  - *Confidence* is the situation-specific trust ingrained in people, whereby they can cope with high-risk or challenging situations and still engage in the new healthy behavior without relapsing.
  - *Temptation* describes the intensity of urges to engage in a specific habit when in the midst of difficult situations. The three most common types of tempting situations are:
    - negative feelings or emotional distress
    - social occasions conducive to the habit
    - cravings

Pre- and early adolescents need support and reminders to deal with temptations, especially when their self-control is poor. They also need support, guidance, and practice on how to redirect their behaviors. Increased confidence will result from this process, but it requires adult involvement. From a developmental perspective, pre- and early adolescents need training in *recognizing* temptations and then developing a plan on how to redirect their behaviors towards healthier alternatives. Constant monitoring of how they deal with daily temptations is also necessary in the case of these age groups.

- *Social liberation* involves the realization, on the part of the adolescent, that social norms are changing in favor of supporting the healthy behavior change. This could be an important process to apply when dealing with socially ambiguous behaviors (e.g., sexual coercion, tobacco use). Adolescents need to be aware of social norms of what is "acceptable" or "desirable" in order to develop healthy lifestyles. This process of social liberation could also be used to help adolescents redefine what is "cool" and what is not, what is "in" and what is "out." This requires an increase in social opportunities or alternatives, especially for young people who are relatively deprived of access to fun healthy alternatives. Advocacy, empowerment exercises, and appropriate policies can produce increased opportunities for health promotion. Examples of these policies include smoke-free zones, salad bars in school lunchrooms, and easy access to condoms and other contraceptives, all of which serve to signify the changing of social norms in favor of healthier alternatives.

The processes listed above are each integral facets of moving from the stage of pre-contemplation to actual behavioral change, and there is a wide variety of studies across a broad range of behaviors and populations that provide empirical support to each of the stages and processes of the Transtheoretical Model. However, if interventionists are to meet the needs of entire populations, they must also know how to distribute the messages and efforts devoted to each stage and process when targeting specific high-risk behaviors. Although there are variations in the distribution of high-risk behaviors, the results of a variety of studies support a general rule of thumb: at any given time, approximately 40% of the population will be in the pre-contemplation stage, 40% in the contemplation stage, and 20% in the preparation stage (Glanz, Rimer, and Lewis 2002).

Decisional balance reflects an individual's weighing of the relative pros and cons of changing a behavior. Findings also suggest several principles in decisional balance for advancing through the stages (Prochaska et al. 1994):

- To progress from pre-contemplation to contemplation, the pros of changing must increase.

Box 9-5. **Processes of Change: Action to Maintenance**
- Helping relationships
- Counter-conditioning
- Contingency management
- Stimulus control (confidence and temptation)
- Social liberation

- To progress from contemplation to action, the cons of changing must decrease.
- Before an individual progresses to action, the pros and cons should cross over, with the pros becoming higher than the cons, as a sign that the person is well-prepared for action.
- Progress from pre-contemplation to action involves approximately a 0.5 standard deviation decrease in the cons of changing; in other words, the perceived barriers to changing decrease by half.

The practical implications of these principles are that the pros of changing must increase twice as much as the cons must decrease. This indicates that perhaps twice as much emphasis should be placed on raising the benefits as on reducing the costs or barriers. With people in pre-contemplation, practitioners would target the pros for intervention and save the cons for people who have progressed to contemplation. Focusing more on the pros than on the cons is particularly effective with adolescents. This decisional balance between pros and cons has been studied for adolescent drinking (Migneault, Pallonen, and Velicer 1997). The relationship was replicated for the stages of acquisition of the drinking behavior, where the pros showed a maximum increase of 1.06 standard deviations and the cons a maximum decrease of 0.63 standard deviation. For cessation, the relationship was not replicated, with the change in the pros and the cons being about equal (0.88 and 0.84 standard deviation, respectively).

The structure of the processes across studies has not been as consistent as the structure of the stages or the pros and cons of changing. In early stages, people tend to apply cognitive, affective, and evaluative processes to progress through the stages. In later stages, people tend to rely more on commitments, conditioning, contingencies, environmental controls, and support for progressing towards maintenance. To help people progress from pre-contemplation to contemplation, practitioners need to apply processes such as consciousness-raising and dramatic relief. In this sense, applying processes such as contingency management, counter-conditioning, and stimulus control to people in the pre-contemplation stage represents a theoretical, empirical, and practical mistake. But for people in action, such strategies represent an optimal matching of process and stage.

Figure 9-1. **Decisional Balance**

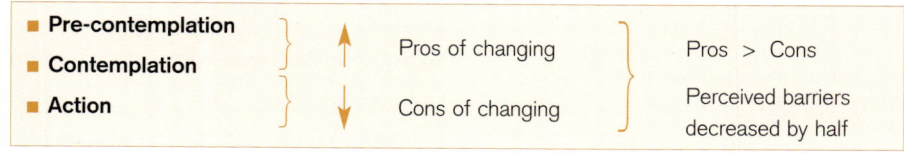

Research and Evidence of Practical Applications of the Transtheoretical Model and Stages of Change to Adolescent Lifestyles

The use of the Transtheoretical Model and stages of change to help design health promotion interventions for adolescents is increasing, particularly in Canada and the United States, but also in Latin America and the Caribbean, as well. It is an easy-to-use theoretical construct for evaluating the effectiveness of interventions. It helps identify baseline behaviors by stages and describes the processes that a health promotion intervention should promote to obtain a behavioral change and progression to the next stage. Post-intervention behaviors can be compared to baseline behaviors by stages to find evidence of effectiveness of the behavior change intervention. The model also provides an opportunity to investigate which factors determine the stage an adolescent is in during different behaviors, as well as the barriers and processes involved when advancing to other stages of behaviors. It includes theoretical constructs described by interpersonal- and community-level theories as an important part of the processes of change (e.g., modeling, social support, empowerment, organizational change). There has been fascinating research in this area, as described in the following paragraphs.

The cross-sectional relationships between weight concerns, weight control behaviors, and initiation of tobacco use among youths have been studied using the Transtheoretical Model of Change in a sample of 16,862 pre- and early adolescents ages 9 to 14 (Tomeo et al. 1999). Contemplation of tobacco use was associated with misperception of being overweight, unhappiness with appearance, and a tendency to change eating patterns around peers. Gender differences were observed. Experimentation with cigarettes was associated with daily exercise to control weight among boys and with periodic purging and daily dieting among girls.

Pallonen and colleagues (1998) analyzed the relationship between temptations to try smoking and stages of smoking acquisition among adolescents. The study showed that nonsmokers' reasons to initiate smoking were related to socializing or to simple curiosity at the very beginning of the acquisition phase. Regulation of negative and positive affective states became prominent at the later acquisition stages when adolescents were prepared to try smoking. Nonsmokers were most tempted to try smoking when they anticipated that smoking would help them reduce negative moods and increase positive ones. The findings in the smokers' temptation level confirmed the importance of affect regulation in maintaining smoking, which is also reported in adolescent drug use.

Mayhew, Flay, and Mott (2000) reviewed empirical studies of predictors of transitions in stages of smoking progression during adolescence. Parent and family influences were found repeatedly to be of major importance in stages of smoking beyond the experimental. Another trend indicated that females who have a smoking and smoking-supportive social network (friends and family members) were more likely to transition from experimental to regular smoking, suggesting that females may display a greater social sensitivity to the smoking environment than males.

Werch and DiClemente (1994) developed a multi-component stage model for matching drug prevention strategies and messages to youth stages when use occurs. The model suggests the most effective use of different channels when motivating youth to avoid drugs. Media and media-related materials such as television, videotapes, comic books, and billboards are believed to be most effective in influencing youth in the pre-contemplation, contemplation, and preparation stages of change. The idea that media can commonly be expected to produce alterations in personal factors such as awareness, knowledge, and motivation is supported by a considerable amount of research. Interpersonal delivery modes such as school classes, health screenings, self-help groups, and student assistance programs are thought to be most effective in influencing youth in the preparation and action stages of change. Personal contacts are believed to significantly increase the reception and integration of communications and are commonly used for teaching and modeling the attitudes and skills needed for behavioral change related to drug use prevention. Lastly, environmental delivery modes, including peer facilitators, parental training, policies, and legislation, are believed to be most effective in influencing youth in the action and maintenance stages of change. Environmental prevention channels are necessary for effecting successful behavioral change in that youth are influenced as much by the physical and social situation in which they function as by personal and behavioral factors. In addition, social support is believed to be essential to the successful maintenance of behavioral change and improvement of health.

The multi-component stage model described by Werch and DiClemente might work with other adolescent health-related behaviors as long as the reasons for not moving from pre-contemplation to the contemplation and preparation stages are lack of awareness and/or information. Raising consciousness through the mass media can definitely increase motivation to move from pre-contemplation to contemplation, particularly since young people enjoy media communications. Nevertheless, if the underlying reasons for not moving from the pre-contemplation stage include strong emotional feelings of avoidance to change (e.g., misperception of being overweight and smoking), which can be conscious or unconscious, media messages will need to create awareness of those feelings and show how to deal with them. These messages might be effective for those adolescents with healthy coping styles, but might not work with adolescents using avoidance coping mechanisms.

The readiness to change the drinking habits of university students who drink heavily was investigated in a recent study (Vik, Culbertson, and Sellers 2000). Two-thirds of the heavy drinkers were found to be at the pre-contemplation stage (67%). Only 20% were at the contemplation stage and 13% at the action stage.

The stage distribution for smoking cessation among adolescents has also been described. A recent study (Prokhorov et al. 2001) involving 1,111 current or former smokers in high school found the following distribution: pre-contemplation 52.5%; contemplation 16%; preparation 7.5%; action 13.2%; and maintenance 10.8%. Pre-contemplators exhibited significantly higher mean nicotine dependence scores than did students in the contemplation or preparation stages. A similar trend was observed for withdrawal symptom scores across the stages of change. Another recent study examined the relationship of nicotine dependence, stress, and coping methods between present and past adolescent smokers aged 12 to 21 and used the Transtheoretical Model of Change to analyze these factors among adjacent smoking cessation stages (Siqueira, Rolnitzy, and Rickert 2001). Smokers were significantly more likely to report smoking additional cigarettes per day as well as have higher levels of physical addiction, greater levels of perceived stress, and less use of cognitive coping methods than former smokers. Three out of 20 withdrawal symptoms (cravings, difficulty dealing with stress, and anger) were reported more frequently among current smokers who had attempted to quit during the past six months than among former smokers ($P = .01$).

A study undertaken with early adolescent girls using the Transtheoretical Model and stages of change to promote higher consumption of fruits and vegetables (Cullen et al. 1998) suggests that to move from pre-contemplation to the action stage for fruit consumption, programs should target fruit preferences and barriers to increased consumption. Finding out which fruits adolescents like and having them available at school and home will increase the effectiveness of the intervention. Skills to choose and prepare fruits and vegetables, problem-solving, and goal-setting activities to reduce perceived barriers also contribute to behavior change.

The "Agita São Paulo" experience, a multi-level, community-wide intervention to promote physical activity among the 34 million inhabitants of São Paulo State, Brazil, applied the Transtheoretical Model, among other theories, in its design. The program developers applied the model to the assessment of changes in the readiness of various subgroups and the selection of change methods and media messages relevant to people in each stage. Focus groups included students from the elementary to university levels, among other population segments.

The Caribbean Food and Nutrition Institute, a PAHO regional center based in

Kingston, Jamaica, and its collaborators analyzed the readiness of the Caribbean population for change in behaviors related to diet and exercise (Caribbean Food and Nutrition Institute 2002). They found that among the obese population, most were between the pre- and contemplation stages for consumption of fruits and vegetables, but among the non-obese population, most were at the pre-contemplation stage. Findings were more encouraging for promoting exercise, where most of the obese population was between the preparation and action stages; however, most of the non-obese population was in the pre-contemplation stage. It would be interesting to analyze this type of information for the different adolescent stages to determine if they behave in the same way as the total population and if there are different cultural barriers to change in behaviors. The compilation of information regarding adult nutritional and physical activity stages of change nonetheless sheds important light on the type of role models parents are being for their children, a value which seems to be deeply rooted in Caribbean culture.

In the sexual and reproductive health arena, Students Together against Negative Decisions (STAND) (Mercer University 1998) is an example of a new genre of HIV prevention that utilizes complementary theoretical models to develop a program that targets both individual and community level change in rural adolescents. STAND is a 28-session teen peer educator training program promoting both abstinence and sexual risk reduction. The theoretical foundation of the curriculum includes the Transtheoretical Model and the Diffusion of Innovations Theory (Chapter Twenty-three) and focuses on individual and community norm change. STAND is teen-centered and skills-based; activities center on active learning and are being implemented in a rural county in the southeastern United States. Acceptance of and participation in STAND suggest that adolescents in rural communities can be accessed through community-based interventions, that they are willing to participate in such intensive programs, and that they perceive the intervention as valuable and enjoyable. Results from a pilot study showed significantly greater increases in self-efficacy and condom use (16% vs. a 1% decrease in the control group) and in consistent condom use (+28% vs. +15%). Adolescent trainees also reported a sevenfold increase in condom use (+213% vs. 31%) and a 30% decrease in unprotected intercourse, compared to a 29% increase in the control group.

These various studies are only a sample of those that have utilized the Transtheoretical Model for behavioral change. Interestingly, in contrast with the findings for the Health Belief Model, sexual health in adolescents is one of the lesser-studied areas using the Transtheoretical Model and stages of change concept. This model could be used to further study the stages and processes of change not only for condom use or negotiation, but also for changing social norms regarding harmful aspects of traditional versions of masculinity and femininity and sexual coercion. The Transtheoretical Model variables can help measure concrete behaviors that should be promoted or changed during pre-adolescence, for example, for a more equitable gender development.

Table 9-1. details the number of studies found using this model according to health behaviors.

Table 9-1. **Most Commonly Researched Adolescent Behaviors Using the Transtheoretical Model and Stages of Change (TTM)**

ADOLESCENT BEHAVIORS	NUMBER OF ARTICLES USING THE TTM	NUMBER OF ARTICLES BY KEYWORDS	
Sexual and Reproductive Health	9	Teen Pregnancy	3
		HIV/AIDS	5
		STIs	2
		Condom Use	6
Tobacco, Alcohol, and Drug Use	27	Tobacco	17
		Alcohol	7
		Drugs	3
Physical Activity and Nutrition	15	Obesity	1
		Physical Activity	8
		Nutrition	7
Violence	0		
TOTAL	**51**		

Box 9-6. Summary of the Transtheoretical Model and Stages of Change and Adolescent Lifestyles

- It is an easy-to-use theory for evaluating the effectiveness of interventions.
- It helps to identify baseline behaviors by stages and describes the processes of change needed to move to the next stage.
- Among pre- and early adolescents, contemplation of tobacco use is associated with the misperception of being overweight, desire to socialize, and simple curiosity.
- Preparation to try smoking is associated with the anticipation of reducing negative moods and increasing positive ones.
- Experimentation with cigarettes is associated with daily exercise to control weight among boys and with daily dieting among girls.
- Girls who have a smoking and smoking-supportive network (friends and family members) are more likely to transition from experimental to regular smoking.
- Media and media-related materials (television, videos, comic books, billboards) are believed to be most effective in influencing youth in the pre-contemplation, contemplation, and preparation stages.
- Interpersonal delivery modes (school classes, health screenings, self-help groups, student assistance programs) are thought to be most effective in influencing youth in the preparation and action stages of change.
- Environmental delivery modes (peer interaction, parental training, policies, legislation) are believed to be most effective in influencing youth in the action and maintenance stages of change.
- Social support is believed to be essential to the successful maintenance of behavioral change.
- One study (Vik et al. 2000) of the readiness to change drinking habits during late adolescence found that 67% of heavy drinkers are at the pre-contemplation stage, 20% are at the contemplation stage, and only 13% are at the action stage.
- Another study of smoking cessation among adolescents found that 52.5% are at the pre-contemplation stage vs. 10.8% in maintenance.
- Pre-contemplators exhibit significantly higher mean nicotine dependence scores than adolescent smokers in the contemplation or preparation stages.
- In a comparison of the consecutive stages of behavior change among smoking adolescents, the most significant difference in cognitive coping skills is between those in the pre-contemplation and contemplation stages.
- Interventions encouraging early adolescent girls to move from pre-contemplation to the action stage for increased fruit consumption should target fruit preferences and reduce barriers to its improved consumption.

[Chapter Ten]

The Theory of Reasoned Action

The Theory of Reasoned Action (Ajzen and Fishbein 1980, Fishbein and Ajzen 1975) states that individual performance of a given behavior is primarily determined by a person's intention to perform that behavior. This intention is determined by two major factors:

- *attitude* (positive or negative feelings) towards performing a behavior. Attitude is determined by:
    - the individual's beliefs about the outcomes of performing the behavior (*behavioral beliefs*) and
    - the value of these outcomes (*evaluation*).

- *subjective norm* associated with the behavior; i.e., the person's perception of other people's opinions regarding the defined behavior. A person's subjective norm is determined by:
    - beliefs about what other people think the person should do (*normative beliefs*) and
    - the person's *motivation to comply* with the opinion of others.

A person who strongly believes that, for the most part, positively valued outcomes will result from performing a given behavior will have a positive attitude towards that behavior. A person who holds strong beliefs that negatively valued outcomes will result from a given behavior will have a negative attitude towards that behavior. These beliefs will differ from population to population, as well as by culture and age. In the case of the adolescent age

> **Box 10-1. The Theory of Reasoned Action: Key Theoretical Constructs**
> - Intention
>   - Attitude
>   - behavioral beliefs
>   - evaluation
>   - Subjective norm
>   - normative beliefs
>   - motivation to comply

group, such emotions as pleasure, joy, anticipation, excitement, or "having fun" are generally considered the most common elements of positively valued outcomes, beyond rational or cognitive evaluations. (Within this context, an interesting possibility for future research might be to determine to what extent, if any, the elements of positively valued outcomes vary through different adolescent developmental stages and by gender.)

A person who believes that certain referents (peers, parents, teachers, etc.) think he/she should perform a behavior, and who is motivated to meet the expectations of those referents, will hold a positive subjective norm. A person who believes certain referents think he/she should not perform the behavior will have a negative subjective norm, and a person who is less motivated to comply with the referents will have a relatively neutral subjective norm. Adolescents who have ongoing nurturing relationships with caregivers, teachers, or other adults tend to respond more to positive or negative subjective norms than adolescents who do not have this type of relationship.

The Theory of Reasoned Action assumes a causal chain: behavioral beliefs and normative beliefs are linked to behavioral intention and behavior via attitude and subjective norm. The authors of the model propose that changes in an individual's behavioral and normative beliefs will ultimately affect the individual's actual behavior. But for adolescents, who devote more time and energy (relative to older age groups) trying to please or displease others (friends, parents, teachers), a change in normative beliefs will most likely be within the context of ongoing nurturing relationships; otherwise, the adolescent will have little or no motivation to comply.

The measurement and computation of model components and causal relationships among those components are clearly specified in Ajzen and Fishbein (1980). The relative weights of attitude and subjective norm depend upon the behavior and the population under investigation. Some behaviors are entirely under attitudinal control, while others are under normative control. The same behavior has been found to be under attitudinal control in one population but under normative control in another population (Fishbein 1990). The relative weights are determined empirically for the particular behavior and population under investigation, and this information suggests whether attitude or subjective norm is the best focus for behavioral change efforts. Correlation and analysis of variance can be used to determine which specific behavioral beliefs or normative beliefs are most

Figure 10-1. **The Theory of Reasoned Action**

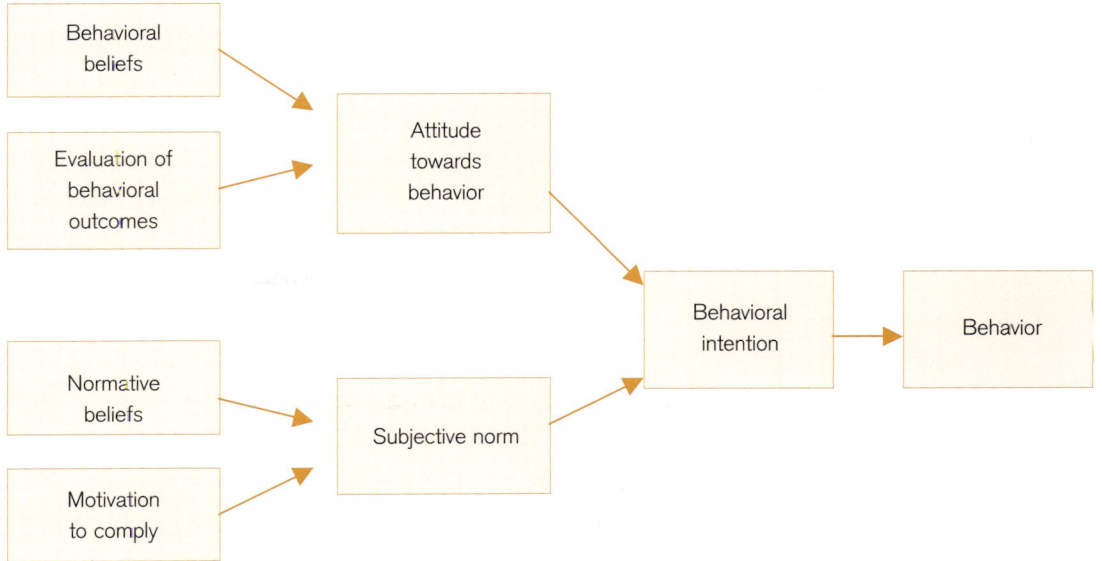

Source: adapted from Ajzen, Icek and Fishbein, Martin; *Understanding Attitudes and Predicting Social Behavior*, 1st Edition, © 1980. Reproduced by permission of Pearson Education, Inc., Upper Saddle River, New Jersey.

strongly associated with intention and behavior, thus providing empirically identified targets for intervention efforts.

The assumption of the Theory of Reasoned Action is that individuals are rational actors. That is, all individuals process information at a cognitive level and are motivated to act upon it. The theory further assumes that there are underlying reasons other than emotions that determine an individual's motivation to perform a behavior. The strength of the theory is that it provides a framework for identifying those underlying reasons and a means to make sense of actions by recognizing, measuring, and combining beliefs that are relevant to individuals or groups. Nevertheless, when working with adolescents, reasons and emotions blend easily. At younger ages (e.g., preadolescence), underlying emotions are probably more determinant than underlying reasons when deciphering behaviors. At this age, many preadolescents still have significant difficulty identifying the underlying emotions and reasons for specific behaviors.

The success of the theory in explaining actual behavior is dependent also upon the degree to which the behavior is under volitional control. It is not clear that the theory's components are sufficient for predicting behaviors in which volitional control is reduced. A person who has high motivation to perform a behavior may not actually perform that behavior due to intervening environmental conditions. A pre- or early adolescent might be highly motivated to adopt a certain sport as a physical activity but might not be able to do so because of lack of opportunities (e.g., economical constraints, lack of parental support and of time). A middle adolescent may have decided to use condoms when having sexual relations but may not be able to buy or obtain free condoms in the local community.

Research and Evidence of Practical Applications of the Theory of Reasoned Action to Adolescent Lifestyles

The use of the Theory of Reasoned Action to change adolescent behaviors has been studied in Africa, Europe, India, and the United States. Instruments to measure adolescents' attitudes and subjective norms have been developed. The predictive value of these constructs has been demonstrated for tobacco and drug consumption. The effect of the subjective norm for condom use behavior has also been studied among adolescents. The effect of the different theoretical constructs (subjective norm, attitude, intention) tends to vary for the different adolescent behaviors being analyzed.

Using data from a diverse statewide sample of tenth grade middle adolescents in California in 1996 and 1997, Unger et al. (2001) investigated the associations between peer influence variables and susceptibility to smoking. Peer influence variables included attitudes about the social consequences of smoking and subjective norms, as described by the Theory of Reasoned Action. Among those who had never smoked ($n = 2,681$) and ever-smokers—those who either had smoked at one time and had quit or continue to smoke—($n = 4,248$), attitudes about social consequences of smoking and subjective norms each were associated with an increased risk of susceptibility to smoking. The model explained a larger proportion of the variance in susceptibility among ever-smokers than among never-smokers. These results are congruent with previous studies using the Theory of Reasoned Action to analyze cigarette use by adolescents and the effects of peer influence (O'Callaghan, Callan, and Baglioni 1999). Another study examined the relationship between beliefs regarding chewing tobacco use and addiction among 473 male university athletes (Hilton et al. 1994). Beliefs were assessed using methods prescribed by the Theory of Reasoned Action. One highlighted finding was that all athletes believed that clinicians, parents, and girlfriends did not approve of their chewing tobacco use, but that male peers, coaches, and professional athletes were fairly indifferent to it. The authors pointed out the importance of strengthening the support of male peers and other athletes who influence the subjects' social norms when planning interventions to help them quit.

Lawson (1994) examined the role of cigarette smoking in the lives of low-income, pregnant adolescents. Based on in-depth interviews, subjects' beliefs and attitudes towards smoking are described in the study. The findings indicated that this population smoked to cope with weight gain, to deliver smaller infants which in turn would decrease the duration of labor and reduce the pain of delivery, to counteract anxiety arising from feelings of abandonment by their families and/or boyfriends, and to establish an identity separate from their parents' and peers' drug abuse. These results suggest that low-income, pregnant adolescents perceive immediate benefits from cigarette smoking that outweigh long-term health consequences. The author argued that smoking prevention programs based on an inaccurate understanding of the social context in which smoking occurs can reinforce the use of tobacco among high-risk, pregnant adolescents.

Laflin et al. (1994) compared the role of self-esteem, attitudes, and subjective norms in the prediction of drug and alcohol use. Measures of self-esteem, drug attitudes, subjective norms, and drug use behaviors were collected from 2,074 U.S. high school and university students. Results indicated that attitudes and subjective norms do predict drug and alcohol use, but self-esteem does not add significantly to the prediction of the drug and alcohol behaviors. O'Callaghan et al. (1997) compared the Theory of Reasoned Action, the Theory of Planned Behavior (reviewed in Chapter Eleven), and an extension of the Theory of Reasoned Action that incorporates past behavior in explaining alcohol use among 122 U.S. university students (82 of whom were female). The results suggested that the extension of the Theory of Reasoned Action provides the best fit to the data. For these students, their intentions to drink alcohol were predicted by their past behavior as well as their perceptions of what others think they should do (subjective norm). In 1999, the authors published the same comparison of theories for cigarette use by adolescents. Respondents consisted of 225 U.S. high school students (O'Callaghan, Callan, Baglioni 1999). Results indicated that the modification of the Theory of Reasoned Action incorporating past behavior provided a marginally better fit than the other models. Nevertheless, they concluded that for this group of high school students, attitudes towards smoking, past behavior in relation to smoking, and perceptions of what others think they should do were significant predictors of their intentions to smoke.

Selvan et al. (2001) studied the intended sexual and condom behavior patterns among higher secondary school students in India using the Theory of Reasoned Action constructs. The results revealed that perceived norms and perceived peer group norms showed significant association with intended sexual behavior and actual sexual behavior and that those children of more highly educated parents are less likely to engage in sexual activities during their adolescent years. Condom use intentions of students at a university in southern Ghana have also been studied using the Theory of Reasoned Action (Bosompra 2001). Subjective norms and the perceived disadvantages of condom use were significant determinants of intention, with the former being more important. The critical difference was that "intenders" consistently held a stronger belief than "non-intenders" that their significant referents approved of condom use. The author proposed shifting from a traditional approach of focusing on individual behaviors to focusing simultaneously on individuals, their sexual partners, and the broader social networks to which the individuals belong in order to enhance perceptions of peer acceptance of condom use. Predictors of intention to be sexually active among Tanzanian middle adolescents were investigated by Klepp et al. (1996). A total of 2,026 students (mean age: 14 years) participated, representing a wide variety of ethnic, socioeconomic, and urban-rural groups. Sixty-three percent of the boys and 24% of the girls reported having already had their first sexual encounter. Attitudes, subjective norms, and self-efficacy were all predictors of intention to have sexual intercourse within the next three months, but prior behavior emerged as the strongest predictor of intention.

Freeman and Sheiham (1997) analyzed the decision-making processes for sugar consumption among adolescents using the Theory of Reasoned Action. One hundred and eighty-seven 16-year-olds in the United States completed a questionnaire on the consumption of sugar using the method developed by Ajzen and Fishbein. The findings suggested that although past dental experiences, behavior, and education, together with the role of parental figures, acted as important influences, *the immediate pleasurable* taste of sugar outweighed and deferred the recognition of dangers associated with its consumption. In another study, Mesters and Oostveen (1994) analyzed the determinants of eating snacks filled with sugar and fats between meals by 560 Dutch adolescents ages 12–15. The results showed that attitude turned out to be more important than the subjective norm in predicting intention to consume such snacks.

The various studies just reviewed are only a sample of those that have used the Theory of Reasoned Action to look at behavioral change. The authors of this book were unable to find any studies applying this theory to change adolescent behaviors which analyzed the theoretical constructs by developmental stages. Most of the research using the theory in adolescents has focused on sexual health and tobacco, alcohol, and drug use. Nevertheless, most of the studies on sexual health were oriented towards condom use and HIV prevention. Unfortunately, no research was found linking condom use, HIV prevention, and changes in normative beliefs or subjective norms regarding sexual coercion or abuse. Table 10-1. shows the number of studies found using the Theory of Reasoned Action according to health behavior.

Table 10-1. **Most Commonly Researched Adolescent Behaviors Using the Theory of Reasoned Action (TRA)**

ADOLESCENT BEHAVIORS	NUMBER OF ARTICLES USING THE TRA	NUMBER OF ARTICLES BY KEYWORDS	
Sexual and Reproductive Health	13	Teen Pregnancy	1
		HIV/AIDS	9
		STIs	0
		Condom Use	6
Tobacco, Alcohol, and Drug Use	14	Tobacco	9
		Alcohol	3
		Drugs	2
Physical Activity and Nutrition	3	Obesity	0
		Physical Activity	1
		Nutrition	2
Violence	1		
TOTAL	**31**		

Box 10-2. **Summary of the Theory of Reasoned Action and Adolescent Lifestyles**

- The theory's use to change adolescent behaviors has been studied in Africa, Europe, India, and the United States.
- Instruments to measure adolescents' attitudes and subjective norms have been developed.
- Attitudes about the social consequences of smoking and subjective norms are associated with an increased risk of susceptibility to smoking.
- Low-income, pregnant adolescents perceive immediate benefits from cigarette smoking: to counteract feelings of abandonment, to establish an identity separate from their parents, to cope with increased weight, and to deliver small infants, which decreases the duration of labor and reduces the pain of delivery. The study (Lawson 1994) suggests that positive attitudes towards cigarette smoking outweigh long-term health consequences.
- Attitudes and subjective norms predict drug and alcohol use among adolescents, but self-esteem does not add significantly to the prediction of this behavior.
- Perceived norms and perceived peer group norms show significant association with intended sexual behavior and actual sexual behavior among middle and late adolescents.
- Subjective norms and the perceived disadvantages of condom use are significant determinants of intention.
- "Intenders" consistently have a stronger belief than "non-intenders" that their significant referents approve of condom use.
- Attitudes, subjective norms, and self-efficacy are all predictors of intention to have sexual intercourse within the next three months.
- The immediate pleasurable taste of sugar outweighs and postpones the recognition of dangers associated with sugar consumption among adolescents.
- Attitude is more important than subjective norm in predicting intention to consume snacks filled with sugar and fats among early and middle adolescents.

[Chapter Eleven]

The Theory of Planned Behavior

Ajzen's Theory of Planned Behavior (Ajzen and Madden 1986) is an extension of the Theory of Reasoned Action (Chapter Ten) that adds *perceived behavioral control* (Figure 11-1.). This accounts for factors outside the individual's control, which may affect his/her intention and behavior. This extension was based in part on the idea that behavioral performance is determined jointly by motivation (intention) and ability (behavioral control). Ajzen indicates that his perceived behavioral control is not really different from Bandura's self-efficacy (i.e., the perceived ability to perform a given behavior, as described in Chapter Eight). According to the Theory of Planned Behavior, perceived control is determined by:

- *control beliefs* concerning the presence or absence of resources for, and impediments to, behavioral performance
- *perceived power*, or the impact of each resource and impediment to facilitate or inhibit the behavior

A person who holds strong control beliefs about the existence of factors that facilitate the behavior will have high perceived control over the behavior. A person who holds strong control beliefs about the existence of factors that impede the behavior will have low perceived control over the behavior.

As in the Theory of Reasoned Action, the particular resources and impediments that are to be measured are not specified by the theory, but instead are identified through inter-

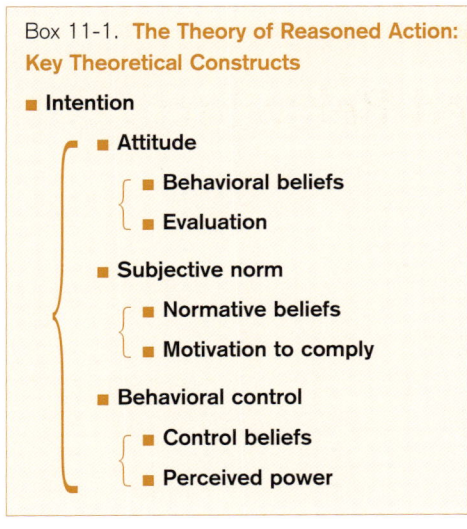

Box 11-1. **The Theory of Reasoned Action: Key Theoretical Constructs**
- **Intention**
  - **Attitude**
    - **Behavioral beliefs**
    - **Evaluation**
  - **Subjective norm**
    - **Normative beliefs**
    - **Motivation to comply**
  - **Behavioral control**
    - **Control beliefs**
    - **Perceived power**

views conducted among the particular population for the behavior under investigation. Once these factors are identified, a person's control beliefs and perceived power regarding each factor are measured.

The theory postulates that perceived control is an independent determinant of behavioral intention along with attitude towards the behavior and subjective norm. Holding attitude and subjective norm constant, a person's perception of the ease or difficulty of behavioral performance will affect his/her behavioral intention. The

Figure 11-1. **The Theory of Planned Behavior**

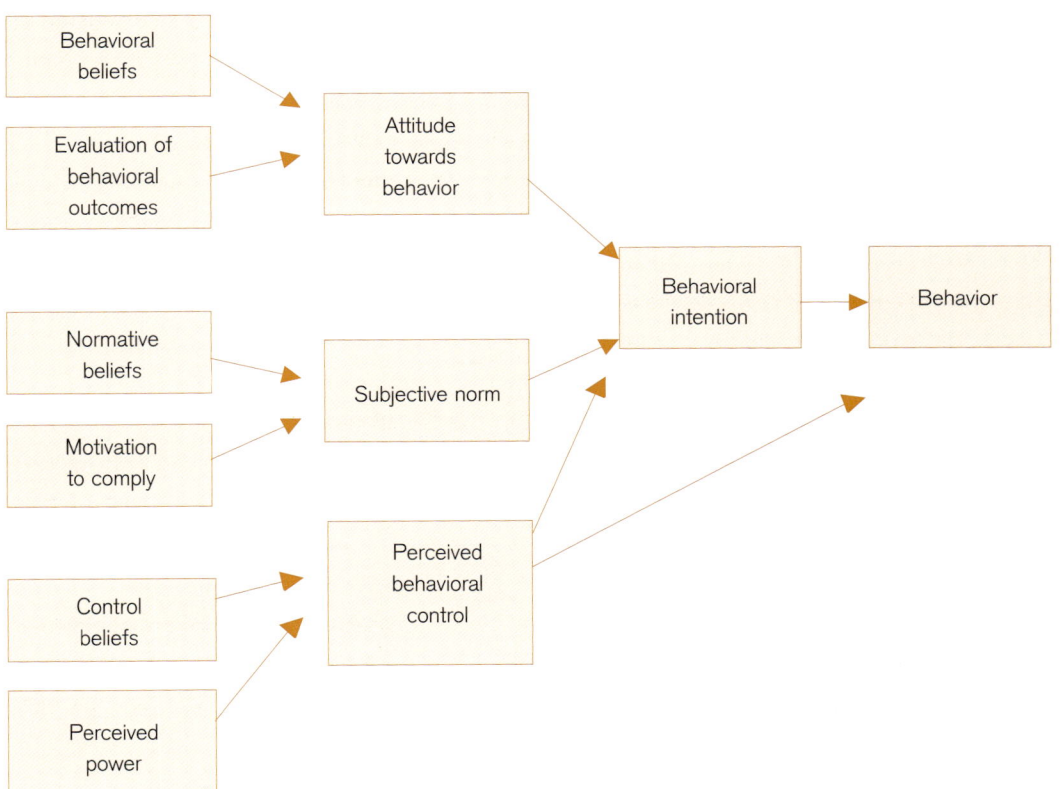

Source: *Health Behavior and Health Education: Theory, Research, and Practice;* by K. Glanz, B.K. Rimer, and F.M. Lewis © 2002. Reprinted by permission of John Wiley & Sons, Inc.

> **Box 11-2. The Theory of Planned Behavior: Key Theoretical Concepts in the Adoption of Healthy Behaviors**
>
> - **behavioral beliefs:** the belief that behavioral performance is associated with certain attributes or outcomes (equivalent to *outcome expectations* in the Social Cognitive Theory, to be presented in Chapter Sixteen)
> - **evaluation of behavioral outcomes:** the value attached to a behavioral outcome or attribute (equivalent to *outcome expectancies* or *incentives* in the Social Cognitive Theory, to be discussed in Chapter Sixteen)
> - **attitude:** an overall evaluation of the defined behavior
> - **behavioral intention:** the perceived likelihood of performing the behavior
> - **normative belief:** the belief about what other people (referents) think the person should do
> - **motivation to comply:** the motivation to follow through in regard to referents' opinions or thoughts about behavior
> - **subjective norm:** the person's perception about referents' feelings about the defined behavior
> - **control belief:** the perceived likelihood of occurrence of each facilitating or constraining condition
> - **perceived power:** the perceived effect of each condition in making behavioral performance difficult or easy
> - **perceived behavioral control:** the overall perceived ability to perform a given behavior (equivalent to *self-efficacy*, as discussed in Chapters Eight and Sixteen)

relative weights of these three factors in determining intention are expected to vary for different behaviors and populations.

Research and Evidence of Practical Applications of the Theory of Planned Behavior to Adolescent Lifestyles

The use of the Theory of Planned Behavior to change adolescent behaviors has been studied in Canada, Europe, and the United States.

One well-researched topic using the theory is the onset of smoking in youth, as described by Kok and colleagues in a chapter entitled "Social Psychology and Health Education" published in the *European Review of Social Psychology* (Kok et al. 1996). Nonsmoking and regular smoking Dutch youth ages 10 to 15 ($n = 219$) were asked questions about smoking, in interviews or open response questionnaires, to elicit salient outcome beliefs, normative beliefs, self-efficacy expectations, and intentions. Based on this eliciting procedure, structured questionnaires were developed, which consisted of the following:

- beliefs and evaluations of the consequences of smoking (e.g., "If I smoke or should start to smoke, this is very [*sociable* versus *unsociable*."])
- normative beliefs and corresponding motivations to comply with respect to various social referents (e.g., mother, father, brothers, sisters, friends, classmates)
- self-efficacy expectations (e.g., student's perceived ability to refuse offers of cigarettes, to provide arguments

against smoking, to resist social pressures to smoke)
- intentions regarding both initial and regular smoking (e.g., smoking with friends, smoking at parties)

The answer to these questions differentiated smoking from nonsmoking youth. Nonsmoking Dutch adolescents are more likely than smokers to:

- endorse that smoking causes negative health consequences (e.g., cancer, coughing, nausea) and has other negative effects (e.g., a bad smell, high cost, tendency to be offensive to others)
- state that there are negative social expectations regarding smoking (e.g., from parents, other relatives, friends, and classmates)
- have higher self-efficacy for not smoking when friends smoke, refusing cigarettes, remaining nonsmokers, and explaining that they do not want to smoke

Dutch smoking students are more likely than nonsmokers to:

- endorse the personal advantages of smoking (e.g., increased sociability, to show off, to relax, or to relieve boredom)
- endorse the importance of belonging to a group and doing what others do
- have negative self-efficacy about stating reasons to refuse a cigarette, not smoking when friends smoke, and becoming a nonsmoker

Hanson (1999) did a cross-cultural study of beliefs about smoking among teenaged females. The Theory of Planned Behavior provided the basis for the development of the research instrument. Participants included 141 African-American, 146 Puerto Rican, and 143 non-Hispanic white females, ages 13 to 19. Logistic regression analysis identified beliefs that were significantly related to smoking behavior in each cultural group. Beliefs related to attitudes about smoking and perceived social pressure regarding smoking *differed among the three cultural groups*. The findings suggest that specific beliefs differentiate between smokers and nonsmokers and that some beliefs differ by culture

One of the limitations of most studies on adolescents is that smoking behavior is measured in a dichotomous manner: that is, a smoker or a nonsmoker. This classification does not allow for an understanding of the process and stages by which adolescents progress from nonsmoking to occasional smoking to smoking on a regular basis. Godin (1996) proposed identifying stages of adoption of a behavior by the intersection of two variables: recent past behavior and the intention to adopt this behavior in a stated time frame (near future). Following this approach, the stages of adopting a smoking behavior would be:

- Stage 1: consists of nonsmokers who do not intend to smoke
- Stage 2: consists of nonsmokers who, contrary to stage 1, intend to smoke

- Stage 3: consists of occasional smokers who do not intend to smoke
- Stage 4: consists of occasional smokers who intend to smoke
- Stage 5: consists of regular smokers who intend to maintain their smoking

In addition, Godin identified a sixth group, known as "quitters," which consists of regular smokers who express the intention to not smoke in the short term. He did not include this group as a stage of behavior, although the intention of this group could serve as the next possible step when and if its members decide to follow through and accompany the intention with actions.

Jomphe Hill et al. (1997) developed a study to identify variables from the Theory of Planned Behavior that differentiated and discriminated among these stages of smoking acquisition in adolescence. The sample consisted of 294 Canadian students, ages 11 to 15. Results showed that the variables of attitude and perceived behavioral control significantly differentiated the students situated in stages 3 and 4. The perceived behavioral control variable significantly differentiated the students situated in stages 4 and 5. Based on the results of the study, the authors suggest that the stages could be characterized in the following manner: students who are situated in stage 1 have an unfavorable attitude towards smoking. Although this attitude remains negative, it is more favorable for students in stages 2 and 3, despite the fact that there is no statistically significant difference. However, compared to stage 3, stage 4 is accompanied by a favorable attitude towards smoking. Stage 5 illustrates an attitude even more favorable towards smoking. A similar profile emerges for the perceived behavioral control variable. The authors propose that the content of smoking prevention programs for adolescents should be based on the beliefs underlying attitude, subjective norm, and perceived behavioral control, and adapted to each stage of smoking acquisition. Students in stages 1 and 2 (nonsmokers) may be influenced by messages that aim to strengthen their unfavorable attitude towards smoking cigarettes. For students at stage 3, messages should aim at the short- and long-term effects of smoking, but also at providing messages that suggest alternatives to the advantages that smokers associate with tobacco smoking, since it was observed that it is at the subsequent stage 4 that students present a favorable attitude towards smoking.

Wall, Hinson, and McKee (1998) used the Theory of Planned Behavior to assess the contribution of alcohol outcome expectancies and attitudes towards drinking in 316 U.S. university undergraduates of legal drinking age who reported drinking at least once a month. Intentions to drink "too much" and self-reported excessive consumption episodes served as criterion measures and attitudes, subjective norm, perceived behavioral control, and the evaluation of behavioral outcomes were employed as predictor variables. The results suggested that the theory appeared to be a valid framework for predicting excessive alcohol consumption among undergraduates. The predictive power of the model, however, was enhanced through the inclusion of gender-specific alcohol outcome expectancies. Specifically, in addition to attitudes and perceived behavioral control, women's expectancies for sociability enhanced the prediction of intentions to drink "too much." Expectancies for sexual functioning (male) and assertiveness (female) improved the prediction of excessive consumption, over and above intentions and perceived behavioral control. The authors concluded that gender-specific alcohol outcome expectancies, unlike attitudes, are proximal predictors of excessive alcohol consumption among undergraduates. These gender-specific determinants are influenced by traditional expectations of masculinity and femininity, in that boys drink to improve their expected sexual functioning and girls drink to improve their otherwise weak assertiveness.

Table 11-1. presents the findings of a Canadian study ($n = 746$) which analyzed how determinants of physical activity could change with adolescent development, using the Theories of Reasoned Action (Chapter Ten) and Planned Behavior (Mummery, Spence, and Hudec 2000).

The authors found significant differences in the importance of the different theoretical constructs in adolescent development. The study shows that addressing the subjective norm will be effective when planning a physical activity promotion program for preadolescents, but will not be influential when planning an activity directed to late adolescents. Perceived behavioral control is equivalent to Bandura's self-efficacy concept; that is to say, in this case, the perceived ability to successfully execute a regimen of physical activity. Perceived behavioral control will be important to consider when planning a program directed to middle or late adolescents, but not necessarily when planning a program for preadolescents.

Schaalma, Kok, and Peters (1993) measured and analyzed the determinants of young people's intentions to use condoms to prevent HIV infection. Their study pro-

Table 11-1. **Changes in Determinants of Physical Activity Intentions during Adolescent Development**

	GRADE 3 (~ 9 YRS.)	GRADE 5 (~ 11 YRS.)	GRADE 8 (~14 YRS.)	GRADE 11 (~17 YRS.)
Subjective Norm	+ + + + + +	+ + + +	+ +	+
Attitudes	+	+ + + + + +	+ +	+ + + +
Perceived Behavioral Control	+	+ +	+ + + +	+ + + + + +

vided detailed information about Dutch youth ages 12 to 18 regarding attitudes, social influences and perceived subjective norms, and self-efficacy expectations or perceived behavioral control, with respect to intentions to use condoms consistently to prevent HIV infection.

Regarding attitudes towards consistent condom use, the results revealed that most young people saw this behavior as sensible and necessary because it provided protection against developing AIDS. On the other hand, they did not regard condom use as something pleasant. Young people who have had intercourse were the least likely to have a positive attitude towards consistent condom use. Although they regarded using condoms consistently as the sensible thing to do, they did not always consider it necessary to do so, especially when having intercourse with a relatively well-known partner. In their opinion, condom use signified an annoying interruption, reduced sensitivity, and reduction in pleasure. These results indicate that in general, young people endorse the preventive advantages of consistent condom use and recognize that these advantages counterbalance the disadvantages and unpleasantness of condom use. However, when young people gain experience with sexual intercourse, the disadvantages of consistent condom use seem to gain increased significance, and the necessity of consistent use seems to become less significant to them.

With respect to social influences, the study revealed that young people did not perceive condom use as a common current practice among their peers, although perceived subjective norms with regard to using condoms consistently were moderately positive. Perceived subjective norms of young people who had not had intercourse were more positive than those of young people who had. When different social referents were considered, the positive social influence of parents was striking.

In regards to self-efficacy or perceived behavioral control, the study showed that young people did expect difficulties regarding their ability to purchase condoms, to carry them regularly, to use them consistently, and to negotiate their consistent use with a (potential) sex partner. Young people who had not had intercourse were most likely to expect difficulties with the purchase of condoms and with carrying them regularly. Young people who had had intercourse were most likely to expect difficulties with the maintenance of consistent use with a relatively well-known partner. Young people who did not form a habit of condom use were more likely to have low self-efficacy expectations regarding the maintenance of condom use and regarding their communicative skills to negotiate condom use with a well-known sex partner.

In addition, the Theory of Planned Behavior has been used to examine the voting intentions of state legislators in North Carolina, Texas, and Vermont. These findings can provide guidance to health educators in planning messages for advocacy efforts. The theory was also used to select messages in the National Anti-Drug Media Campaign, developed in the United States in 1997 (Capella et al. 2001).

Table 11-2. summarizes the number of studies found using the Theory of Planned Behavior according to health behaviors.

Table 11-2. **Most Commonly Researched Adolescent Behaviors Using the Theory of Planned Behavior (TPB)**

ADOLESCENT BEHAVIORS	NUMBER OF ARTICLES USING THE TPB	NUMBER OF ARTICLES BY KEYWORDS	
Sexual and Reproductive Health	13	Teen Pregnancy	2
		HIV/AIDS	7
		STIs	2
		Condom Use	10
Tobacco, Alcohol, and Drug Use	12	Tobacco	6
		Alcohol	5
		Drugs	1
Physical Activity and Nutrition	4	Obesity	0
		Physical Activity	4
		Nutrition	0
Violence	0		
TOTAL	**29**		

Box 11-3. Summary of the Theory of Planned Behavior and Adolescent Lifestyles

- Attitudes and perceived behavioral control significantly differentiate occasional adolescent smokers who intend to smoke from those who do not.

- Perceived behavioral control differentiates regular adolescent smokers from occasional adolescent smokers who intend to smoke.

- Attitudes, perceived behavioral control, and expectancies for sociability enhance the prediction of intentions of late adolescent girls to drink alcohol.

- Gender-specific outcome expectancies—better sexual functioning among boys and more assertiveness among girls—improve the prediction of excessive alcohol consumption, over and above intentions and perceived behavioral control in late adolescence.

- Subjective norm is effective when planning a physical activity promotion intervention for preadolescents, but is less influential when planning an activity directed to late adolescents.

- Perceived behavioral control is important to consider when planning a program directed to middle or late adolescents, but not when planning a program for preadolescents.

- When young people gain experience with sexual intercourse, the disadvantages of consistent condom use seem to become more significant, and the necessity of consistent use seems to become less significant to them.

- Young people with intercourse experience are the least likely to have a positive attitude towards consistent condom use, especially when having intercourse with a relatively well-known partner.

- The positive social influence of parents regarding condom use is striking.

- Regarding perceived behavioral control of condom use, young people expect difficulties regarding their ability to purchase condoms, to carry them regularly, to use them consistently, and to negotiate their consistent use with a sex partner.

- Young people without intercourse experience are most likely to expect difficulties with the purchase of condoms and with carrying them regularly.

- Young people who do not form a habit of condom use are likely to have low self-efficacy expectations regarding the maintenance of condom use and regarding their communicative skills to negotiate condom use with a well-known sex partner.

[Chapter Twelve]

The Goal-Setting Theory

The setting of goals leads to better performance because individuals with goals exert themselves more, persevere in their tasks, concentrate more, and, as the situation requires, develop strategies for carrying out the behavior (Bartholomew et al. 2001). The Goal-Setting Theory is clearly a theory of action and describes a particular method for achieving behavior change. In teaching about HIV/AIDS prevention, for example, the health educator might attempt to associate safer sex with other important goals the students have chosen, such as future careers, which might be threatened by the consequences of practicing unsafe sex. In this way, safer sex becomes part of the strategy to attain long-term goals young people have set for themselves.

A main criticism of the traditional behavior change theories (e.g., Health Belief Model, Stages of Change, Theory of Planned Behavior) is that they do not take into account the fact that individuals may differ with respect to the goals they pursue (Buchanan 2000) and, as a result, may vary in the extent to which they value their health (Gebhardt and Maes 2001). According to this criticism, these theories also overrate rational decision-making about pros and cons as the main process underlying health behavior. Historically, health promotion program developers have been trained to identify the behavior goals of a given intervention according to the health outcome they wish to achieve (e.g., to decrease HIV infection as the health outcome and increase condom use as the behavioral goal).

Goal theories, on the other hand, which have been applied more recently in psychological research, *do* lead researchers to focus on variances in the goals individuals pursue and differences in the relative value assigned to personal health. The theories assert that behavior is effectuated to achieve one's previously set goals, whatever the nature of these might be. These goals are the result of personal processes that are related to one's self-concept and/or an analysis of the personal desirability and feasibility of a potential goal. From this goal-oriented approach, behavior is believed to be initiated only when it is expected to serve a highly valued goal. Goal selection, the consecutive choice of behavior, and the control mechanisms to accompany the behavior change all determine whether a change in behavior will occur. Gebhardt (1997) and Maes (Maes and Gebhardt 2000) developed the "Health Behavior Goal Model" based on these considerations. A basic tenet of the model is that progression towards the target health behavior is dependent upon the degree of compatibility between the target behavior and other personal goals of the individual. The concept of personal goals, which is at the core of the model, encompasses all that is important to the person; that is, the things a person wants to do with his or her life. As Martin E. Ford notes, "Facilitating personal goals and not coercing humans should be the guiding principle in motivating humans to change their behaviors" (Ford 1992, also cited in Maes and Gebhardt 2000, and in Gebhardt and Maes 2001). He further notes that *motivation* is the combination of three psychological functions: *goals*, *emotions*, and *personal agency beliefs*, or the expectations about whether one can achieve a goal (Ford 1992).

Facilitating personal goals is a key contributing element to the consolidation of identity development during the adolescent period. Goal-setting has been traditionally encouraged among middle and late adolescents, but it is also crucial to include this approach in programs and interventions targeting pre- and early adolescents. Goal-setting helps to develop an "ego ideal," which permits young people to model, evaluate, and picture themselves in the future. This "ego ideal" enables early adolescents to envision and project a sense of self over time instead of merely reacting to daily events in which they respond to the needs of the moment (pleasure, need for affiliation and acceptance) and exhibit high vulnerability to peer pressure (Greenspan 1993). In this sense, the assumption that behavior will be initiated only if it is expected to serve a highly valued goal is a particularly promising one within the context of adolescent health research.

A goal should be behaviorally specific and measurable or observable. Strecher and colleagues (1995) advise that goals should be stated in terms of behavior (e.g., exercise and food intake) instead of health outcomes (e.g., weight loss). Locke and Latham (1991) have demonstrated that setting a challenging goal, one that is difficult but nonetheless feasible, leads to a better performance than does setting an easy goal or no goal at all. This positive

> Box 12-1. **The Goal-Setting Theory: Key Concepts in the Adoption of Healthy Behaviors**
> - Facilitating personal goals motivates humans to change behaviors.
> - The choice and pursuit of individual goals is a key element of adolescent identity development.
> - Goal-setting should be encouraged not only during middle or late adolescence, but also during pre- and early adolescence.
> - Behavior will be initiated only if it is expected to serve a highly valued goal.
> - Compatibility between the target behavior and other personal goals of the individual is crucial for behavior change.
> - A goal should be behaviorally specific and measurable.
> - Goals should be stated in terms of behavior instead of health outcomes.
> - Goal-setting may be not effective when the task is too complex.
> - Setting a challenging goal—one that is difficult but nonetheless feasible—leads to better performance than setting an easy goal or no goal at all.
> - It is important for health educators to provide small, incremental goals leading to the overall goal and to suggest viable strategies for reaching it.
> - Social support for developing strategies and reaching self-set goals is particularly critical for younger adolescents lacking in experience and self-efficacy.

effect of difficult goals occurs only if a person accepts the challenge and has sufficient experience, self-efficacy, and feedback to perform adequately. Because adolescents may lack experience and self-efficacy, this positive effect will usually depend on social support received from parents, teachers, other adults, and/or more experienced friends who are willing to guide them through the process of learning, adhering to the goal, and overcoming barriers. The rewards for reaching the goal are not only the expected outcomes but also a sense of self-satisfaction. Although goal-setting may not be effective when the task is relatively complex, the educator can still work to help identify smaller, incremental goals leading to the overall goal and suggest viable strategies for reaching it, especially when working with younger adolescents.

Research and Evidence of Practical Applications of the Goal-Setting Theory to Adolescent Lifestyles

The Goal-Setting Theory helps adolescents organize their dreams and design a corresponding plan of action. Scales and Leffert (1999) describe the "sense of purpose in life" as one of the important Positive Identity Assets in their Developmental Assets Framework (further described in Chapter Nineteen). The ability to plan for the future is part of the *executive functions*, which are instrumental in self-regulation activities and emanate from the brain's prefrontal lobes. As noted in Chapter Nine and as will be discussed further in Chapter

Thirteen, this asset does not reach maturity until the last stage of adolescence (ages 16 to 19).

Goal-setting can also be an effective way of capturing child and adolescent motivation, since the ability to face challenges and competition is an important ingredient in the development of personal identity. This is especially true for the 9-to-12 age group, when engaging in competition with others is the primary means by which a child figures out what he or she does and does not excel at in relationship to others. Although more so for males than for females, competition in sports and games is particularly attractive at this stage of development. In the later stages of adolescent development, the need for success is a constant given; therefore, efforts to compete against one's own goals can become an effective way to obtain behavioral change. Thus, creating opportunities for adolescents to feel competent and successful, especially in areas they highly value, is an important way to encourage health-promoting behaviors.

The Goal-Setting Theory has demonstrated that adolescents who target a behavior (physical activity or eating habits) tend to improve more than those who do not (Cullen, Baranowski, and Smith 2001; Patrick et al. 2001; Schnoll and Zimmerman 2001). The University of California has pioneered once such successful example of this with EatFit, an educational intervention targeted to middle school students living in low income communities. Personally guided goal-setting is the pivotal strategy, and computer technology is employed to assist adolescents with diet assessment and "guided" goal-setting as they make their own healthy lifestyle choices. The program's nine lessons address three messages previously identified by the middle school students' focus group as motivators for changing eating and physical activity behaviors: increased energy, improved appearance, and greater independence.

In a crossover controlled field trial, the EatFit intervention was evaluated for effectiveness. Students made positive changes in dietary behaviors ($p = .03$) and physical activity self-efficacy (paired T-test: $p = .02$). When students set a dietary goal, they increased positive dietary behaviors specific to that goal ($p = .04$). Participants rated themselves as making at least one lasting improvement in dietary (74%) and physical activity (69%) choices, respectively. A randomized controlled field trial investigated the effect of the guided goal-setting component of EatFit. Seventy-three percent of the participants in the treatment group (intervention with goal-setting) made improvements in their dietary practices compared to the control group (intervention without guided goal-setting) with 53% ($p = .04$). Treatment participants also improved significantly compared to control participants (44% vs. 29%) on the physical activity self-efficacy variable ($p = .01$). In 2003, 10,000 middle school students in California participated in the

EatFit program (University of California 2004).

Sanderson and Cantor (1995) examined whether late adolescents bring different goals to bear in social dating by applying a "Social Dating Goals Scale" to 905 students in the United States. The study identified two different prevailing dating goals: *intimacy goals* related to open communication and mutual dependence and *identity goals* related to self-reliance and self-exploration. These different prevailing dating goals were also associated with different patterns of dating and sexual behavior: adolescents with predominant identity goals had more casual dating and sexual partners and those with more intimacy goals had longer dating relationships.

Sanderson and Cantor further hypothesized that adolescents with predominant intimacy goals would be particularly likely to identify with educational activities that emphasize effective communication with a partner about safer sex. On the other hand, those with predominant identity goals may gravitate towards activities that facilitate self-reliance by focusing on technical and eroticizing skills relevant to condom use. The study suggests that tailoring activities that teach about safer sex to fit these different dating goals should increase the impact and effectiveness of such education.

The authors developed a second study in which to test this hypothesis. One hundred and thirty-six U.S. undergraduates (mean age of 19.8 years) were randomly assigned to one of three education conditions: technical skills, communication skills, or a no-education control group. The communication skills group included activities focused on negotiation with partners about condom use and training in role-playing. The technical skills group included activities focused on proficiency with condoms and eroticizing skills training. The results of a one-year follow-up indicated the long-term effects of participation in goal-relevant safer sex education for greater intentions of using condoms. These results provided evidence that individuals are most likely to learn and follow through on intentions about safer sex in educational and naturally occurring dating situations that are most relevant to their predominant dating goals.

Kaldmae and colleagues (2000) described their experience with three prevention projects that were carried out with young people by the Estonian Anti-AIDS Association from 1997 to 1999. The idea of preventive strategies was to promote young people's own decision-making about risk behavior. The authors highlight the importance of maintaining the continuity of preventive projects that will help young people to develop personal insight and enable them to establish goals regarding their sexual and general health.

The Goal-Setting Theory also has been used to address teen pregnancy (Montgomery 2001; Perrin et al. 2000; Brown, Saunders, and Dick 1999; Walsh and Corbett 1995). The Dollar-A-Day program in the U.S. state of North Carolina was established in 1990 to discourage subsequent pregnancies in girls under 16 years of age who had already given birth to one child (Brown, Saunders, and Dick 1999). Weekly meetings featured education on nutrition, an informal program to consider needs identified by members, the setting of short-term goals, and an award of a dollar for each day the participants did not become pregnant. After five years of operation, only 15% of the 65 girls enrolled in the program experienced subsequent pregnancies. The program remains a model for similar initiatives.

Although the Goal-Setting Theory is described as an individual behavior change theory, it could also be applied to promote changes at the interpersonal and community levels. MacDonald and Green (2001) studied the implementation of a school-based alcohol and drug prevention project in secondary schools in British Columbia, Canada. The authors explain that one of the main focuses of the project workers after establishing their credibility in the school was to reconcile the *goals*, values, and philosophy of the project with those of the school.

The Goal-Setting Theory has been less commonly researched in adolescent behaviors than the other theories described in previous chapters, although it appears to play a critical underlying role in the planning, implementing, and monitoring of health promotion interventions for adolescents. The theory helps to foster development of an "ego ideal," an important developmental task of early adolescence, as we have seen. It also allows for the encouragement and monitoring of specific behavior changes during adolescence.

Table 12-1. details the number of studies found using the Goal-Setting Theory according to health behaviors.

Table 12-1. **Most Commonly Researched Adolescent Behaviors Using the Goal-Setting Theory (GST)**

ADOLESCENT BEHAVIORS	NUMBER OF ARTICLES USING THE GST	NUMBER OF ARTICLES BY KEYWORDS	
Sexual and Reproductive Health	10	Teen Pregnancy	6
		HIV/AIDS	2
		STIs	1
		Condom Use	1
Tobacco, Alcohol, and Drug Use	5	Tobacco	4
		Alcohol	3
		Drugs	4
Physical Activity and Nutrition	8	Obesity	1
		Physical Activity	1
		Nutrition	6
Violence	0		
TOTAL	**23**		

Box 12-2. **Summary of the Goal-Setting Theory and Adolescent Lifestyles**

- Possessing a sense of purpose in life, as it relates to establishing personal goals, is an important internal developmental asset and has been associated with health-promoting lifestyles among adolescents.
- Goal-setting helps to develop an "ego ideal," which allows young people to model, evaluate, and picture themselves in the future.
- Setting individual goals can be an effective way of capturing child and adolescent motivation, since the ability to face challenges and competition is an important ingredient in the development of personal identity.
- Adolescents who target a behavior (e.g., physical activity or eating habits) tend to improve more than those who don't.
- Adolescents can have two different prevailing dating goals:
  - Intimacy goals (longer dating relationships)
  - Identity goals (casual dating with different partners)
- Goal-relevant safer sex education will increase intentions of using condoms among adolescents.

[Chapter Thirteen]

The Self-Regulation Theory

Recently, a new theoretical perspective has emerged emphasizing the importance of self-regulation, whose development, as we have already seen in previous chapters, reaches its peak during late adolescence. The Self-Regulation Theory underlines the dynamic processes involved in setting, striving toward, and achieving health goals. These processes encompass the consequences of both successes and failures and also how to deal with obstacles to change health-compromising behaviors and adopt new, healthier ones.

Self-regulatory conceptualizations deal with how individuals can correct personal behaviors on their own (Bartholomew et al. 2001). The basic elements are:

- accurately identifying and recording a specific type of behavior;
- setting acceptable objectives;
- evaluating the response; and
- changing the previous behavior according to assessment of the response or reinforcing the response if the standard is met.

The above process is cyclical and based on monitoring. The ability to self-regulate is an extremely important developmental task to learn during adolescence. It is more easily achieved by some adolescents and presents greater challenges for others, due to biological and environmental differences. Self-regulatory capabilities include self-demands in goal-setting, self-motivation, and self-direction in reaching the proposed goals, and self-evaluation in assessing errors, shortcomings, and obstacles. Self-regulation is achieved when individuals are able to monitor their own behavior through cues and feedback from the outside world as well as through internal cognitive assessment and affective processes. While self-regulation capacity increases with age, actual functioning nonetheless is always determined by biological considerations (i.e., the state of development of the prefrontal lobes in the brain) and objective external forces, as well as by socio-environmental consequences (Muss 1996).

As noted in Chapters Nine and Twelve, the term *executive functions* refers to self-directed actions the individual employs for self-regulation purposes. Analysis and understanding of these functions can provide unique information about how human behavior becomes self-regulated or internally guided. Russell Barkley (1997) reviewed different models of prefrontal lobe executive functions (Damasio 1995, 1994; Goldman-Rakic 1995a, 1995b; Fuster 1995, 1989; Bronowski 1987, 1978, 1977; Vygotsky 1962) and suggested the following functions as necessary for self-regulation:

- behavioral inhibition
- working memory
- internalization of speech
- motivational appraisal system
- reconstitution (behavioral synthesis)

Behavioral inhibition:

Behavioral inhibition requires the acquisition of a system that provides for the inhibition of responses that have as their function the maximization of immediate consequences. The development of the behavioral inhibition function is critical in enabling delayed consequences to affect behavioral control. The teaching of self-regulatory skills has been demonstrated in the school setting (Schunk 1998). Most young people train their behavioral inhibition capacity to not disrupt a classroom through constant reinforcement from their teachers, for example. Over time, they gradually learn to suppress the impulse to speak loudly or out of turn and engage in other disruptive classroom behaviors. This inhibitory system also provides adolescents with the power to interrupt ongoing behavioral patterns, should information from immediately past behaviors in the sequence be indicating errors or the ineffectiveness of the ongoing pattern. For example, in this system, children will interrupt disruptive behavior if the response of the teacher is a silent, but stern facial expression. Finally, it appears that this inhibitory system functions to control potential sources of interference that could disrupt, subvert, or preempt the activities taking place within working memory. The end result is that over time children learn to keep their attention focused on the classroom and to filter out extraneous environmental distractions.

The development of behavioral inhibition ability is crucial in helping adolescents effectively face and learn to deal with the numerous temptations and dangers that are part of their daily lives. Unfortunately, the achievement of behavioral inhibition is increasingly challenged in today's world by the pervasiveness of media messages, such as those found in musical videos, radio and television advertisements, and movies, which encourage the enactment of impulsive behaviors related to the consumption of unhealthy foods, as well as tobacco and alcohol, and sexual experimentation and to the resolution of conflicts through violence. This situation is further abetted by the fact that adolescents find themselves acquiring increasing levels of autonomy at the same time that parental supervision is decreasing. Particularly in those cases in which parents spend a great deal of time outside the home due to work schedules and other nonfamily commitments, valuable opportunities to provide adolescents with constant reinforcements and feedback about their behavioral inhibition abilities are missed.

The acquisition of behavioral inhibition abilities by adolescents sets the stage for the development of the capacity to engage in self-regulation via the four other executive functions that are discussed below.

■ Working memory:

In most real-life situations, individuals will store and be able to recall information not for the purpose of recall itself, but as a prerequisite for solving a problem at hand. These memory recalls involve deciding which types of information are useful for dealing with the situation at hand and then selecting this information out of the totality of all available knowledge stored in the brain. Furthermore, as the nature of our activities changes, we can make a smooth, instantaneous switch from one selection to another, and then are able to repeat the process. Memory that is based on such ever-changing, fluid decision-making, information selection, and information switches back and forth is guided by the frontal lobes and is called *working memory*. It is closely linked to the critical role the frontal lobes play in the temporal organization of behavior and in controlling the proper sequence in which various mental operations are enacted to meet the individual's objective.

Goldman-Rakic (1995a) described two temporally symmetrical functions within this system, one of which permits the recall or re-sensing of the past and which in turn gives rise to the second, which is the construction of hypothetical futures, the preparation of plans for attaining those future scenarios as envisioned, and the construction of behavioral structures that are associated with them.

When adolescents are confronted by temptations and pressures, they need to not only possess behavioral inhibition abilities, but also the skills to make decisions on how to react to those temptations. In this way, the working memory system appears to shift behavioral response away from the immediate stimulus and away from external control and focus it more towards the future by way of internally-generated information arising from private, covert mental activity.

■ Internalization of speech:

Research in developmental psychology suggests that this process of turning speech inward in a form of internal dialogue with oneself, which becomes progressively more private, covert, or internalized, is a major contributor to the development of self-control (Berk 1994, 1992; Kopp 1982). Therefore, speech internalization will need to be included in any model of executive functions that is used to account for the development of human self-regulation. Adolescents facing temptations and dangers will be able to increase their possibilities of making a mindful and healthy choice if they have the capacity to activate an internal dialogue and think through the array of different response alternatives, instead of merely reacting upon impulse.

■ Motivational appraisal system:

This system provides for the affective and motivational appraisal of past events being held in the working memory and of the hypothetical futures created from them. By providing such affective and motivational color or tone to these events, the motivational appraisal system permits them to be immediately retained or discarded depending upon their affective and motivational value to the individual. Such a system, as Damasio (1994) notes, provides the constraints that must be placed on decision-making when a variety of past events and hypothetical option-outcome pairs are being considered. The reactivation of past sensory-motor information automatically brings with it the affective/motivational aspects linked to those events in the past (their *somatic markers*), and these markers are then inherently linked with those plans or hypothetical futures constructed from the past. For example, if an adolescent has a pleasurable experience with his or her friends when participating together in a physical activity, it is more likely that he or she will be motivated to exercise again with those friends in the future.

■ Reconstitution (behavioral synthesis):

Bronowski (1977) asserted that the power to synthesize novel and complex behavioral structures arises out of the ability to analyze and dismember past behavioral structures and their hierarchy. One can then reorganize them into new structures and sequences, all of which is done mainly for the purpose of attaining a specific goal. Such a function grants humans a tremendous capacity for diversity, flexibility, and creativity in the formulation of behavioral structures aimed at the future. For example, as we saw in Chapter Nine, role-playing can be an effective technique of dramatic relief to help move individuals from the pre-contemplation to contemplation stage because it facilitates the acknowledgment of the underlying emotions that accompany unhealthy behavioral risks and their consequences. In this sense, when adolescents are taught drug-resistant skills through role-playing, they will be better able to reconstitute those previously learned skills when a real-life situation occurs that is charged with similar emotions to those they have come to recognize and understand through the role-playing exercises.

Studies of the development of executive functions in children and adolescents illustrate the probable differential timing for the maturation of these functions. Levin et al. (1991) found significant increases as a function of age on a number of executive function measures. Differences in sensitivity to feedback, problem-solving, concept formation, and impulse control between 7- to 8-year-old and 9- to 12-year-old age groups of normal children were found. Further significant developmental advances were noted in memory strategies, memory efficiency, planning of time, problem-solving, and hypothesis-seeking between 9-to-12-year-old and 13-to-15-year-old age groups of normal adolescents.

Research and Practical Applications of the Self-Regulation Theory to Adolescent Lifestyles

Griffin et al. (2000a) studied psychosocial and behavioral factors in early adolescence as predictors of heavy drinking among high school students. As part of a school-based survey, seventh-grade students ($n = 1,132$) reported varying degrees of experimentation with alcohol and cigarettes. Several psychosocial factors

---

Box 13-1. **Executive Functions Needed for Self-Regulation**

- **Behavioral inhibition:** the ability to inhibit responses and delay immediate gratification
- **Working memory:** the ability to store and recall information useful for problem-solving
- **Internalization of speech:** the ability to turn speech inward in a form of dialogic conversation with oneself
- **Motivational appraisal system:** the affective and motivational assessment of past events being held in the working memory for their applicability to the creation of hypothetical futures
- **Reconstitution (behavioral synthesis):** the ability to synthesize novel and complex behaviors, analyze and/or dismember past behavioral structures and their hierarchy, and combine and reorder both past and novel behaviors into new structures and sequences

deemed to be important in the etiology of drinking were also assessed. Students were followed up in the 12th grade, when 16% were categorized as heavy drinkers. Logistic regression analysis revealed that heavy drinking was predicted by having experimented with alcohol or cigarettes, having had a majority of one's friends who also drink, and having had poor behavioral self-control during early adolescence. Tarter et al. (1995) analyzed the association between childhood irritability and liability to substance use during early adolescence. The follow-up results indicated that family dysfunction, the stress state of the child, and low behavioral self-control added up to a significant proportion of variance on irritability scale scores two years later, and that this trait, in conjunction with family discord, was associated with substance use being adopted during early adolescence as a coping response.

Wills et al. (2001a) examined the relationship between temperament dimensions and substance use in 1,810 U.S. public school students (mean age 11.5 years). The presence of good self-control led to higher academic competence and had direct effects on lowering individual substance use; poor self-control led to more deviant peer affiliation.

Novak and Clayton (2001) looked at the influence of school environment and self-regulation on transitions between stages of cigarette smoking. The analyses of the multilevel interactions between self-regulation and school context revealed that students possessing low emotional regulation were more likely to initiate experimental smoking in schools with poor levels of discipline and involvement (i.e., less caring for the students and showing a less active interest in their well-being) than similar types of students in schools with higher levels of these characteristics. This study illustrates how psychological risk factors for substance use may vary across school social environments.

Wills, Sandy, and Yaeger (2002a) tested predictions, derived from the self-regulation model, about variables moderating the relationship between level of substance use (tobacco, alcohol, and marijuana) and problems associated with use (interpersonal relationships, school performance, and difficulties with the legal/justice systems) in middle adolescence. It has been proposed that some individuals have difficulty in coping with problems and regulating emotions and that several aspects of these self-regulation characteristics would make individuals more prone to experience substance-related problems. The authors hypothesized that variables related to poor self-control and negative affectivity would increase the relationship between substance use level and these problems. The presence of good self-control and positive affectivity would have protective moderation effects, reducing the relationship between substance use level and the problems. The predictions were tested in two samples ($n = 1,699$ and $n = 1,225$) of U.S. adolescents. Mean age was 15.5 years (middle adolescence). The results confirmed the prediction that variables indicative of good self-control had protective moderation effects, reducing the relationship between level and problems. Variables indicative of poor self-control had risk-enhancing moderation effects, increasing the relationship between level and problems. These findings help to emphasize the importance of fostering self-regulation and self-control as developmental capacities in the earlier stages of adolescent development.

Hernández and DiClemente (1992) analyzed HIV-related knowledge, attitudes, moral development, psychosocial factors, and behaviors among U.S. male university students. They found that late adolescents who had low scores for ego-development (goal-directedness) and self-control were significantly more likely to engage in sex without condoms. In another study of gender differences and sexual behavior (MacKellar et al. 2000), low self-control was also associated with non-use of condoms among homeless and runaway youths, but only among males.

The studies just described are only a sample of those that have used the Self-Regulation Theory to analyze adolescent health behaviors. Generally, the theory has been utilized to understand tobacco, alcohol, and drug consumption among adolescents, yet has scarcely been taken into consideration when examining sexual and reproductive behaviors. Self-regulation and self-control abilities are extremely important developmental tasks to master during the pre- and early adolescent developmental stages. They allow, among other things, for a better regulation of sexual arousal in boys in today's society which encourages sexual experience in young males and which is characterized by high rates of sexual coercion and gender abuse.

Table 13-1. presents a breakdown of the number of studies found using the Self-Regulation Theory according to health behaviors.

Table 13-1. **Most Commonly Researched Adolescent Behaviors Using the Self-Regulation Theory (SRT)**

ADOLESCENT BEHAVIORS	NUMBER OF ARTICLES USING THE SRT	NUMBER OF ARTICLES BY KEYWORDS	
Sexual and Reproductive Health	4	Teen Pregnancy	1
		HIV/AIDS	2
		STIs	0
		Condom Use	3
Tobacco, Alcohol, and Drug Use	31	Tobacco	13
		Alcohol	27
		Drugs	16
Physical Activity and Nutrition	3	Obesity	3
		Physical Activity	
		Nutrition	
Violence	4		
TOTAL	**42**		

Box 13-2. **Summary of the Self-Regulation Theory and Adolescent Lifestyles**

- Poor behavioral self-regulation and self-control during adolescence are associated with heavy drinking, substance use, experimentation with tobacco, deviant peer affiliation, and increased likelihood of engaging in sex without condoms.

- Good self-control and positive affectivity have protective moderation effects, reducing the relationship between substance use level (tobacco, alcohol, and marijuana) and problems associated with substance use (interpersonal relationships, school performance, and difficulties with the legal/justice systems).

- The presence of good self-control leads to higher academic competence and has direct effects on lowering adolescent substance use.

[Chapter Fourteen]

The Sensation-Seeking Theory

Why are some adolescents more temperamental, active, risk-taking, and/or "difficult" than others? Individual differences have been described as being present at birth and influenced—but not determined—by postnatal experience. The concept of temperament has been widely recognized as one of the basic aspects of the psychological component of behavioral functioning. Findings of a systematic study by Stella Chess and Alexander Thomas in their long-term investigation, the New York Longitudinal Study (NYLS), led to the establishment of an extensive body of research on temperament and other individual differences (*see* Kohnstamm et al. 1989). Chess and Thomas (1996) described nine categories of individual variance that determine temperament: (1) activity level; (2) "rhythmicity" or regularity of biological functions and predictability; (3) tendency to approach or withdraw when confronted with new stimuli; (4) adaptability to new situations; (5) threshold of responsiveness; (6) intensity of reaction; (7) quality of mood; (8) distractibility; and (9) attention span and persistence.

Chess and Thomas also described three main temperament constellations:

- *Easy temperament*, which is characterized by regularity, positive approach responses to new stimuli, high adaptability to change, and mild or moderately intense mood that is preponderantly positive;
- *Slow-to-warm-up temperament*, which is a combination of negative responses of mild intensity to new stimuli with slow adaptability after repeated contact, as well as some irregularities of biological functions (e.g., sleep patterns and feeding schedules); and

- *Difficult temperament*, which is characterized by significant irregularities in biological function, negative withdrawal responses to new stimuli, nonadaptability to change, and intense mood expressions that are frequently negative.

The NYLS showed that infants with difficult temperaments tended to evolve into "difficult children and adolescents," characterized by an oppositional, defiant style of interaction with others. Chess and Thomas have insisted that although "difficult children" display behavior disorders (e.g., aggressiveness, delinquency), this behavior only occurs as the result of interaction in an inappropriate caretaking environment or otherwise inadequate social environment. Furthermore, according to an earlier study (Thomas, Chess, and Birch 1968), parent-child interaction should be analyzed not only for parental influences on the child but equally for the influence of the child's individual characteristics upon the parent. The term *goodness of fit* was coined by these authors to explain how the consonance between the child and his/her environment potentiates optimal positive development, and how the dissonance between the capacities and characteristics of the child, on the one hand, and the environmental opportunities and demands, on the other, lead to maladaptative functioning and distorted development (*poorness of fit*). Carey (1989) introduced the concept of *temperament risk factors* as any temperament characteristics predisposing a child to a poor fit with his or her environment, to excessive interactional stress and conflict with his/her caretakers, and to secondary clinical problems manifesting themselves in the child's physical health, development, and/or behavior.

One of the important individual differences described by the temperament studies is the tendency to approach or withdraw when confronted with new stimuli. According to Zuckerman (1994), this general dispositional approach involves three distinctive individual traits: *sensation-seeking*, *impulsivity*, and *sociability*. Sensation-seeking represents the optimistic tendency to approach novel stimuli and explore the environment. Impulsivity is a style of rapid decision-making when faced with a given stimulus. Sociability is the tendency to approach others in social situations, whether familiar or strangers, with few or no reservations. Persons with low sociability, on the other hand, tend to withdraw under circumstances where the stimuli are too novel or the anticipated outcome is too uncertain. All three components of approach—sensation-seeking, impulsivity, and sociability—have a genetic basis accounting for 40% to 60% of the variance in the approach trait. The model suggests that underlying this trait, at the biological level, are the monoamine neurotransmitters and the gonadal hormones.

Sensation-seeking is a trait describing the tendency to seek novel, varied, complex, and intense sensations and experiences and the willingness to take risks for the sake of participating in the experience.

The idea of "novelty" presupposes that the given situation or event is something not previously experienced. The need for complexity in perceptual stimuli and cognitive challenges is a salient feature of the sensation-seeking trait. In those situations that entail risk, *high sensation-seekers* find the sensations or experiences well worth the risk, whereas *low sensation-seekers* either do not value the sensations of the activity as highly or do not think the experience is worth the risk involved.

The end goal of sensation-seeking behavior is the increase of stimulation. Generally, human beings enjoy a large variety of stimulation emanating from the different senses: sight (e.g., provocative images, whether witnessed first-hand or through the media); smell (e.g., perfumes, aromas); taste (e.g., sweet, salty, or spicy foods); tactile (e.g., gentle touch, caresses) and deep proprioception, or the reception of heightened pressure by cells located between the skin and muscles (e.g., massages); sound (e.g., music, nature); and movement in space (e.g., riding roller coasters, water slides). Some people are highly reactive to these types of stimulation and prefer to enjoy them at a lower intensity, while others are less reactive and desire a higher intensity. During preadolescence (ages 9–12), young people increasingly complain of being "bored." The reason for this is that the need for high sensation-seeking increases during the preadolescent period, accompanied by an increase in the cognitive, verbal, motor, and social developmental skills, while at the same time, the lack of complete autonomy from parents, teachers, and other adults presents restraints to the adolescent's ability to react to these sensory stimulations as fully and intensely as he or she would like to.

Sensation-seeking is a normal trait of personality. Sensation-seekers have a strong capacity to focus attention on a particular stimulus or task. Cognitive styles associated with sensation-seeking include a tendency for broad cognitive generalization and an inclination toward employing more complex cognitive categories. Low sensation-seekers, on the other hand, use a narrower range of simpler constructs. Openness to new experiences is a requisite for creativity in any field. Sensation-seekers tend to be original and innovative in open-ended problem-solving. However, particularly in the case of preadolescents, when high sensation-seeking is combined with other negative traits or affective experiences (e.g., lack of positive socialization), the situation can result in a severe health-compromising lifestyle, which in turn could become a serious clinical condition affecting the adolescent's physical and mental health and development.

The Sensation-Seeking Scale (SSS), originally developed by Zuckerman and colleagues (Zuckerman et al. 1964), has become the basic method of identifying high versus low sensation-seekers in the population in order to study their behaviors and biology (Zuckerman 1994). It consists of four subscales: "thrill- and adventure-seeking," "experience-seeking," "disinhibition," and "boredom susceptibility." The first three subscales have shown good cross-gender and cross-cultural replicability, and the SSS as a whole has been translated from English into 15 other languages.

Research and Practical Applications of the Sensation-Seeking Theory to Adolescent Lifestyles

Russo et al. (1993, 1991) developed a children's version of the Sensation-Seeking Scale (SSS-C) that includes three subscales: "thrill- and adventure-seeking," "social disinhibition," and "drug and alcohol attitudes." In this study, the three subscales and the total score significantly increased as a function of age in groups between 9 and 14 years old. Gender differences were also found, with males presenting higher scores than females. Findings indicating a decline in general sensation-seeking, and in the forms of thrill- and adventure-seeking and social disinhibition, beginning in late adolescence or during the early 20s, have been widely demonstrated through cross-sectional studies.

A significant relationship between adolescent risk behaviors and sensation-seeking has been described in the literature. Adolescents who rank high in their tendency to seek sensation (high sensation-seekers), relative to those who rank low (low sensation-seekers), are much more at risk of using a variety of drugs and of experiencing an earlier onset of use. Zuckerman (1988) described the relationship between sensation-seeking and past or current smoking in students at the University of Delaware in the 1980s. The relationship is highly significant. Among the high sensation-seeking students, 43% were current smokers or had smoked in the past, compared to 32% of the medium sensation-seeking group and 22% of the low sensation-seeking group. The relationship between smoking and sensation-seeking has also been found for U.S. high school students (Dinn et al. 2004, Andrucci et al. 1989), British male college students (Golding, Harpur, and Brent-Smith 1983), Norwegian high school students (Pederson, Clausen, and Lavik 1989), and Israeli adolescents (Teichman, Barnea, and Rahav 1989).

Although this relationship between sensation-seeking and smoking was found in both genders, females who were current heavy smokers, smoking two or more packs a day, were as low as nonsmokers on the Sensation-Seeking Scale. Zuckerman suggests that in this group, smoking may be more related to anxiety than to sensation-seeking. Teichman and colleagues found that those who started at a younger age had the highest scores on the Sensation-Seeking Scale, followed by those who started later, while those who consistently abstained had the lowest scores.

Sensation-seeking is also related to alcohol and drug use in adolescence and preadolescence, and early adolescent sensation-seeking traits can predict later substance use (Crawford et al. 2003, Stanton et al. 2001). This relationship has been found in many countries. Marijuana tends to be the first illegal drug used and is favored by young high sensation-seekers. In all of these studies of adolescent drug use, sensation-seeking is strongly implicated, whereas anxiety and depression seem to have little or no predictive value. Only the use of depressants in the Israeli sample (Teichman, Barnea, and Rahav 1989) was associated with anxiety and depression. In another study done in 20 U.S. middle schools (n = 3,127 eighth graders) the author was able to demonstrate that peer pressure and perceived peer marijuana use had only a relatively trivial effect on low sensation-seekers and a much greater effect on high sensation-seekers (Slater 2003). In another study conducted in Spain, Comín Bertrán and colleagues (Comín Bertrán, Torrubia Beltri, and Mor Sancho 1998) found not only an association between tobacco and alcohol use and sensation-seeking scores in sixth graders (mean age: 11.4) and eighth graders (mean age: 13.2), but also high scores among those who were actively involved in sports and exercise. These results support the need for alternative experiences for youth exhibiting high levels of sensation-seeking and refocusing this tendency on healthier, but still novel and intense experiences.

High sensation-seekers' needs for stimulation are associated with distinct preferences for high sensation-value media messages that elicit greater sensory, affective, and arousal responses. Such messages contain elements that are novel, dramatic, emotionally powerful, physically arousing, graphic, explicit, unconventional, fast-paced, and/or suspenseful. High sensation-value messages have proven to be more effective than low sensation-value messages among high sensation-seeking teenagers and young adults in helping them decide to call a prevention hotline, in improving media message recall, in having more negative attitudes towards drugs, and in lowering behavioral intentions to use drugs (Palmgreen et al. 2001). The same study showed that antidrug public service announcements placed in high sensation-value television programming also elicit significantly greater attention from high sensation-seekers than do those placed in low sensation-value programs.

These findings led Philip Palmgreen, professor of communications at the University of Kentucky in Lexington, to develop the Sensation-Seeking Targeting (SENTAR) prevention approach. This approach incorporates four principles: (1) use sensation-seeking as a targeting variable; (2) conduct formative research with target audience members; (3) design high sensation-value prevention messages; and (4) place messages in program contexts that are attractive to the target audience.

The SENTAR prevention approach was effectively used in a recent television campaign to reduce marijuana consumption among high sensation-seeking adolescents in two different communities (Palmgreen et al. 2001). Five televised public service announcements (PSAs) appeared between January and April 1997 in Fayette County, Kentucky. Similar campaigns were launched there again and in Knox County, Tennessee, between January and April 1998. The PSAs were designed to appeal to adolescents who had tested high on a Brief Sensation-Seeking Scale and were placed during television programs (such as *The Simpsons* and *StarTrek: The Next Generation*) that were most likely to be watched by this group of teens, as determined by a survey before the spots aired. Effects from the single campaign in Knox County were still evident several months after its conclusion. There, the estimated drop in the relative proportion of high sensation-seeking adolescents using marijuana was 26.7%. In Fayette County, the drop in marijuana use among this group was estimated to be approximately 38%. For low sensation-seeking adolescents, both marijuana usage rates and reactions to the PSAs were much lower than for their high sensation-seeking counterparts. The campaign effects were specific to marijuana use, however, with no effects seen in the use of tobacco, alcohol, and other drugs.

The four SENTAR principles are currently being applied in the U.S. Office of National Drug Control Policy's five-year National Youth Anti-Drug Media Campaign (Office of National Drug Control Policy 2002b), in conjunction with other proven cognitively-oriented theoretical frameworks, such as the Social Cognitive Theory, the Health Belief Model, the Theory of Reasoned Action, and the Theory of Planned Behavior (Chapters Sixteen, Eight, Ten, and Eleven, respectively, in this book).

The newest wave in information technology, media communications, and commercial advertising is the presentation of highly compressed visual and auditory images and stimuli displays, a product partly of economics and partly of recently expanded digitalization capacities. The advent of video games and cutting-edge musical programming on cable network television has created an entirely different way of processing information through "sight bites" and "sound bytes," and today's young people have come to expect and prefer this type of high-paced stimulation from the media.

Substantive research indicates an increase in sensation-seeking during the pre- and early adolescent periods (9–14 years of age), which reaches its peak during middle adolescence (ages 15–16 years) and tends to decline in late adolescence, around the age of 20. These findings, combined with the reality that adolescents respond to targeted messages on a spontaneous and visceral level, provide a strong argument for the need to "use what works" when developing health-promoting media campaigns directed towards adolescents and youth.

In this sense, effective program design should not only target behaviors to adopt or change, but also seek to satisfy adolescent needs and wants (Chapter Five), appropriately tailor interventions to the adolescents' developmental stage (Chapter Six), and take into account gender and cultural considerations, which will be discussed further in Chapter Twenty-seven. The research shows that adolescents *want* novelty and fun, and they will search for ways to satisfy their increasing *need* for sensation-seeking. Additionally, what might be considered exciting to the senses will be different for boys and girls, for preadolescents and late adolescents, and for youth living in Argentina, Jamaica, Panama, and the United States (as well as in different communities within each of these countries). PAHO recommends that program designers keep these ideas in mind when planning all types of health promotion and prevention interventions. It is also crucial that the team developing the interventions be highly creative, young in spirit, and empathetic to the intensified need for novelty during adolescence.

Given that adolescents find the elements of novelty, drama, fast pacing, emotional arousal, unconventionality, suspense, etc., to be highly appealing, another important aspect in designing successful health promotion and behavior change interventions is discussing the reasons behind adolescent preferences and concerns with the participants themselves. In this sense, program developers should seek to actively engage adolescents from the beginning and encourage their input and feedback, thereby winning their trust, helping them to see the relevancy of the process, and building their confidence in their ability to become agents of their own change.

As all parents and teachers of "bored" adolescents will agree, young people, as they become older, need to gradually shift from expecting the world to entertain them to learning to entertain themselves, overcome feelings of boredom, and seek sensations in healthy ways. Part of this shift will occur naturally as the adolescent moves through the different developmental stages, faces new challenges and experiences, and gains increased self-confidence in his or her decision-making ability. But this shift also needs to be accompanied by support from the surrounding social environment in which the adolescent lives, studies, plays, and works. Families, schools, and other key community members need to work together in formal and informal partnerships to provide positive forms of stimulation to adolescents that enable them to discover the world around them and embrace new and healthier activities on their own terms.

The studies just described are only a sample of those that have used the Sensation-Seeking Theory to analyze adolescent health behaviors. Generally, the theory has been utilized to understand tobacco, alcohol, and drug consumption among adolescents, yet has scarcely been taken into consideration when examining sexual and reproductive behaviors, physical activity, eating behaviors, and violence. The few studies examining risky early sexual activity have been in relationship with other risky behaviors, such as alcohol and drug abuse. Unfortunately, the theory has mostly been used to identify youth at risk for alcohol and drug abuse, tailoring high-sensation value messages to prevent these behaviors. Only two studies (Stanton et al. 2001; Comín Bertrán, Torrubia Beltri, and Mor Sancho 1998) have identified the high sensation-seeking trait as an opportunity for developing health promotion and prevention programs that would offer youth healthy alternatives (e.g., sports involvement) for the types of novel and intense experiences they find most appealing.

Table 14-1. presents a breakdown of the number of studies found using the Sensation-Seeking Theory according to health behavior.

Table 14-1. **Most Commonly Researched Adolescent Behaviors Using the Sensation-Seeking Theory (SST)**

ADOLESCENT BEHAVIORS	NUMBER OF ARTICLES USING THE SST	NUMBER OF ARTICLES BY KEYWORDS	
Sexual and Reproductive Health	6	Teen Pregnancy	
		HIV/AIDS	
		STIs	
		Condom Use	6
Tobacco, Alcohol, and Drug Use	52	Tobacco	19
		Alcohol	33
		Drugs	33
Physical Activity and Nutrition	2	Obesity	
		Physical Activity	2
		Nutrition	
Violence	5		
TOTAL	65		

Box 14-1. Summary of the Sensation-Seeking Theory and Adolescent Lifestyles

- Sensation-seeking is a trait describing the tendency to seek novel, varied, complex, and intense sensations and experiences and the willingness to take risks for the sake of participating in the experience.

- There is an increase in sensation-seeking during the pre- and early adolescent periods (9–14 years of age), which reaches its peak during middle adolescence (ages 15–16 years) and tends to decline in late adolescence, around the age of 20.

- A significant relationship between adolescent risk behaviors and sensation-seeking has been described in the literature.

- Adolescents who rank high in their tendency to seek sensation (high sensation-seekers), relative to those who rank low (low sensation-seekers), are much more at risk of using a variety of drugs and of experiencing an earlier onset of use (tobacco, alcohol, and illegal drugs).

- Peer pressure and perceived peer marijuana use have only a relatively trivial effect on low sensation-seekers and a much greater effect on high sensation-seekers.

- High sensation-seekers' needs for stimulation are associated with distinct preferences for novel, high sensation-value media messages that elicit greater sensory, affective, and arousal responses.

- High sensation-value messages have proven to be more effective than low sensation-value messages among high sensation-seeking teenagers and young adults in helping them decide to call a prevention hotline, in improving media message recall, in having more negative attitudes towards drugs, and in lowering behavioral intentions to use drugs.

- Research shows that adolescents *want* novelty and fun, and they will search for ways to satisfy their increasing *need* for sensation-seeking. Therefore interventions will be more effective if they are highly creative, young in spirit, and empathetic to the intensified need for novelty during adolescence.

[Chapter Fifteen]

At a Glance: The Individual Level Theories and Models for Behavior Change

Of all the theories and models reviewed in Chapters Eight through Fourteen to promote change at an individual level, the Health Belief Model (Chapter Eight) has been the most utilized when addressing adolescent behaviors, particularly those involving sexual and reproductive health. This finding must be taken with caution, however, since, as noted in Chapter Eight, the studies of adolescent behaviors using the model usually lack a developmental perspective, and, in essence, represent the extrapolation of a theory developed to change adult health behaviors to this younger age group. Furthermore, most of the interventions to reduce HIV-risk-associated sexual behavior among adolescents in community settings using the model have been conducted with youth in late adolescence (Jemmot and Jemmot 2000). Interestingly, tobacco, alcohol, and drug prevention efforts have relied more on the Self-Regulation Theory and Sensation-Seeking Theory to explain underlying factors and have used the Stages of Change Model to promote healthy behaviors. This model has also been the one most used to promote physical activity and healthy nutrition among adolescents. While there have been a few efforts to understand aggressive behaviors at the individual level using the Self-Regulation Theory and Sensation-Seeking Theory, this adolescent behavior has been the least studied through individual change theories.

Table 15-1. summarizes the number of studies found using the theories and models discussed in Chapters Eight through Fourteen according to health behaviors.

One interesting observation that may be gleaned from Table 15-1. is the fact that comparatively little research has been conducted on adolescent sexual and reproductive health utilizing the Self-Regulation and Sensation-Seeking Theories, compared to their application to studies of tobacco, alcohol, and drug use, even though the two classifications are intimately related as risky behaviors—particularly the link between alcohol use and unprotected sexual activity.

Table 15-2. provides a summary of the behavior change theories and models discussed in Chapters Eight through Fourteen and the most salient characteristics of each.

Table 15-1. **Summary of Most Commonly Researched Theories and Models for Changing Individual Adolescent Behaviors**

Number of Articles on Adolescence and Individual Behavior Change Theories and Models	Sexual and Reproductive Health	Tobacco, Alcohol, and Drug Use	Physical Activity and Nutrition	Violence	Total
Health Belief Model	37	18	9	2	66
Transtheoretical Model and Stages of Change	9	27	15	0	51
Theory of Reasoned Action	13	14	3	1	31
Theory of Planned Behavior	13	12	4	0	29
Goal-Setting Theory	10	5	8	0	23
Self-Regulation Theory	4	31	3	4	42
Sensation-Seeking Theory	6	52	2	5	65
Total	92	159	44	12	307

Table 15-2. Individual Level Theories and Models and Their Application to Adolescent Behavioral Change: A Comparison of Conceptual Frameworks, Applications, and Benefits

Theory/Model	Conceptual Framework	Application	Benefits
Health Belief Model (Chapter Eight)	This theory proposes that adolescents will change their health-compromising behaviors and/or adopt health-promoting behaviors if they consider themselves vulnerable to a disease, believe it has serious consequences, and feel that changing their behavior will reduce their susceptibility to the disease or its severity.	This theory is a very useful one when working with adults, but it should be used with caution with adolescents. Because of the assumption that the person must feel threatened by their current behavior, the model may be used for certain adolescent concerns (e.g., body image and fat consumption for girls), but not necessarily for all risk behaviors, especially if the individual does not feel threatened or dissatisfied with his or her current behavior. The majority of research using this model to address different adolescent lifestyles and behaviors has been in the area of sexual and reproductive health, such as efforts to reduce teen pregnancy, STIs, and HIV/AIDS. One important finding is that the severity of the HIV/AIDS disease, more than fear of contracting an infection and barriers to taking action, is a significant predictor of the adoption of HIV-preventive behaviors among adolescents (Yep 1993). The results of the only known study to analyze the Health Belief Model with a developmental perspective (Petosa and Jackson 1991) suggest that the model variables can be useful when designing educational programs to promote safer sex intentions in younger adolescents; however, its effectiveness decreases as they grow older.	This model can be useful for program developers when designing interventions and messages encouraging pre- and early adolescents to delay sexual initiation and protect themselves from contracting STIs or HIV/AIDS or getting pregnant. However, evidence suggests that these types of messages are not long-lasting among the adolescent population, and their effectiveness decreases for middle and late adolescents and young adults. The model may be considered when choosing the conceptual framework for pre-adolescent interventions, but should not be the only theory chosen to guide program interventions because of its limited effect.

Table 15-2. **Individual Level Theories and Models and Their Application to Adolescent Behavioral Change: A Comparison of Conceptual Frameworks, Applications, and Benefits**–*(continued)*

Theory/Model	Conceptual Framework	Application	Benefits
Transtheoretical Model and Stages of Change (Chapter Nine)	This model conceives behavioral change as a process and not as an isolated event, involving progress through a series of stages: pre-contemplation, contemplation, preparation for action, action, and maintenance. According to this model, tailoring interventions to match the adolescent's readiness or stage of change is essential. This model states that people use a variety of different processes (e.g., dramatic relief, environmental reevaluation, self-efficacy and social support, modeling, coping with barriers, counter-conditioning) as they move from one stage of change to another. Efficient behavior change thus depends on the individual doing the right thing (processes) at the right time (stages).	The use of the Transtheorical Model and Stages of Change to help design health promotion interventions for adolescents is increasing, particularly in Canada and the United States, but also in Latin America and the Caribbean, as well. It has been applied to study the relationship between weight concerns, weight control behaviors, and initiation of tobacco use among youths and the relationship between temptations to try smoking and stages of smoking acquisition. It has also been adopted to match drug prevention strategies and messages to youth stages when use occurs and to study the readiness to change drinking habits among university students. Finally, the model has been used to encourage higher consumption of fruits and vegetables among early adolescent girls, to promote physical activity in large populations (Brazil), to analyze population readiness to change diet- and exercise-related behaviors (the Caribbean), and to develop innovative HIV prevention interventions for rural adolescents targeting both individual and community level change.	The model is an easy-to-use theoretical construct for evaluating the effectiveness of interventions. It helps identify baseline behaviors by stages and describes the processes that a health promotion intervention should promote to obtain a behavioral change and progression to the next stage. Post-intervention behaviors can be compared to baseline behaviors by stages to find evidence of effectiveness of the behavior change intervention. Another benefit of this model, from a developmental perspective, is that it can serve as a planning guide for how to change behaviors step-by-step, particularly when adolescents have not yet developed sufficient skills to plan ahead on an independent basis. The model also provides an opportunity to investigate which factors determine the stage an adolescent is in during different behaviors, as well as the barriers and processes involved when advancing to other stages of behavior. A final benefit is that the model may be used to promote change not only at the individual level, but also at the interpersonal and community levels.
Theory of Reasoned Action and Theory of Planned Behavior (Chapters Ten and Eleven)	The Theory of Reasoned Action states that an adolescent's intention to adopt or change a behavior predicts his or her final behavior. Intention can be affected by influencing the adolescent's attitude towards a behavior and/or the adolescent's subjec-	The use of the Theory of Reasoned Action to change adolescent behaviors has been studied in Africa, Europe, India, and the United States. It has been applied in the study of the associations between peer influence variables and susceptibility to	The messages designed under these two theoretical frameworks seem to be more successful at encouraging adolescents to adopt healthy behaviors than messages designed with the Health Belief Model. Because these theories help to identify

Table 15-2. **Individual Level Theories and Models and Their Application to Adolescent Behavioral Change: A Comparison of Conceptual Frameworks, Applications, and Benefits**–*(continued)*

Theory/Model	Conceptual Framework	Application	Benefits
Theory of Reasoned Action and Theory of Planned Behavior *(continued)*	tive norm associated with the behavior. The Theory of Planned Behavior is an extension of the Theory of Reasoned Action which additionally considers that there are factors outside the adolescent's control that can affect his or her intention to adopt a behavior and that these need to be addressed, as well, in the design of interventions.	smoking; the role of smoking in the lives of low-income pregnant adolescents; in comparisons of self-esteem, attitudes, and subjective norms in the prediction of drug and alcohol use; the intended sexual and condom behavior patterns among high school students; and in the analysis of the decision-making processes for sugar consumption among adolescents. The use of the Theory of Planned Behavior to change adolescent behaviors has been studied in Canada, Europe, and the United States. Research applying the theory includes the onset of smoking in youth, a cross-cultural study of beliefs about smoking among female teenagers, the identification of variables that differentiate and discriminate among the various stages of cigarette smoking, the contribution of alcohol outcome expectancies and attitudes towards drinking, how determinants of physical activity change with adolescent development, and the measurement and analysis of the determinants of young people's intentions to use condoms to prevent HIV infection.	determinants of behaviors that can be targeted to change adolescents' behavioral intentions, and, ultimately, their actual behaviors, it is important that program developers give careful consideration to the particular sociocultural context within which the interventions will take place. At the same time, program planners and developers should keep in mind that there can be significant differences in the role that different theoretical constructs (e.g., subjective norm and behavioral control) can play at different adolescent stages.
Goal-Setting Theory (Chapter Twelve)	Adolescents with goals exert themselves more, persevere in their tasks, apply greater concentration, and, as the situation requires, develop the necessary strategies for carrying out the behavior (Bartholomew et al. 2001). From this goal-oriented approach, behavior is believed to be initiated only when it is	The theory has been used to demonstrate that adolescents who target a behavior for improvements (e.g., physical activity, eating habits) tend to achieve greater success than those who do not. It has also been utilized to examine the different goals (intimacy vs. identity) late adolescents bring to bear in social	Although described as an individual behavior change theory, the Goal-Setting Theory may also be applied to promote changes at the interpersonal and community levels. It is a crucial theory to consider when planning, implementing, and monitoring health promotion interventions for adolescents in that it helps to foster

Table 15-2. Individual Level Theories and Models and Their Application to Adolescent Behavioral Change: A Comparison of Conceptual Frameworks, Applications, and Benefits—*(continued)*

Theory/Model	Conceptual Framework	Application	Benefits
Goal-Setting Theory (*continued*)	expected to serve a highly valued goal. Goal selection, the consecutive choice of behavior, and the control mechanisms to accompany the behavior change all determine whether a change in behavior will be achieved.	dating considerations, to promote young people's own decision-making about risky sexual behavior choices, and to address teen pregnancy. The Goal-Setting Theory has been less commonly researched in adolescent behaviors than the Theories of Reasoned Action and Planned Behavior and the Health Belief and Transtheorical Models.	an important developmental goal of early adolescence: the emergence of an "ego ideal" and a "sense of purpose in life," which have been identified as protective internal assets that help ward off risk-taking behaviors. A strong advantage of this theory is that it encourages health providers and program developers to facilitate adolescents' personal health goals, rather than employ strategies which youth might find too coercive in nature and thus have greater difficulty identifying with.
Self-Regulation Theory (Chapter Thirteen)	Self-regulation conceptualizations focus on how individuals can monitor and correct personal behaviors on their own. Mastering self-regulatory techniques is an extremely important developmental task to be learned during adolescence. It requires the ability to make self-demands in goal-setting, as well as the development of skills in self-motivation, self-direction in reaching the proposed goals, and self-evaluation in assessing errors, shortcomings, and obstacles. While self-regulation capacity increases with age, actual functioning is determined by the extent of the adolescent's biological growth process, objective external factors, and socio-environmental consequences (Muss 1996).	The theory has been utilized to better understand tobacco, alcohol, and drug consumption among adolescents, yet has scarcely been taken into consideration when examining sexual and reproductive health behaviors. Issues studied using this theory include psychosocial and behavioral factors in early adolescence as predictors of heavy drinking among high school students; the association between hyperactivity and executive cognitive functioning in childhood and substance abuse in early adolescence; the influence of school environment and self-regulation on transitions between stages of smoking; predictions regarding variables moderating the relationship between substance abuse level and problems (interpersonal, academic, and legal) associated with use in middle adolescents; and HIV-related knowledge, attitudes, moral development, psychosocial factors, and behaviors among university-age males.	The success of self-management interventions, obviously, depends upon the level of the individual adolescent's skills. Evidence shows that adolescent males have greater difficulties acquiring self-regulation and self-control than their female counterparts. Yet these are extremely important developmental goals to master during pre- and early adolescence, particularly among males, because they will allow for a better regulation of boys' sexual arousal in a society that encourages sexual experience in young males and which is characterized by high rates of sexual coercion and gender abuse.

Table 15-2. **Individual Level Theories and Models and Their Application to Adolescent Behavioral Change: A Comparison of Conceptual Frameworks, Applications, and Benefits**—*(continued)*

Theory/Model	Conceptual Framework	Application	Benefits
Sensation-Seeking Theory (Chapter Fourteen)	Sensation-seeking is a normal trait of personality describing the tendency to seek novel, varied, complex, and intense sensations and experiences and the willingness to take risks for the sake of experience. Openness to new experiences is a requisite for creativity and personal growth. Sensation-seekers tend to be original and innovative in open-ended problem-solving. However, particularly in the case of preadolescents, when high sensation-seeking is combined with other negative traits or affective experiences, the situation can result in a severe health-compromising lifestyle, which in turn may become a serious clinical condition affecting the adolescent's physical health and development.	A version of the Sensation-Seeking Scale has been developed for adolescents (Russo et al. 1993). A significant relationship between adolescent risk behaviors and sensation-seeking has been described, particularly for tobacco, alcohol, and drug use (Zuckerman 1994). These findings have led to the development of the Sensation-Seeking Targeting (SENTAR) prevention approach (Palmgreen 2001), which utilizes sensation-seeking as a target variable, designs high-sensation-value messages, and seeks to place messages within contexts that are attractive to the adolescent target audience. Substantive research indicates an increase in sensation-seeking during the pre- and early adolescent periods (9–14 years of age), which reaches its peak during middle adolescence (ages 15–16) and tends to decline in late adolescence, around the age of 20.	The studies conducted on sensation-seeking among adolescents have shed much light on the reasons behind this group's need for novelty, adventure, and intense stimulation, including the adoption of new (and potentially risky) sexual behaviors. It has also helped developers of interventions and programs to better understand and design "what works"—i.e., what adolescents will find appealing and will attract their attention. In this sense, activities will have a better chance of reaching young people and satisfying their need for sensation-seeking if they offer elements of novelty and non-conventionality, a variety of physical, mental, and/or emotional stimulation, heightened intensity, and age-appropriate complexity. In this sense, it is critical that the intervention team be highly creative and "cutting edge" in its collective thinking and sincerely empathetic and responsive to the needs and wants of adolescents. At the same time, program designers should bear in mind that what is considered exciting and new might be different for boys and girls, for preadolescents and late adolescents, and for young people living in different socioeconomic and cultural settings.

Theories and Models that Promote Change at the Interpersonal Level

Individuals are social beings who derive their sense of self and of personal efficacy from others through interpersonal exchanges. This interpersonal environment provides the means, models, reinforcements, and resources with which people can learn more about themselves and is also critical in affecting and predicting an individual's health behavior and, in turn, health outcomes. Consideration of the social influences on health behaviors and outcomes during adolescence is crucial. Most recent reviews on resiliency to adversity (Infante 2001) and other human development literature (Greenspan and Shanker 2003, 2002) also highlight the crucial role of the ongoing interplay between the characteristics of the individual, the family, the community, and the broader culture. While the adolescent's gradual separation from the parents allows for the development and strengthening of individual identity, there may be less of a buffer as he/she experiences increased exposure to the larger social environment.

In Chapters Sixteen through Twenty-one, the following theories and models of interpersonal health behavior will be reviewed within the context of working with adolescents:

- the Social Cognitive Theory
- the Social Network and Social Support Theories
- the Authoritative Parenting Model
- the Resiliency Theory
- the Stress and Coping Theories

[Chapter Sixteen]

The Social Cognitive Theory

Bandura's (1986) Social Cognitive Theory encompasses both determinants of behavior and the methods of promoting behavioral change. The theory explains behavior in terms of a triadic, dynamic, and reciprocal model in which *socio-environmental*, *personal* or *cognitive*, and *behavioral* factors all interact.

This theory provides a particularly useful theoretical framework for understanding and describing the potential impact of the social environment on health behaviors among adolescents.

Three basic principles emerge from this framework. The first, according to this theory, is that behavior is influenced by both socio-environmental and personal factors. This principle emphasizes the multifaceted nature of adolescent behavior. Therefore, a behavior such as high-risk sexual activity is not the result of a single factor (e.g., lack of knowledge about the consequences of unprotected sexual activity), but rather the result of numerous factors within the adolescent's social environment and his/her individual disposition.

The second principle is that socio-environmental factors play a significant role in the onset of behaviors, but their influence is mediated via personal cognitions. In other words, the adolescent does not respond automatically to socio-environmental factors (e.g., pressures to be thin) but instead makes personal choices as to whether or not he/she will engage in a particular behavior.

Thirdly, adolescent behavior is not only influenced by socio-environmental and personal factors, but also influences these factors. This simultaneous influence is called *reciprocal determinism* and posits that a change in one component holds implications for the others.

Figure 16-1. illustrates the triangular relationship between socio-environmental, personal (cognitive), and behavioral factors.

The environment is important in this theory in part because it provides *models* for behavior. Bandura and Walters (1963) proposed that children could watch other children learn a new behavior and did not need to be rewarded directly. Thus, a child learns by observing (*observational learning*) the behaviors of others (*modeling*) and the rewards these others receive (*vicarious reinforcement*). In other words, people learn what is appropriate by observing the behaviors, successes, and mistakes of others. Specifically, adolescents observe their parents when they eat, drink, smoke, and use seat belts, and they see the various rewards or penalties the parents receive for these activities.

In the same way, adolescents observe their peers smoking and notice the rewards and punishments that the smokers receive. If the observers consider the consequences of smoking to be rewarding (e.g., acceptance from peers, the creation of a desirable image), the observers become more predisposed to smoke. Observational learning presents the greatest impact when the person being observed is powerful, respected, and/or considered to be like the observer (in age, interests, background, etc.).

Figure 16-1. **Reciprocal Determinism of the Social Cognitive Theory**

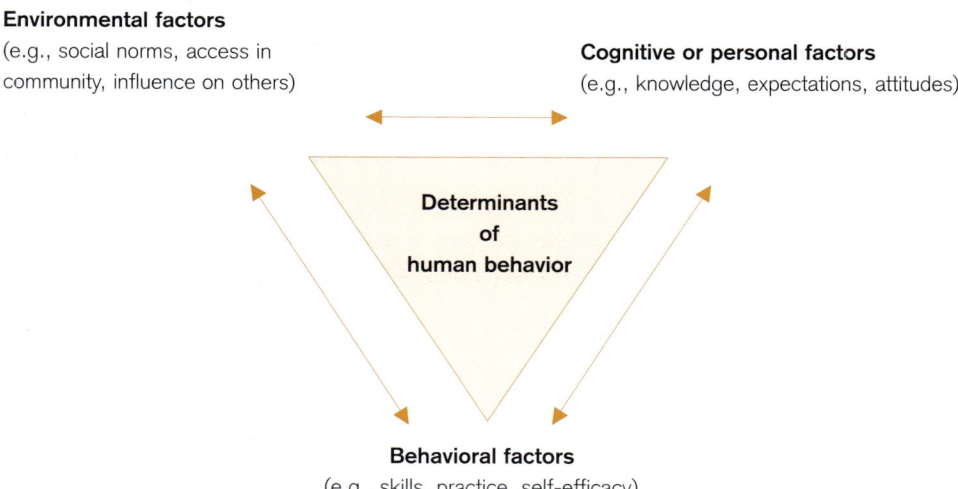

Environmental factors
(e.g., social norms, access in community, influence on others)

Cognitive or personal factors
(e.g., knowledge, expectations, attitudes)

Behavioral factors
(e.g., skills, practice, self-efficacy)

Source: Resource Center for Adolescent Pregnancy Prevention 2000. [Internet site] Available at: www.etr.org/recapp/theories/slt/Index.htm

Within the Social Cognitive Theory context, the mass media provides adolescents with heavy doses of vicarious learning experiences. Media today surrounds youth. As the media increasingly shapes society's images of reality, we learn a great deal by the consequences media characters experience as a function of their behavior. The content featured in these technologies is increasingly graphic, interactive, provocative, and commercially manipulative in nature, and media corporations are increasingly recognizing and targeting youth as a profitable group of consumers. UNESCO recently reported that today's average 12-year-old spends three hours a day watching television (Groebel 1999). In addition to traditional television programming, music, magazines, and movies catering to the youth market, new kinds of media such as interactive CD-ROMs, video games, e—mail, chat rooms, and Web sites offer everything from instructions on how to form anonymous friendships to information on how to lose weight overnight to access to electronic displays of virtual sex and violence. A recent survey in the United States found that 8-to-18-year-olds spend six to eight hours a day exposed to some form of media (Roberts 2000). Furthermore, this media use is becoming more private as children recede to their bedrooms to watch television or listen to music alone and unsupervised. Research by PAHO in the area of adolescent health and media exposure has yielded results that closely parallel those of other international studies. In 2003, a study of 11 Latin American countries revealed that adolescents ages 12 to 19 are permanently engaged with one or another type of media communication (particularly television and radio), except when they are in the school classroom or interacting with friends and/or parents (Organización Panamericana de la Salud 2003a).

It is important to note at this juncture that while Albert Bandura and other learning theorists stress the context in which behavior takes place, they are not especially developmental in their approach. For learning theorists, the basic processes of human behavior are the same during adolescence as they are during other periods of life. Although Bandura included in his model the mediation of personal cognitions to respond to socio-environmental factors, the principal emphasis of his theory is on how the socio-environment may affect behavior, and it has tended to overlook or ignore developmental and emotional aspects that will affect personal cognitions to respond to these social influences.

Within the framework of the Social Cognitive Theory, before performing a new behavior, people anticipate many aspects of the situation in which the behavior might be performed. They develop and test strategies for dealing with the situation and anticipate what will happen as a result of their behavior in this situation. People develop expectations about a situation and *expectations for outcomes* of their behavior before they actually encounter the situation ("If I use a condom consistently, I will prevent STIs"). These anticipatory outcomes of a behavior are known as *outcome expectations*. This anticipatory behavior reduces anxiety and increases one's ability to handle the situation. Outcome expectations are observed in adolescents in the process of exploring a new behavior, except when the behavior is performed impulsively. Outcome expectations are comparable to the *behavioral beliefs* described in the Theories of Reasoned Action and Planned Behavior (Chapters Ten and Eleven).

In considering the Social Cognitive Theory, health promotion project designers should be cautioned about automatically assuming that anticipatory behavior is a developed ability in adolescence. In the earlier stages of adolescence, such as pre- and early adolescence, these age groups are still developing their cognitive abilities to anticipate what will happen as a result of a behavior, and consequently, many of their exploratory behaviors will have an impulsive component, and they will be learning more by experience than by anticipation.

Other aspects involved in the process of engaging in a new behavior are the *outcome expectancies* or *incentives*, meaning the values that individuals place on a certain outcome. Expectancies influence the behavior according to the level of pleasure experienced; that is, if all other things are equal, a person will choose to perform an activity that maximizes a positive outcome or minimizes a negative outcome. Outcome expectancies are comparable to *evaluations* (outcome values) in the Theories of Reasoned Action and Planned Behavior. A person's positive expectancies should be assessed very early on in any project designed to promote changes in health behavior in order to identify motivators for that behavior. An emphasis on immediate positive expectancies, for example, is more likely to influence the initiation of some desired behaviors than an emphasis on long-range expectancies. McAlister et al. (1980) provided strong evidence for this when it was shown that smoking prevention programs for adolescents are more successful if they emphasize avoidance of the immediate negative effects of smoking, such as bad breath or unattractiveness, rather than the long-term effects such as morbidity and mortality from cancer and heart disease.

The types of outcomes people anticipate depend largely on their judgments of how well they will be able to perform in given situations. *Self-efficacy*, as noted in Chapters Eight and Eleven, is the level of confidence a person feels about performing a particular activity, including confidence in overcoming the barriers to performing that behavior. Bandura proposed that self-efficacy is the most important prerequisite for behavioral change, because it affects how much effort is invested in a given task and what level of performance is attained. When a person is in a situation in which outcome expectations are positive and strong, but self-efficacy for that behavior is low, avoidance or denial may occur, and the person is unlikely to attempt to achieve the new behavior. A meta-analysis of the research literature published between 1983 and 1991 (Gillis 1993) showed that self-efficacy was the strongest predictor of a health-promoting lifestyle. In an example of a specific behavior, self-efficacy has been identified as a primary predictor of intention to make healthier food choices among third- and fourth-grade students (Parcel et al. 1995a).

Complex behaviors usually involve a sequence (steps) of simple tasks that all together might seem difficult for an adolescent to perform. Bandura and other learning theorists propose that repetition of the performance of a single task builds a person's self-efficacy by changing the person's performance expectations. For example, when learning to play basketball, repetitions of a single task (e.g., dribbling) build the adolescent's self-efficacy by changing his/her performance expectations every time he/she experiences better control of the ball. The goal, then, is to break down any particular challenge or multi-step complex new behavior so that the adolescent can have a sense of success as he/she masters one step at a time. Learning theorists state that through the repeated successful enactment of incremental tasks (e.g., the first step as learning to master dribbling, the next step as learning to pass and catch the ball, the third step as learning to run and dribble simultaneously, and the final step as running, catching, dribbling, and shooting) the person acquires enhanced expectations of success in the tasks to be learned, which in turn affects task initiation, persistence, and endurance, and thus serves to promote and reinforce behavioral change.

Simplifying a complex new behavior into small steps of incremental tasks and allowing individuals to practice each one in isolation, with many repetitions, enables them to build self-efficacy about performing each task. When people are self-confident about each step, they can progressively put the steps together and build self-efficacy about the entire behavior. The strategy of breaking down complex new behaviors into small steps is particularly useful when working with adolescents to the degree that it keeps them motivated and avoids mechanical and boring repetition. It should not be assumed that adolescents will stay motivated repeating a single task just because they will improve self-efficacy by changing their performance expectations. The key to success, therefore, becomes the structuring of the more mechanical and/or repetitive aspects leading to mastery of a new behavior—whether it be to play basketball or tennis, learn mutiplication tables or verb conjugations in a foreign language, adopt the use of a condom or healthier eating, etc.—in such a manner that the adolescent's motivation and interest levels are always kept high.

Furthermore, in order to actually assume a new behavior (behavioral change), tasks must not only be learned by adolescents with a desire to perform them, but they must also be actually *performed*. A task may be learned yet not performed, whereas performance presumes learning. The concept of *behavioral capability* maintains that if a person is to perform a particular behavior, he or she must know what the behavior is (knowledge of the behavior) and how to perform it (skill). Self-efficacy is the person's perception; capability is the real thing. Behavioral capability is the result of the individual's training, intellectual capacity, and learning style. The skills training, called *mastery learning*, provides cognitive knowledge of what is to be performed, practice in performing activities, and feedback and reinforcement to refine successful performance until the person performs the behavior at a predefined level of acceptability.

The Social Cognitive Theory incorporates different types of reinforcement: direct reinforcement (as in operant conditioning), vicarious reinforcement (as in observational learning), and self-reinforcement. It also describes *external reinforcement* as the occurrence of an event or act known to have predictable reinforcement value and *internal reinforcement* as a person's own experience or perception that an event has some value. Educational programs that are *intrinsically reinforcing* result in more learning, interest in, and retention of the subject matter. Program designers and health practitioners may also choose to use external rewards to encourage the adoption of behaviors that are part of a behavioral change program. These may be discontinued by the end of a program, when the intrinsic rewards of the behavioral change itself are strong enough to maintain the new behavior. *Self-control of performance* refers to a person's behavior focused on the achievement of self-set goals. One of the most important goals of this type of health education is to bring the performance of health behavior under the control of the individual.

Bandura recognized that excessive emotional arousal inhibits learning and performance. Yet while Social Cognitive Theory constructs and methods are often employed to learn behavioral management of emotional and physiological arousal, they usually ignore the underlying reasons for those emotions.

The principles of reciprocal determinism may be useful in developing adolescent behavioral change programs that do not focus on behavior in isolation, but rather on changes in the environment and in the individual himself/herself. Examples of the social environment include family members, friends, neighbors, and classmates and peers. The physical environment might include the availability of highly nutritious and healthy foods, a playground and/or gymnasium to encourage adequate physical activity, acceptable indoor and outdoor air quality, and public restrictions on smoking.

The Social Cognitive Theory describes a number of crucial *personal factors* that are

> **Box 16-1. The Social Cognitive Theory: Key Theoretical Concepts in the Adoption of Healthy Behaviors**
>
> - **reciprocal determinism:** the simultaneous influence between socio-environmental, cognitive, and behavioral factors
> - **observational learning:** learning by observing the behaviors of others
> - **modeling:** the illustration by positive role models of how to effectively overcome barriers and achieve behavior change; also the **modeling of behavior**, in which adolescents are shown by others, step-by-step, how to perform a new behavior, such as the correct way to put on a condom
> - **vicarious reinforcement:** through observational learning, the gaining of increased awareness regarding the rewards received as a result of specific behaviors enacted by others
> - **external reinforcement:** the occurrence of an event or act known to have predictable reinforcement value
> - **internal reinforcement:** a personal experience or individual perception that an act or event has some value
> - **outcome expectations:** the expectations that are developed prior to the occurrence of a given situation and about the outcomes of the behavioral response to it (e.g., "If I use a condom consistently, I will prevent STIs.")
> - **outcome expectancies:** the values that individuals place on a certain outcome; also the incentives to perform the behavior; comparable to *evaluations* (outcome values) presented in the Theories of Reasoned Action and Planned Behavior (Chapters Ten and Eleven)
> - **behavioral capability:** the capability to perform a given behavior that results from possession of knowledge about the behavior and of skills in how to perform it
> - **self-efficacy:** the degree of confidence a person feels about performing a particular activity, including confidence in overcoming the barriers to performing that behavior; also a key theoretical concept in the Health Belief Model (Chapter Eight) and the Theory of Planned Behavior (Chapter Eleven)
> - **self-control of performance:** the possession of self-determined or self-regulated behavior that is focused on the achievement of self-set goals

part of the process of analyzing influences, messages, and/or models from the environment before an adolescent makes the choice to engage or not engage in the new behavior. These factors are the adolescent's capacity to:

- symbolize behavior (*cognition*)
- anticipate the outcomes of behavior (*outcome expectations*)
- possess confidence in performing a behavior, including overcoming any barriers to performing the behavior (*self-efficacy*)
- possess self-determined or *self-regulated* behavior (*self-control of performance*)
- reflect upon and analyze experiences
- learn by observing others (*observational learning*)

The capacity for observational learning, in turn, will be affected by:

- *attention to and perception of* the relevant aspects of modeled behaviors (including characteristics of the observer and the model)

- *retention, representation, and remembering* of learned knowledge
- production of appropriate behavior (*behavior capability*)
- motivation as a result of observed positive incentives and reinforcement

What is not sufficiently emphasized in Bandura's model is that the proficiency in use of these *personal factors* will vary through the different developmental stages and need to be *fostered* by adolescents, rather than assumed as current capabilities. Messages and models that capture the adolescent's *attention* and *perception* will vary by age, gender, learning style, and personal interests. These aspects and the level of attention given to the message or model will also affect *retention*, *representation*, and *remembering*. The capacity to *symbolize behavior*, *anticipate the outcomes of behavior*, *self-regulate*, and *reflect upon and analyze* experiences will also vary by individual personality differences, gender, and age.

Recent Additions to and Refinements of the Social Cognitive Theory

During the past two decades, Bandura has continued to permanently review and refine his theory to respond to the passage of time and the emergence of new concepts. As a result, over the past five years or so, he has shifted the focus of the Social Cognitive Theory from the domain of mechanistic constructs of human behavior to the views of the person as an agent in control of his or her own life (Glanz, Rimer, and Lewis 2002; Bandura 2001, 1997). He states in one of his more recent articles that "the capacity to exercise control over the nature and quality of one's life is the essence of humanness," whereby "consciousness is the very substance of mental life that not only makes life personally manageable, but worth living" (Bandura 2001). These statements are similar to those expressed by David Buchanan in his work *An Ethic for Health Promotion: Rethinking the Sources of Human Well-Being* (2000), in which he encourages "collective consciousness-raising and strengthening people's capacity toward mindful, responsible choices."

Along this same line of thought, Bandura's article "Social Cognitive Theory: An Agentic Perspective," published in the 2001 *Annual Review of Psychology*, describes core features of "human agency," or operation, which he called *intentionality*, *forethought*, *self-reactiveness*, and *self-reflectiveness*. He defines *intentionality* as a representation of a future course of action to be performed, in which "intentions center on plans of action." *Forethought* refers to people setting goals for themselves, motivating themselves, and guiding their actions in anticipation of future events. *Self-reactiveness* refers to the ability to give shape to appropriate courses of action and to motivate and regulate their execution. Bandura incorporates concepts of the Self-Regulation Theory (Chapter Thirteen) recognizing that "this multifaceted self-directness operates through self-regulatory processes that link thought to action." With *self-reflectiveness*, "people evaluate their motivation, values, and the meaning of their life pursuits."

All of these core features of human agency described by Bandura are essential goals to achieve during adolescent development. Most young people enter adolescence without a full development of these capacities and need help in mastering them. PAHO encourages program developers to incorporate these latest additions to the Social Cognitive Theory and not operate within the older versions that carry a more limited, mechanistic view of human behavior.

Research and Evidence of Practical Applications of the Social Cognitive Theory to Adolescent Lifestyles

A number of principles similar to those in the Social Cognitive Theory are incorporated in Jessor's model (Jessor 1993) aimed at explaining adolescent risk/lifestyle. The tendency for behaviors to cluster together provides support for the concept of lifestyle. This concept directs our attention away from the specific behaviors (substance abuse, risky sexual practices, etc.) towards the adolescent as a whole person. In Jessor's model, *personal*, *socio-environmental*, and *behavioral factors* are shown to influence the adolescent's lifestyle with reciprocal relationships among all of the factors (reciprocal determinism). Personal factors are separated into biological and personality domains, while socio-environmental factors are divided into actual domains (e.g., socioeconomic status) and perceived domains (e.g., *models* for deviant or conventional behavior). Both risk factors and protective factors may exist within each domain.

Consideration of the Social Cognitive Theory and the concepts of risk and protective factors and adolescent lifestyle have a number of significant implications for the development of intervention programs for adolescents. Jessor summarized these as follows:

- The complexity of causation suggests that interventions that are comprehensive promise to yield greater successes than those that are limited in scope.
- Programs should aim to simultaneously reduce risk and promote protection.
- Programs directed at lifestyle change may be more appropriate than programs focusing on specific behaviors.
- Programs need to acknowledge the salience of the social environment, where young people growing up in adverse social environments may experience more risk factors and less protective factors.
- Programs should not only focus on the individual but also need to aim for social change because risk is embedded in the larger social context of adolescent life (Neumark-Sztainer 1999, Jessor 1992).

In many ways, the contribution of Jessor's model represents an integration of the Social Cognitive Theory with an ecological approach (Chapter Four) and evidence coming from resiliency studies (Chapter Nineteen). However, in this work, as in many others discussed in this book, there appears to be little or no emphasis on the changing developmental aspects of adolescent health which PAHO considers to be so critical to the relevancy and effectiveness of targeted interventions.

In a review of the literature, the Social Cognitive Theory has been identified as the underlying theoretical framework for a number of adolescent health promotion and prevention programs, probably because of its consideration of socio-environmental factors affecting individual behaviors. However, one of the drawbacks of such a broad theoretical formulation (environmental, personal, and behavioral factors) is that program designers might feel pressured to explain almost any phenomenon using one or more of the constructs without a complete understanding of how they operate separately and together. They might even adopt the theory as their theoretical framework even if the interventions include actions only at the environmental and personal level and do not include a focus on specific behavioral variants, such as the target group's capacities in observational learning, self-efficacy, and self-control of performance. At the same time, there is considerable conceptual confusion about how to apply, measure, and analyze constructs of health behavior theories (Glanz, Rimer, and Lewis 2002).

One example of this problem is the work of Pender (1998), who conducted a research literature review of 20 studies aimed at encouraging children and adolescents to adopt more active lifestyles. He found that although the Social Cognitive Theory provided the theoretical basis for most of the studies reviewed, specification of how theory concepts were operationalized in the interventions was often unclear. In his conclusions, he proposed that in the future, the rigor of theoretically-based intervention studies aimed at promoting physical activity be increased in order to provide the much-needed answers to this question.

Moreover, it is not only important that program designers possess a clear understanding of how theoretical constructs operate in practical interventions, but also about the people who implement the intervention itself (e.g., facilitators of a workshop, teachers in a school sexual education program). In one study, the Social Cognitive Theory was used to define the reasons why fourth- and fifth-grade preadolescents were not consuming sufficient amounts of fruit, vegetables, and 100% juice products. The reasons, according to the theory, were due to environmental, personal, and behavioral factors. A creative school curriculum called "Gimme Five!" was designed to help remedy these influencing factors and thereby increase consumption of these healthy foods. Outcome analyses of this project revealed no change in consumption patterns by the end of the fifth grade (Baranowski et al. 2000). Yet, as a process evaluation of the project revealed (Davis et al. 2000), classroom teachers implemented only about 50% of the "Gimme Five!" curriculum tasks and only 22% of the curriculum tasks shown most likely to result in behavior change. Teachers might not have fully implemented the curriculum for a variety of reasons. The Diffusion of Innovations Theory, as we will see in Chapter Twenty-three, helps to anticipate and avoid failures due to low implementation when planning health promotion and prevention projects, because it focuses on the need for a strong linkage system between those who develop innovative messages and tasks, those who are charged with adopting and diffusing them (in this example, schoolteachers), and those who are to be the recipients (the students). In this sense, the inclusion of this theory in the overall theoretical framework design would perhaps have ensured the project's greater success.

The Social Cognitive Theory also has been used to understand the determinants of physical activity in children and adolescents as they relate to the prevention of obesity in these age groups. Strauss et al. (2001) conducted a study with 92 pre-, early, and middle U.S. adolescents, aged 10 to 16 years. Health beliefs, self-efficacy, social influences, and time spent in sedentary behaviors were determined through questionnaires. There was a significant decline in physical activity levels between ages the ages of 10 and 16, particularly in girls. In their responses, the children reported spending 75.5% of each day in sedentary activities—watching television, sitting at the computer, and preparing homework assignments. In contrast, this group replied that only 1.4% of their day was spent in vigorous physical activity. Among other findings, Strauss and colleagues conclude that health promotion programs that enhance adolescents' self-efficacy—their belief in their ability to successfully adhere to a regular regimen of exercise—increase the motivation to be physically active.

Wallace et al. (2000) applied the Social Cognitive Theory and the Stages of Change Model (Chapter Nine) to determine the personal, behavioral, and environmental characteristics associated with exercise behavior and intentions among 937 youth between the ages of 17 and 24. Among females, exercise self-efficacy and family social support for physical activity were the best predictors of the stage of exercise behavior change. Social support from friends, the history of physical activity, and exercise self-efficacy were significant predictors of the stage of exercise behavior change among males. Exercise self-efficacy was associated with the stage of behavioral change, but the source of significant social support (family vs. friends) was different for males and females.

From the perspective of the Social Cognitive Theory, substance use is conceptualized as a socially learned, purposeful, and functional behavior which is the result of the interplay of socio-environmental and personal factors. By the mid-1980s, detailed analyses of research results indicated that *social influence programs*, most of them designed under the concepts of the

Social Cognitive Theory (Clubb 1991), were consistently more effective than programs based on the information deficit or affective education models (discussed in Chapter Two) in preventing cigarette smoking. Several of the most successful smoking prevention programs included components designed to increase adolescents' ability to resist the various pro-use social pressures, particularly pressure from their peers. Social influence strategies have typically been applied in the United States through school-based programs for students in the sixth through eighth grades.

Although several of these programs have had significant and substantial short-term impacts on smoking behavior (U.S. Department of Health and Human Services 2000), the effects have tended to dissipate over time (Wakefield and Chaloupka 2000). A meta-analysis of Project D.A.R.E. (Drug Abuse Resistance Education) outcome evaluations concluded that the initiative's effect on tobacco use was small at best (Ennet et al. 1994) and substantially less than that of other, more interactive prevention programs. The Hutchinson Smoking Prevention Project, also in the United States, provides more evidence that pure "social influence" programs are not effective over time (Hatcher and Scarpa 2002, Peterson et al. 2000).

Several health promotion programs have tried to increase adolescents' problem-solving capacities through role-playing activities, also with mixed results. Although strengthening these capacities during adolescence is crucial to help young people in their decision-making, formulas that have no meaningful reference points in the adolescents' personal experience are learned in a rote manner and cannot readily be transferred from one situation to another. On the other hand, programs that have demonstrated greater effectiveness in improving adolescents' problem-solving abilities have been those that have been most successful in coupling the participants' prior intense emotional experiences with the skills needed to successfully address those experiences.

Langlois, Petosa, and Hallam (1999) used the Social Cognitive Theory to examine the impact of participating in a school-based smoking prevention program in improving several variables related to smoking initiation reduction. The study's theory constructs included behavioral capability to resist positive images of smoking, skills efficacy in refusal to smoke, total positive refusal expectations and importance, and total negative refusal expectations and importance. The smoking prevention program had a significant impact on the students' refusal skills efficacy, along with total positive refusal expectations and importance. However, the program did not affect behavioral capability to resist positive images of smoking and total negative refusal expectations and importance.

The 2000 report of the U.S. Surgeon General (U.S Department of Health and Human Services 2000), *Reducing Tobacco*

Use, concludes that attempts to reduce the scope of smoking prevention programs to skills training alone are likely to be ineffective. More complex and intensive programs combining interventions within and outside of schools are needed to overcome the powerful pro-smoking cultural images fostered by the larger social environment.

Sargent et al. (2002) employed various Social Cognitive Theory constructs, such as observational learning and modeling, to study the association between viewing tobacco use in movies and attitudes toward smoking among early adolescents ($n = 3,766$) who had never tried cigarette smoking. The results showed that greater exposure to depictions of tobacco use in movies significantly increased the number of positive expectations endorsed by the adolescent and the perception that most adults smoke, but not the perception that most peers smoke.

Chen et al. (2002) studied the receptivity to pro-tobacco media and its impact on early and middle adolescent cigarette smoking for African-Americans, Asian-Americans, Hispanic, and non-Hispanic whites in California ($n = 20,332$). The results showed that receptivity to pro-tobacco media is associated with a higher prevalence of cigarette smoking among California youth from diverse ethnic backgrounds. Hawkins and Hane (2000) studied adolescent perceptions of smoking in U.S. print advertising. The authors concluded that students who smoked at least occasionally were more likely to believe messages conveyed by print cigarette ads than were students who had never smoked. Hawkins and Hane attribute this difference to the *vicarious reinforcement* portrayed in print cigarette advertising. Furthermore, the authors propose that the Social Cognitive Theory can help to increase the efficacy of anti-smoking advertising campaigns.

A cross-country study by the Global Youth Tobacco Survey Collaborative Group (2002) showed that in Latin America and the Caribbean, exposure of middle adolescents to pro-tobacco advertising is extremely high, reaching over 90% in Argentina, Bolivia, Costa Rica, Mexico, and Uruguay. Padgett, Selwyn, and Kelder (1998) investigated adolescent attitudes and behaviors toward cigarette smoking in Ecuador. Using the Social Cognitive Theory as a basis, the cross-sectional survey focused attention on such social influences as the smoking habits of family members and peers, as well as on the role of cigarette advertisements. The smoking status of family members and peers significantly predicted student-smoking status. The Global Youth Tobacco Survey Collaborative Group study (2002) found that in Latin America and the Caribbean, the percentage of middle adolescents exposed to smoke from others at home reaches over 60% in Argentina, Chile, Cuba, and Uruguay, and that of this group, two out of every three definitively think smoke from others is harmful to their health.

Project Northland (2003), a large randomized community trial conducted for the prevention of adolescent alcohol use, involved approximately 2,400 students from the graduating class of 1998 from 24 school districts in northeastern Minnesota during their sixth-, seventh-, and eighth-grade years (1991–1994). Based on the social cognitive theoretical concept of reciprocal determinism, Project Northland utilized an understanding of the environmental, intrapersonal, and behavioral factors that influence alcohol as a basis for designing school and community-level activities. The project's intervention involved three years of behavioral curricula in the classrooms, parental involvement programs, extracurricular peer leadership, and community-wide task force activities. After three years, when students were at the end of eighth grade, reports of monthly drinking were 20% lower among students in the intervention school districts compared with students in the reference districts, and reports of weekly drinking were 30% lower. Project Northland was effective in changing peer influence to use alcohol, normative expectations about how many young people drink, and parent-child communication about consequences of alcohol use, while at the same time reinforcing the importance of reasons for not using alcohol (Komro et al. 2001, Perry et al. 2002).

Project Northland is an excellent example of an intervention in which the Social Cognitive Theory has been identified as the successful underlying theoretical framework (Glanz, Rimer, and Lewis 2002), in the sense that it incorporated the environmental, intrapersonal, and behavioral factors that influence alcohol as a basis for designing school and community-level interventions. However, the project's development was not limited solely to constructs described by the Social Cognitive Theory; namely, role-playing, rewards, and the use of parents and peers as role models. Other elements, borrowed from a variety of other constructs, included intensive group discussions on problem-solving, entertaining classroom games, strengthening of parenting skills, youth development, and community organization components (Bernstein et al. 1999, Veblen-Mortenson et al. 1999). In assessing the long-term outcomes to community actions such as Project Northland, Perry and colleagues emphasize, however, that developmentally appropriate, multi-component, community-wide programs should be developed to remain in place throughout the adolescence period to reduce and maintain low levels of alcohol use (Perry et al. 2002).

The Social Cognitive Theory states that health behavior essentially results from a judgment of self-efficacy. The 1993 Gillis review of research literature published between 1983 and 1991, mentioned earlier in this chapter, focused on identifying the determinants of a health-promoting lifestyle. From 23 studies reviewed, six dealt with children and adolescents. A meta-analysis of these studies showed that self-efficacy was the strongest predictor of a health-promoting lifestyle, followed by social support, perceived benefits, self-concept, perceived barriers, and health definition.

Although it was Bandura who first introduced the concept of self-efficacy as the most important prerequisite for behavioral change, it was also added later by Rosenstock, Stretcher, and Becker (1988) to the Health Belief Model. The literature published on self-efficacy and adolescent behaviors is extensive. The impact of the self-efficacy construct has also been widely studied for several behaviors related to sexual health and reproduction among adolescents, particularly condom use. In a Medline search focusing exclusively on sexual behaviors among adolescents, the authors of this book were able to retrieve 86 articles addressing self-efficacy issues and condom use. Research indicates that this behavior may depend on critical factors such as the expected consequences of condom use, perceived social support for condoms, perceived barriers to condom use, perceived susceptibility to HIV infection, and perceived self-efficacy in condom use (Zamboni, Crawford, and Williams 2000; Adih and Alexander 1999).

Adih and Alexander studied the determinants of condom use to prevent HIV infection among youth in Ghana ($n = 601$ men, ages 15–24). The study used constructs from the Health Belief Model and Social Cognitive Theory and adopted them to the Ghanaian sociocultural context. Findings from multiple logistic regression analysis indicate that perceived susceptibility to HIV infection, perceived self-efficacy to use condoms, perceived barriers to condom use, and perceived social support were significant predictors of condom use. Young men who perceived a high level of self-efficacy to use condoms and a low level of barriers to condom use were nearly three times more likely to have used condoms during their last intercourse when compared to others who did not hold these perceptions. Self-efficacy scales for HIV risk behaviors have been developed for different adolescent populations (Smith et al. 1996; Bilodeau, Forget, and Tetreault 1994).

Richard, Van der Plight, and DeVries (1995), based on previous research findings indicating that sexual behavior is heavily influenced by emotions that might interfere with rational decision-making (Gerrard et al. 1993), decided to investigate whether anticipated, post-behavioral, affective reactions influence sexual behaviors among 822 Dutch adolescents between 15 and 19 years of age. Their study found that adolescents are more likely to refrain from sexual intercourse or to use condoms in casual sexual encounters if they believe themselves capable of managing sexual situations (perceived self-efficacy). They also found that anticipated affective reactions predict a significant proportion of variance in behavioral expectations, over and above components of the Theory of Planned Behavior (e.g., attitudes, subjective norm, perceived behavioral control). The authors stress the importance of emphasizing not only cognitive but also affective issues when designing AIDS prevention campaigns aimed at adolescent sexual behavior. They suggest that social modeling could easily combine efforts to increase self-efficacy and the salience of negative feelings that may be experienced following risky sexual activities and the positive feelings that may be experienced after safe sex.

The Social Cognitive Theory and the Theory of Gender and Power (Wingood and DiClemente 2002, Connell 1987) were used as theoretical models to guide the development of a five-session social skills intervention. Its effectiveness was tested through a randomized, single blind controlled trial among economically disadvantaged youth and young adult African-American women. Compared with the delayed HIV education control condition, women in the social skills intervention demonstrated increased consistent condom use and the adoption of norms supporting this practice by their partners and greater sexual self-control, sexual communication, and sexual assertiveness (DiClemente and Wingood 1995). The authors concluded that the effectiveness of this intervention might be attributed to the use of the Social Cognitive Theory constructs (e.g., positive role models facilitating the acquisition of social skills through modeling exercises that emphasized skills mastery training) within a gender-appropriate model useful for understanding relationship dynamics, as is stressed in the Theory of Gender and Power.

The studies reviewed in this section are only a sample of those that have utilized the Social Cognitive Theory to analyze adolescent health behaviors. It has been by far mostly used to understand tobacco, alcohol, and drug consumption among adolescents, as Table 16-1. illustrates. The theory's concepts have also been used to understand and develop violence prevention programs for early and middle adolescents (Durant, Barkin, and Krowchuk 2001; Orpinas et al. 2000). Research to date in this behavior indicates that observational learning and role modeling are key elements to be considered when designing interventions oriented to promote nonviolent anger expression and conflict resolution, particularly among younger age groups before violent behavioral patterns have been adopted.

Table 16-1. presents a breakdown of the number of studies found using the Social Cognitive Theory according to health behaviors.

At this juncture, it is interesting to note that the Social Cognitive Theory has been utilized more frequently to understand and develop interventions to change adolescent behaviors than any of the individual level theories and models introduced in Chapters Eight through Fourteen. Table 16-2. shows a comparison of the total number of published articles using the Social Cognitive Theory and each of the individual level theories and models to address four categories of adolescent lifestyles and behaviors.

Table 16-1. **Most Commonly Researched Adolescent Behaviors Using the Social Cognitive Theory (SCT)**

ADOLESCENT BEHAVIORS	NUMBER OF ARTICLES USING THE SCT	NUMBER OF ARTICLES BY KEYWORDS	
Sexual and Reproductive Health	19	Teen Pregnancy	3
		HIV/AIDS	11
		STIs	1
		Condom Use	15
Tobacco, Alcohol, and Drug Use	48	Tobacco	17
		Alcohol	17
		Drugs	14
Physical Activity and Nutrition	9	Obesity	0
		Physical Activity	7
		Nutrition	2
Violence	9		
TOTAL	**85**		

Table 16-2. **A Comparison of the Social Cognitive Theory and the Individual Level Theories and Models for Adolescent Behavioral Change**

Number of Articles on Adolescence and Individual Behavior Change Theories and Models	Total	Sexual and Reproductive Health	Tobacco, Alcohol, and Drug Use	Physical Activity and Nutrition	Violence
Social Cognitive Theory	85	19	48	9	9
Health Belief Model	66	37	18	9	2
Sensation-Seeking Theory	65	6	52	2	5
Transtheoretical Model and Stages of Change	51	9	27	15	0
Self-Regulation Theory	42	4	31	3	4
Theory of Reasoned Action	31	13	14	3	1
Theory of Planned Behavior	29	13	12	4	0
Goal-Setting Theory	23	10	5	8	0

It should be further noted that the number of research articles listed on adolescent health and the Social Cognitive Theory would increase significantly if the articles addressing self-efficacy alone (i.e., without specifying or focusing on the specific theory/theories utilized) were included. There are, for example, several articles using other theories or models to research behavioral change among adolescents (e.g., the stages of change model) that specifically identify the self-efficacy construct as being among the variables studied.

> **Box 16-2. Summary of the Social Cognitive Theory and Adolescent Lifestyles**
>
> - This theory explains behavior in terms of a triadic, dynamic, and reciprocal model in which *socio-environmental*, *personal* or *cognitive*, and *behavioral* factors all interact.
> - The environment is particularly important in this theory in part because it provides *models* for behavior. Thus, an adolescent learns by observing (*observational learning*) the behaviors of others (*role models*) and the rewards these models receive (*vicarious reinforcement*).
> - Within the Social Cognitive Theory context, the mass media provides adolescents with heavy doses of vicarious learning experiences.
> - The Social Cognitive Theory incorporates different types of reinforcement: direct reinforcement (as in operant conditioning), vicarious reinforcement (as in observational learning), and self-reinforcement.
> - Health promotion programs that enhance adolescents' self-efficacy—their belief in their ability to successfully adhere to a regular regimen of exercise—increase the motivation to be physically active.
> - Attempts to reduce the scope of smoking prevention programs to skills training alone are likely to be ineffective. More complex and intensive programs combining interventions within and outside of schools are needed to overcome the powerful pro-smoking cultural images fostered by the larger social environment.
> - Social influences, such as the smoking habits of family members and peers, as well as cigarette advertisements, significantly predict student-smoking status.
> - Self-efficacy is the strongest predictor of a health-promoting lifestyle.
> - Young men who perceive a high level of self-efficacy to use condoms and a low level of barriers to condom use are nearly three times more likely to use condoms during their last intercourse when compared to others who do not hold these perceptions.
> - Adolescents are more likely to refrain from sexual intercourse or to use condoms in casual sexual encounters if they believe themselves capable of managing sexual situations (perceived self-efficacy).
> - Safe sex health promotion and HIV prevention campaigns directed towards adolescents will be more effective if they combine social modeling with efforts to increase self-efficacy and the salience of negative feelings that may be experienced following risky sexual activities and positive feelings that may be experienced after safe sex, along with a gender-appropriate model useful for understanding relationship dynamics, such as the Theory of Gender and Power.

[Chapter Seventeen]

The Social Networks and Social Support Theories

Social relationships are the foundation for human existence and interdependency. In particular, the adolescent lives in a number of social worlds, many of which overlap and interact with each other. The concept of the *social network* is an analytical framework for understanding relationships among members of various social systems. Networks are classified as personal, based on ties that an individual has with other persons, or as an integrated network, based on the relationship among a defined group of people. Sociologists have referred to the actual and potential resources available to an individual through a network as *social capital*. Within the health education community, Green and Kreuter (1999) have defined social capital as the structures and processes developed among people and organizations that lead to accomplishing goals with outcomes of mutual societal benefit. Understanding the role of social networks and social support in adolescent life and their impact on adopting healthy or unhealthy behaviors is crucial to the design of effective health promotion and prevention interventions.

The personal *social network*, defined as a person-centered web of social relationships, is the structure through which *social support* may be provided. Social support is defined as "aid and assistance exchanged through social relationships and interpersonal transactions" (Israel 1982). Four main types of social support have been identified:

- *emotional*:   the provision of love, caring, and/or empathy;
- *instrumental*: the provision of aid or a service (e.g., babysitting or lending money);
- *informational*: the provision of information, advice, and/or suggestions; and

- *appraisal*: the provision of information that is useful for self-evaluation purposes, such as constructive feedback, affirmation of beliefs, and social comparison.

Social networks have structural and relationship properties, as shown in Box 17-1. The structure can be described as consisting of nodes (individuals, groups, or organizations) and the relationships as the ties among these nodes (Bartholomew et al. 2001).

An individual, group, or organization may play any of several roles in a network: serving as a member, as a linking agent that brings information across network boundaries, or as an isolate with few ties to other network members (Bartholomew et al. 2001, Fulk and Boyd 1991). Furthermore, different types of social networks are associated with specific types of social support. Small, dense, geographically close, intense networks provide more emotional and appraisal support. On the other hand, large, diffuse, and less intense networks provide more informational support and social outreach.

Box 17-1. Structural and Relationship Properties of Social Networks

Structural Properties

- **Range:** the number of network members
- **Geographic dispersion:** the extent to which network members live in close proximity to one another and to the individuals of interest to the network analysis
- **Homogeneity:** the extent to which network members have similar characteristics (age, race, gender, economic status, etc.)
- **Boundedness:** the proportion of all ties of network members that stay within the network's boundaries
- **Density:** the extent to which network members know and interact with each other and are connected; measured by the proportion of direct ties that exist among network members out of all possible ties that could exist among them
- **Reachability:** the average number of ties required to link any two network members
- **Degree:** the extent to which a network member has direct ties with other network members
- **Cliques:** the portions of networks in which all members are tied directly
- **Clusters:** the portions of networks in which not all members are tied directly

Relationship Properties

- **Frequency:** the quantity of contact between two network members
- **Duration:** the length of time a relationship has existed
- **Intimacy or intensity:** the perceived emotional closeness between two network members
- **Symmetry:** the extent to which social support is both given and received between two network members
- **Reciprocity:** the extent to which resources and support are both given and received in a relationship
- **Multiplexity:** the number of different types of social support exchanged between two network members
- **Complexity:** the extent to which social relationships serve many functions

The extent and nature of social relationships have been linked to a person's health status in a number of studies (Heaney and Israel 1997). The mechanisms underlying these epidemiological findings have been hypothesized to include modeling and reinforcement of positive health-related behaviors, the buffering of the effects of stress on health, and providing access to resources to cope with stress. John Cassel (1976), a social epidemiologist whose work has served to highlight the importance of social support to physical and mental well-being, states that social support constitutes a key protective factor that reduces individual vulnerability to the harmful effects of stress on health. Among the four types of social support described above, emotional support is known to be the most strongly and consistently associated with good health and well-being (Heaney and Israel 2002). Michael and colleagues (1999) demonstrated that having at least one strong intimate relationship is an important predictor of good health. There is also increasing evidence that negative interpersonal interactions (e.g., mistrust, criticism, and excessive demands) are more strongly related to negative mood (Fleishman et al. 2000) and cigarette smoking (Burg and Seeman 1994) than is lack of social support (Heaney and Israel 2002).

Heaney and Israel also suggest that any proposed support-enhancing intervention needs to begin with an assessment of the social networks that are maintained by the study population; in this case, adolescents of different ages, genders, and cultural backgrounds. These authors recommend assessing the weaknesses as well as the strengths of existing networks in terms of their abilities to meet the needs of the targeted (i.e., focal) individuals (i.e., adolescents). In recent years, several different social network mapping and assessment tools have been developed for this purpose. The software package UCINET allows users to undertake sophisticated networks analysis. Other programs, such as KrackPlot and Pajek, also map networks for visual display and analysis (see Barrera 2000 and Berkman and Glass 2000 for reviews of these tools).

Heany and Israel (2002) identify four ways in which social networks and social support may be strengthened.

(1) *Developing new social network linkages* might be called for when the existing social support is ineffective or insufficient. The strategies include:

- introducing *mentors* or *advisers*; i.e., individuals who have already coped with the situation being experienced by the focal individual;
- providing *buddies*; i.e., individuals who are experiencing the same or a similar stressor or life transition at the same time as the recipient; and
- coordinating *self-help groups*, in which the roles of support provider and support recipient are mutually shared among the various members.

(2) *Enhancing existing social network linkages* might be called for when existing net-

works are ignored because they are not perceived as being useful. The perceived value of the networks may be improved by changing the attitudes and behaviors of support providers, including:

- strengthening network members' skills to provide effective support; and
- training focal points who become in charge of mobilizing and maintaining social networks.

Heany and Israel point out several special challenges that might arise when attempting to enhance existing social networks. These include identifying existing network members who are committed to providing support and who possess the necessary resources to sustain their commitment, identifying the changes in provider attitudes and behaviors that might improve perceived support by the support recipient, and intervening in ways that are consistent with the network's established norms and styles of interaction.

(3) *Enhancing networks at the community level through participatory problem-solving processes*, or involving network members' participation in the identification and resolution of community problems, helps to collectively strengthen social network ties and to stimulate the creation of new ones. This process also promotes the network's identification and assessment of overlapping networks within the community and increases its own understanding of how the network members seek social support and how this is provided in the community.

(4) *Enhancing networks through the use of natural helpers* provides a community-based system of care and social support that complements, but does not replace, the more specialized services of health professionals (Eng and Smith 1995). Natural helpers are members of social networks to whom other network members spontaneously turn for advice, emotional support, and concrete help. Natural helpers are different from lay health advisers (e.g., outreach workers), who also provide social support, but who may not be part of the recipient's social network. Improving social networks through natural helpers calls for:

- identifying natural helpers in the community;
- identifying existing social networks of natural helpers;
- training natural helpers to provide improved advice, assistance, and referrals within their existing helping networks;
- linking natural helpers with health service providers and community leaders to facilitate an ongoing dialogue on local health problems; and
- supporting natural helpers in implementing short-term and long-term self-help actions in response to local health needs.

According to Eng and Parker (2002), forming a partnership between natural helpers and health professionals increases community competence in two important ways: it improves health practices, and it enables a more effective coordination of community services.

Although a variety of social networks and resources most likely already exist in any given community, effective social network programs must nonetheless be tailored to the needs and goals of the targeted participants. Thus, establishing participatory assessment processes during which members and participants may identify and discuss the strengths and weaknesses of their social networks will help structure and further fine-tune truly supportive programs.

Heany and Israel (2002) list a series of characteristics for health-enhancing social support among members of the general population. They hold equal relevance in the case of the adolescent population, as well:

- Interactions between helpers and individuals receiving social support should facilitate expressions of trust, closeness, and caring.
- Helping relationships should be founded on a basis of mutual interdependence and exchange.
- People who are socially similar to the support recipient and who have experienced similar stressors or situations have a better chance to provide effective support (Thoits 1995).
- It is crucial that the support provider understands, and can be empathetic to, the needs and values of the support recipient.
- Social support will be most effective if it takes into consideration the recipient's own perception of support needs.

Heany and Israel also note that it is not clear whether professional helpers (e.g., health care providers) are effective sources of social support. Professional-lay relationships (e.g., physicians or nurses and adolescents) usually involve asymmetry in terms of information management and power, which may result in a poor empathic understanding of the adolescent's needs and wants. Additionally, professional helpers are rarely available to provide support over long periods of time, and, particularly in the case of primary health care settings, personnel availability follows a highly rotational structure. These authors suggest that a combination of formal and informal helpers may be most effective, then, in cases in which both informational and emotional support are needed.

Adolescence can be a challenging period of life for parents, adolescents, and all others with whom they normally interact within the community at large. Rapid physical and emotional changes that accompany this period ensure that the future will always be unpredictable. To better cope with and derive maximum benefit from this time of growth and maturity, both adolescents and parents need social support. The participatory assessment should therefore include as many of the community actors who form part of the adolescent's social world as possible. Heaney and Israel (1997), in recognizing the need for and the value of ecological approaches to adolescent health promotion, note that social network interventions that combine strategies across multiple units of practice (e.g., family, friends, neighbors, institutions) deserve the greatest attention.

Research and Evidence of Practical Applications of the Social Networks and Support Theories to Adolescent Lifestyles

Adolescents grow up establishing new social relationships with *peers* and *adults* within their *schools*, *neighborhoods*, and *workplaces*. The *peer group* can be crucial in adolescent development by responding to the adolescent's need to be accepted, belong to a group, and develop identity. Ennett and Bauman (1993) pioneered use of the Social Networks Theory in assessing *peer social networks* among 1,092 ninth graders in five different high schools within a large North Carolina school district in the United States. Based on interviews with students over a one-year period, the authors described three categories of social network affiliation among adolescents:

- *clique members*: adolescents who carry out most of their interactions within their small group of peers. Cliques are usually composed of four to six adolescents (but may be as small as two or as large as 12 members) who are generally of the same sex and age. The clique is the social setting in which adolescents share together in informal and leisure-time activities, frequently communicate via telephone, e–mail, etc., and form close relationships.
- *liaisons*: adolescents who interact with two or more adolescents who are members of a clique, but who are not themselves part of the clique
- *isolates*: adolescents who have few or no linkages to others via a social network

Figure 17-1. depicts the spatial differences between these three categories.

Social network analysis also permitted Ennett and Bauman in this study to describe the proportion of adolescents occupying each social position. Although this varied among the five studied schools, in all of them less than half of the adolescents were members of cliques. The percentage of isolates ranged from 17.5% to 38.2%. The study also examined the relationship between peer group structure and cigarette smoking, in order to better understand the assumption at the time of the study that peer group plays a crucial role in the initiation and maintenance of smoking. Surprisingly, the authors found that at four of the five schools, the odds of being a current smoker were significantly higher for isolates than for clique members and liaisons. The authors concluded that emphasis in smoking prevention programs perhaps should be placed more on helping adolescents join and participate in cliques and not only on resisting peer influence, at the same time that isolates should be considered as possible high-risk targets.

Ennett, Bauman, and Koch (1994) also used network analysis to understand cigarette smoking within and between adolescent friendship cliques in the same sample of

Figure 17-1. **Map of an Adolescent Social Network: Cliques, Liaisons, and Isolates**

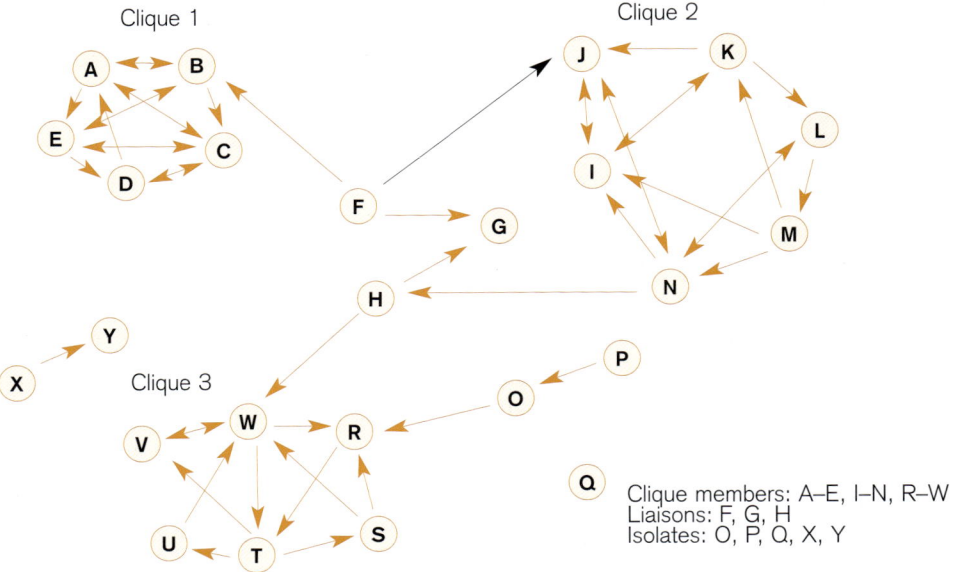

Clique members: A–E, I–N, R–W
Liaisons: F, G, H
Isolates: O, P, Q, X, Y

Source: reproduced with permission from the American Sociological Association and authors. From the *Journal of Health and Social Behavior*, Vol. 34 (September 1993); "Peer Group Structure and Adolescent Cigarette Smoking: A Social Network Analysis" by S.T. Ennett and K.E. Bauman.

ninth graders described above. The authors found intra-clique homogeneity and inter-clique heterogeneity in current cigarette smoking patterns: i.e., smokers tended to belong to cliques in which other members smoked, while nonsmokers tended to be grouped with other nonsmokers. Ennett, Bauman, and Koch highlighted the fact that most cliques (68%) were composed entirely or mostly of nonsmokers (89.9%), suggesting that friendship cliques contribute more to the maintenance of non-smoking than to the onset and maintenance of smoking. They also confirmed, however, that smoking has a greater social significance for girls than boys.

Using data from 10,030 Californian adolescents, Unger and Chen (1999) found that age of smoking initiation was earlier among those whose friends, siblings, and/or parents were smokers, and among those adolescents who had a tobacco advertisement they particularly liked, who had received tobacco promotional items, or who would be willing to use tobacco promotional items. Alexander and colleagues (2001) studied the effect of popularity, best-friend smoking, and cigarette smoking within peer networks on the current smoking patterns of seventh- through 12th-grade students in the United States. Adjusting for age, gender, race/ethnicity, parent education, school, and availability of cigarettes at home, the risk of current smoking was significantly associated with peer networks in which at least half of the members smoked, or one or two best friends smoked, and with increasing rates of school smoking prevalence.

In a literature review of adolescent alcohol use, Monica Gaughan (2003) found that the most important predictor of this behavior is the use pattern of peers. She found significant evidence supporting the fact that adolescents whose peers consume alcohol are more likely to drink than adolescents without friends who drink, and that adolescents with friends who drink heavily are more likely to engage in this type of behavior as well. Thomas Valente (2003) points out in the introductory article for a journal review on social network influences on adolescent substance use: "We find in these results, and other studies, that *social network matters*. Adolescents select friends like themselves, those friends influence their behavior, and they often engage in risky behavior together." The analysis by Gaughan (2003) published in the same journal also demonstrates that adolescent friends not only influence one another to establish and maintain alcohol use patterns over time, but that healthy friends can also create social dynamics that exert protective effects to help reduce the frequency of excessive drinking.

The strong influence of peers on adolescent behavior has led to the increased use of *peer education* in health promotion programs. Other theories have also been identified as supporting the development of peer education: the Social Cognitive Theory (Chapter Sixteen) because of its contribution of using peers to serve as behavioral models, the Theory of Reasoned Action (Chapter Ten) because of the influence exerted by individual perception of social norms or beliefs on behavioral change, the Diffusion of Innovations Theory (Chapter Twenty-three) because of its use of opinion leaders who serve as agents of behavioral change by disseminating information and influencing group norms in their community, and the Theory of Participatory Education (Freire 1970) because of its empowerment component (Joint United Nations Programme on HIV/AIDS 1999b). However, peer education in practice has differed in its definition of *who* constitutes the most appropriate kind of peer and *what type* of education this peer ideally should provide (e.g., counseling, distributing materials, providing support, making referrals to services, facilitating discussions, etc.) (Shoemaker et al. 1998; Flanagan, Williams, and Mahler 1996).

The Social Networks and Social Support Theories provide a natural framework to understand the person-centered *network* of social relationships through which *social support* may be provided. The description of health-enhancing social support characteristics and how social networks and social support may be strengthened (Heany and Israel 2002) are useful contributions that will most likely improve the effectiveness of peer education in the future, especially among adolescents. Unfortunately, much of the evidence of peer education and HIV/AIDS in the last decade, for example, comes from experiences among the adult population (e.g., commercial sex workers, men who have sex with men, factory workers, people living with HIV/AIDS) (Joint United Nations Programme on HIV/AIDS 1999b). On the other hand, however, over the past five years a growing evidence base of peer education effectiveness among youth has been developing.

Albrecht and colleagues (1998) studied the use of *peer support* in smoking cessation programs in the United States for pregnant adolescents (ages 12–20). Participants were randomized to one of the following groups: Teen FreshStart with a buddy program (TFSB), a Teen FreshStart program (TFS) without peer support (a standardized cognitive behavioral group model developed by the American Cancer Society specifically for adolescents), and the usual care control group. The group that received peer support (TFSB) achieved consistently higher smoking cessation rates across all measures when compared to the subjects in the other two groups. Furthermore, peer education programs have been found to offer benefits to adolescent peer leaders by increasing their knowledge, teaching them new skills, encouraging them to assume greater responsibility for their own health, and improving their self-perception as an agent of positive change in their community (Pearlman et al. 2002, Neumark-Sztainer 1999).

However, a few studies have shown contradictory findings regarding the effectiveness of peer education. Kirby et al. (1997) found that although a peer-led interactive HIV/AIDS and pregnancy prevention curriculum significantly increased HIV/AIDS-related and reproductive health-related knowledge, it did not significantly change actual sexual or contraceptive behaviors. A study by Dishion, McCord, and Poulin (1999) found that high-risk youth are particularly vulnerable to peer group interventions when they are grouped together, a situation that can lead to increased occurrences of substance abuse and acts of violence.

Greydanus and colleagues (1990) have described the gang phenomenon as the extreme use of a negative peer group for the purpose of securing self-identification and note that adolescents are more likely to join a gang if their families and communities do not offer them the security, structure, and opportunities that they need. According to Dishion and colleagues (1991), the process of antisocial peer group formation begins at home with problematic parent-child relationships that are coercive and hostile. This is also mentioned in a survey of 938 youth *maras* (gangs) living in El Salvador, where almost half of them described their early family relationships as bad or very bad and reported having witnessed domestic violence against their mothers and/or siblings, and one-third reported being the recipient of physical violence coming from their fathers (Santacruz Giralt and Concha-Eastman 2001). *Mara* members describe their fellow gang members as their family, a reference group from which they receive social support, establish a sense of belonging, exercise mutual loyalty and protection, and share positive affects, freedom from obligations, and the opportunity to "hang out" together.

Moraes and Reichenheim (2002) estimated the prevalence of domestic violence during pregnancy and its principal risk groups among public health care users in Rio de Janeiro, Brazil. The authors found that physical violence mainly occurred among adolescent women with comparatively fewer years of schooling, who did not work outside the home, who had fewer prenatal care visits, and who reported having little social support. Families with proportionately more children under age 5 in the household, who reported alcohol and drug abuse, and who held low socioeconomic status were also more likely to report the presence of domestic violence.

Several studies have reported associations between neighborhood conditions and levels of parent-to-child physical aggression (Limber and Nation 1998). Molnar and colleagues (2003) conducted a multilevel study to understand the association between several neighborhoods' characteristics and parent-to-child aggression. Data used in the analysis came from the Project on Human Development in Chicago Neighborhoods and from cohorts in the 3-, 6-, 9-, 12-, and 15-year-old age groups and their caregivers. In 30% of the households, the primary caregiver was a female single parent. The authors found that concentrated disadvantage (using several poverty-related neighborhood indicators) and community violence (using the 1995 neighborhood murder rate as an indicator) significantly predicted higher use of parent-to-child physical aggression, controlling for sex and age of the child. However, the authors also found that for Hispanic families only, the size of the social network was significantly associated with lower use of physical aggression by caregivers. In this interaction model, the existence of family social support also predicted lower rates of parent-to-child physical aggression.

Familias Unidas (Coatsworth, Pantin, and Szapocznik 2002) is a multilevel, family-centered intervention designed to prevent problem behaviors in Hispanic adolescents. The intervention rests on building a strong parent-support network and then uses that network to increase knowledge and improve practice of culturally relevant parenting skills to reduce behavioral risks frequently found in poor, urban environments. The intervention found that some neighbors may be less inclined to feel it is their role to watch out for the safety of neighborhood adolescents and may even think that this role is an inappropriate one for them. However, in other instances, communities have created formalized opportunities to reach out to high-risk youth via block parties, regular activities at local community centers, the creation of community newsletters, and adult mentoring programs (Neumark-Sztainer 1999).

One successful program, based on developing new social network linkages by matching adolescents with adult mentors, has been the Big Brothers/Big Sisters program (Furano et al. 1993). The program provides mentors to young people between ages 10 and 16 living in single-parent households in the United States. Participants in the intervention group had statistically significant better attitudes toward school and better school attendance, improved relationships with their parents and peers, and less likelihood of antisocial behavior and of initiating drug and alcohol use. The benefits were particularly strong among minority youths. Mentors who believed that their major role was to support the growth and development of their mentees were more successful than mentors who believed that their major role was to change their mentees (Glantz, Rimer, and Lewis 2002). These results have been used to inform the development of successful mentoring guidelines (Jucovy 2001) for broader use in other types of similar health promotion and prevention activities.

There is also increasing evidence of the critical role that social networks and social support play in the school environment. Adolescents who feel part of their school, and who feel cared for by people in this environment, are less likely to use substances, engage in violence, or initiate sexual activity at an early age (McNeely, Nonnemaker, and Blum 2002). The authors analyzed data from the in-school and school administrator surveys of the National Longitudinal Study of Adolescent Health (75,515 students in 127 U.S. schools) to estimate the association between school characteristics and the average level of school connectedness in each school. Positive classroom management climates, participation in extracurricular activities, tolerant disciplinary policies, and small school size were associated positively with higher school connectedness. Laufer and Harel (2003) studied the relative importance of family, peers, and school in predicting youth violence among a nationally representative sample of 8,394 students from grades 6–10 in Israel. The authors found that lack of parental support in the family regarding school, a lack of social integration by peers, and perceptions of frequent acts of violence in school were variables that predict violence.

Primary health care services in the community could play a potentially important role in enhancing social support for adolescents and their families. However, in many countries, adolescents do not use health services as often as they might because they feel that their needs have not been appropriately targeted. Young males in particular are in need of services addressing their particular needs and concerns. Andrew, Patel, and Ramakrishna (2003) surveyed 811 students in India to generate information regarding their health needs. The findings revealed that there is not only an unmet need for sexual and reproductive health information, but also for psychosocial support on issues ranging from violence in schools to poor relationships with caregivers, educational difficulties, and stress-related health symptoms, which are often perceived by adolescents to be of primary importance.

Results from a survey (Pan American Health Organization 2000a) conducted with 10–19-year-old adolescents from nine Caribbean countries (n = 15,695) reveals the perception of this group of poor confidentiality received from health care services providers and others in their community. The least-trusted adults are physicians, followed by teachers, nurses, counselors, and parents. Surprisingly, parents were more trusted than their own peers. Table 17-1. presents the findings of the PAHO study.

Guzmán and colleagues (2003) examined the impact of comfortable communication about sex on intended and actual sexual behavior of 1,039 Latino adolescents ages 11 to 17 living in California. Results showed that these adolescents have a broad communicative network, including friends, dating partners, and extended family members, with whom they talk about sex. Daughters feel more comfortable communicating with their mothers about sex, and sons are more likely to communicate and feel comfortable communicating with their fathers. Regression analysis suggests comfortable sexual communication is predictive of less likelihood of being sexually active, of being older at first intercourse, and of increased intentions to delay intercourse. However, comfortable mother-adolescent sexual discussions, but not father-adolescent communication, were related to abstinence among adolescents. The study also showed that while comfortable communication with nonparental others was related to safer sexual behaviors, comfortable communication with

Table 17-1. **PAHO Survey of Caribbean Adolescents' Perception of Confidentiality**

	TOTAL	FEMALE	MALE	< 12 YEARS	13–15 YEARS	16–18 YEARS
"If I tell the physician something personal, my parents will find out."	**33.2%**	31.3%	36.3%	38.7%	32.1%	26.5%
"If I discuss sex with the teacher, others will find out."	**26.0%**	24.2%	28.9%	26.4%	26.3%	25.1%
"If I tell the peer counselor something personal, others will know."	**21.4%**	20.1%	23.5%	23.6%	21.0%	18.6%
"If I tell a problem to the nurse, others will know."	**20.8%**	19.7%	22.6%	22.5%	19.6%	20.9%
"If I tell the guidance counselor I am having a problem, others will know."	**20.1%**	18.7%	22.2%	23.4%	19.2%	16.7%
"If I tell my parents, the neighborhood will find out."	**14.0%**	12.1%	17.1%	17.0%	13.3%	9.6%

Source: Pan American Health Organization and WHO Collaborating Center on Adolescent Health, University of Minnesota 2000.

dating partners predicted being sexually active and was related to less intention to delay intercourse.

Breidablik and Meland (2001) compared the social networks and health-related behaviors of late adolescent students living at home and outside the home in Norway. The results showed that students living on their own reported more health risk than their at-home counterparts. The difference was higher for adolescents ages 15–17 compared with adolescents over age 18. Differences were found for cigarette smoking, alcohol use, unhealthy diet, and age of sexual debut. Health-risk behavior was most prevalent among students in vocational program curricula living alone. The authors propose that greater efforts be made to create bridges for students leaving home that can transition into the formation of new social networks to support the student in his/her new environment. These recommendations might be applicable to the increasing numbers of rural adolescents migrating to urban areas, as well as those coming from neighboring countries in search of new opportunities.

Table 17-2. presents a breakdown of the number of studies found using the Social Networks and Social Support Theories according to health behaviors.

Most of the research on social networks and social support has been related specifically to parental support (various parenting models will be described in Chapter Eighteen), and much less attention has been focused on identifying, creating, and

Table 17-2. **Most Commonly Researched Adolescent Behaviors Using the Social Networks and Social Support Theories (SNSS)**

ADOLESCENT BEHAVIORS	NUMBER OF ARTICLES USING THE SNSS	NUMBER OF ARTICLES BY KEYWORDS	
Sexual and Reproductive Health	21	Teen Pregnancy	6
		HIV/AIDS	13
		STIs	1
		Condom Use	2
Tobacco, Alcohol, and Drug Use	45	Tobacco	24
		Alcohol	30
		Drugs	15
Physical Activity and Nutrition	19	Obesity	1
		Physical Activity	14
		Nutrition	4
Violence	20		
TOTAL	**105**		

strengthening protective social networks for adolescents and tailoring these to the adolescent's changing development needs and wants and including a gender perspective.

As young people enter into adolescence, they need—and most of them want—increasing amounts of social interaction. They want to spend time with their friends in the neighborhood and other public spaces, enjoy "sleep-overs" at their friends' houses, maintain frequent phone contact when not together, and, if they have access to a computer, interact back and forth through "instant messaging" and other similar modern technologies. Research shows that parental support is critical to the adoption of healthy behaviors, but there coexists a natural tendency toward separation and individuation during this second decade of life. Parents often have difficulties in redefining how best to continue providing support in terms that respect the adolescent's need for exploration and separate identity formation. In this struggle, parents sometimes give up, and others purposefully spend less time with their sons and daughters, relying on their growing independence to help them make the best choices. The peer network becomes crucial at this point. Research shows in this regard that healthy friends can act as protective factors helping adolescents to adopt and maintain healthy behaviors, just as friends exploring risky behaviors can act as risk factors in the adoption of health-compromising behaviors. Parents and other adults in the community can play a pivotal role by offering developmentally appropriate social support to adolescent networks that promotes the adoption of healthy behaviors and acknowledges the members' particular needs and wants.

The number of articles found on social networks and social support within the context of adolescent health is higher than for the other behavioral theories and models discussed thus far in this book, particularly in the area of violence and adolescence (Table 17-3.). Although a few articles analyzed the impact of social networks and community social support on adolescent violent behaviors, most of them provided compelling evidence for the relationship between lack of parental support, violence in the home, and the expression of adolescent violent behaviors.

Parental skill and support is perhaps the single-most important key to the successful transitioning of adolescents through the different stages of physical and emotional development. Yet at times, parents need special guidance in developing effective parenting styles, and there is strong evidence linking the development of protective adolescent health behaviors with what has been described as *authoritative parenting*, which will be discussed at further length in the following chapter. Programs that enhance existing social network linkages both for adolescents and their parents; develop new social network linkages, particularly through the training of natural helpers in parenting styles; and facilitate parental involvement in ongoing community problem identification and problem-solving will also contribute to protect adolescents from adopting health-compromising lifestyles.

Table 17-3. **A Comparison of the Social Networks and Social Support Theories, the Social Cognitive Theory, and the Individual Level Theories and Models for Adolescent Behavioral Change**

Number of Articles on Adolescence and Individual Behavior Change Theories and Models	Total	Sexual and Reproductive Health	Tobacco, Alcohol, and Drug Use	Physical Activity and Nutrition	Violence
Social Networks and Social Support Theories	105	21	45	19	20
Social Cognitive Theory	85	19	48	9	9
Health Belief Model	66	37	18	9	2
Sensation-Seeking Theory	65	6	52	2	5
Transtheoretical Model and Stages of Change	51	9	27	15	0
Self-Regulation Theory	42	4	31	3	4
Theory of Reasoned Action	31	13	14	3	1
Theory of Planned Behavior	29	13	12	4	0
Goal-Setting Theory	23	10	5	8	0

Box 17-2. Summary of the Social Networks and Social Support Theories and Adolescent Lifestyles

- Peer social networks may be characterized by *clique members* (a small group of adolescent peers generally of the same sex and age), *liaisons* (adolescents who interact with two or more adolescents who are members of a clique, but who themselves are not part of the clique), and *isolates* (adolescents who have few or no linkages to others via a social network).

- The odds of being a current smoker are significantly higher for isolates than for clique members and/or liaisons.

- Adolescent smokers tend to belong to cliques in which other members smoke, while non-smoking adolescents tend to belong to cliques with other nonsmokers.

- The risk of current smoking is significantly associated with peer networks in which at least half of the members smoke, or one or two best friends smoke, and with increasing rates of school smoking prevalence.

- Adolescents whose peers consume alcohol are more likely to drink than adolescents without friends who drink. At the same time, adolescents with friends who drink heavily are more likely to engage in this type of behavior, as well.

- Adolescent friends not only influence one another to establish and maintain alcohol use patterns over time, but healthy friends can also create social dynamics that exert protective effects such as reducing the frequency of excessive drinking.

- The strong influence of peers on adolescent behavior has led to the increased use of peer education in health promotion programs. However, in practice, there remain differences in definition of *who* constitutes the most appropriate kind of peer and *what type* of education this peer ideally should provide.

- Among Hispanic families, the size of the social network is significantly associated with lower use of physical aggression by caregivers, and family social support also predicts lower rates of parent-to-child physical aggression.

- Building parent-support networks and then using these networks to increase knowledge and improve practice of culturally relevant parenting skills help to reduce adolescent risks frequently found in poor, urban environments.

- Lack of parental support in the family regarding school, lack of social integration by peers, and perceptions of frequent acts of violence in school are variables that predict violence.

- Adolescents who feel part of their school, and who feel cared for by people in this environment, are less likely to use substances, engage in violent behavior, or initiate sexual activity at an early age.

- Comfortable mother-adolescent sexual discussions, but not father-adolescent communication, are related to abstinence among adolescents.

[Chapter Eighteen]

The Authoritative Parenting Model

Educators Ralph DiClemente, Richard Crosby, and Michelle Kegler include in their 2002 book *Emerging Theories in Health Promotion Practice and Research: Strategies for Improving Public Health* (2002) a chapter dedicated to the link between the Authoritative Parenting Model and adolescent health behavior. This parenting style approach, originally attributed to Diana Baumrind (1978) and refined by Maccoby and Martin (1983), has gained wide acceptance in the field of adolescent health education because of the growing evidence showing inverse relationships between what has been labeled as "authoritative parenting" and the adoption of risky health behaviors among children and adolescents.

Baumrind (1971, 1967) explored the parenting practices that related to children's adjustment. She found that parents whose children were self-reliant, self-controlled, buoyant, and approach-oriented were themselves firm, loving, demanding, and understanding. Parents whose children were disruptive and not willing to comply were firm, punitive, and unaffectionate. Maccoby and Martin (1983) expand this line of thinking by analyzing parenting styles along two dimensions:

- *demandingness*: the extent to which parents demand mature behavior, supervise activities, and discipline transgressions
- *responsiveness*: the extent to which parents are attuned to their children's physical, social, and emotional needs and support their increasing autonomy

Figure 18-1. **A Classification of Parenting Style Approaches**

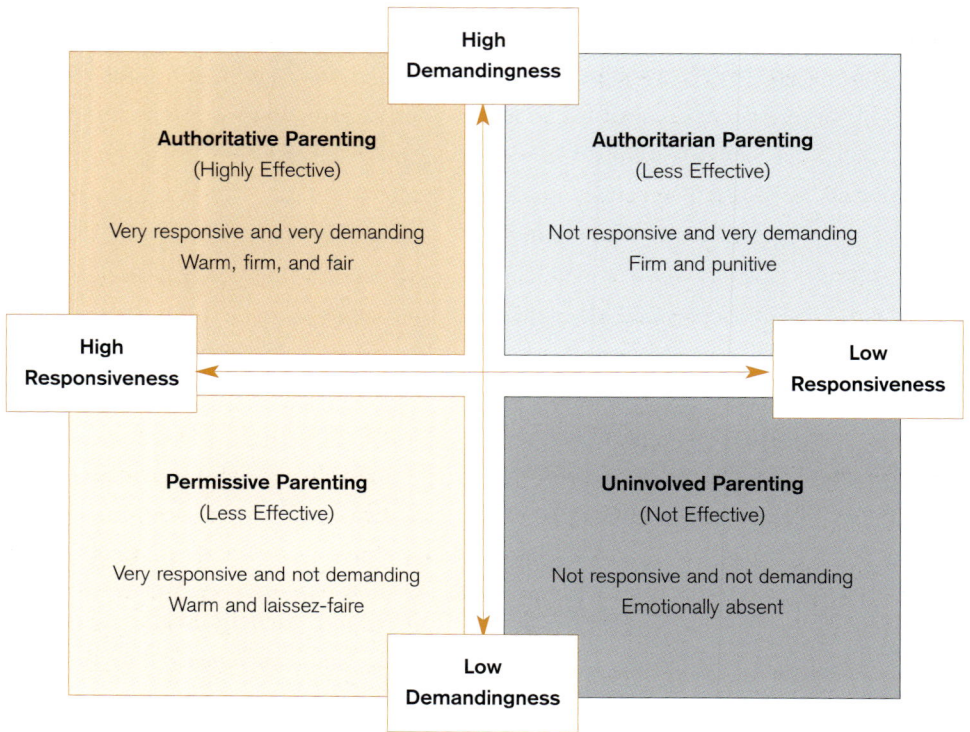

Source: adapted from the *Handbook of Child Psychology, Fourth Edition,* by P. H. Mussen (series editor) and E.E. Maccoby and J.A. Martin (volume authors) © 1983. Reprinted by permission of John Wiley & Sons, Inc.

Figure 18-1. illustrates four different parenting styles. This classification does not consider the presence of abusive parenting, which nonetheless is a frequent reality in today's world. Abusive parenting behavior as a form of discipline is most often seen linked to the authoritarian parenting styles. If emotional, verbal, and/or physical abuse accompanies other manifestations of this style, the approach can result in noneffective and detrimental parenting with long-term consequences for the child (Kim et al. 2001, Champion 1999, Stevenson 1999).

Maccoby and Martin observed that demandingness and responsiveness could be relatively independent of each other. It is possible, for example, for a parent to be very responsive without being very demanding and vice versa. Many studies give support to the description of the four different parenting styles presented in Figure 18-1. by combining these two dimensions.

Maccoby and Martin's model also enables the quantification of parental responsiveness and demandingness. Measures of parental responsiveness seek to quantify how frequently, consistently, and successfully parents attend to their children. Measures of demandingness seek to quantify how frequently, consistently, and concisely parents supervise and monitor their children, set standards for their behavior, and encourage specific, goal-directed behaviors (Simons-Morton and Hartos 2002). Studies show a positive relationship between parental demandingness and adolescent behavioral adjustment, as well as between parental responsiveness and adolescent psychosocial development. The presence of both in balance contributes to the adolescents' positive behavioral adjustment and psychosocial development.

The Components of Authoritative (Effective) Parenting

Authoritative parents are warm, firm, and fair. Although the literature refers to this type of parenting with the original term "authoritative" given by Baumrind and Maccoby and Martin, the authors of this book prefer to use the term "effective parenting," whenever appropriate, in order to avoid confusion with the similar term "authoritarian parenting," which has significantly different manifestations and outcomes. Most researchers agree that *authoritative*, or *effective*, *parenting* is composed of three main components (Steinberg 1999): *warmth*, *structure*, and *autonomy support*. Following is a description of each of these components, with the addition of a fourth, *development support*, which PAHO also considers to be a key aspect of effective parenting.

- *Warmth (responsiveness)* is the degree to which a parent successfully communicates to the adolescent that he/she is loved and accepted. Authoritative or effective parents are *warm* in their relationships with their children. When adolescents have developed an earlier strong attachment to their parents, they are more willing to please them and be more open to their influence. But parents need to be cautious and not take this relationship for granted when conflicts arise during adolescence. Instead, they need to constantly nurture existing positive bonds by spending quality time with their adolescents, sharing in their interests, and participating in activities of mutual enjoyment. Parents should also be empathetic when intense negative emotions arise due to frustrations and disappointments and maintain a permanent *positive emotional climate*, even at times of high environmental stress and parent-child disagreements.

Anger, aggression, rivalry, and competition are healthy emotions that become part of the daily affective experiences of adolescents, which are then expressed to parents in a variety of ways. Very often this process becomes a mechanism through which adolescents attempt to define their individuality and differentiate themselves from parents, siblings, and even peers. These intense negative emotions can sometimes be difficult for parents to tolerate and react to with calm and patience. Yet, as most parents come to realize, ignoring these feelings or pretending that they do not exist will not make them go away and often only increases their intensity or the frequency with which they are expressed. Parents do not really have a choice about whether or not adolescents have these emotions. Yet, if they are counterbalanced with expressions of warmth and empathy by the parent, this reaction can serve as a model to enable children and adolescents to learn more appropriate and healthy ways to express negative feelings.

- *Structure (demandingness)* is the degree to which the adolescent has expectations and rules for his or her behavior. Authoritative or effective parents are *firm* in the limits set for their sons and daughters. Effective parents set standards for the child's conduct but form expectations that are consistent with the child's developing needs and capabilities. The authoritative parents are effective in protecting adolescents from negative influences not only because they set clear limits and enforce consequences when these limits are trespassed, but also because they maintain an even balance between restrictiveness and autonomy by monitoring the adolescent's behaviors and choices and anticipating risky situations. Effective parents also enforce limits by redirecting adolescents' behaviors before they trespass.

In order to increase their autonomy, adolescents frequently attempt to "push" set limits. Authoritative parents recognize that there are *negotiable limits*, which teach responsibility, and *nonnegotiable limits*, which protect young people from harm. Adolescents occasionally will trespass negotiable limits (e.g., agreed time to arrive home) and learn through enforcement of the previously agreed-upon consequences. Authoritative or effective parents monitor closely the early signs of risky situations that could tempt adolescents to trespass nonnegotiable limits (e.g., consume illegal drugs) and anticipate these by redirecting behaviors, offering other alternatives to satisfy the need for exploring those risky behaviors, and increasing communication with their adolescents about the involved risks. Which limits are negotiable and which are not will vary from family to family and will also be influenced by cultural differences.

- *Autonomy support* is the degree to which parents accept and encourage the adolescent's individuality. Authoritative or effective parents are *fair* in exercising their authority. Authoritative parents are more likely than authoritarian parents to give children more independence gradually as they get older, providing adolescents with opportunities to develop self-reliance, but also providing clear standards and limits for behaviors, along with their respective guidelines. Effective parents place a high value on the development of autonomy and self-direction but continue to assume ultimate responsibility for their child's behavior. Authoritative or effective parents increase the amounts of negotiable limits gradually, according to the child's developing needs and capabilities. They also closely monitor the adherence to nonnegotiable limits. Although there is a continuum from childhood to adolescence, authoritative parenting is extremely important during pre- and early adolescence, during which periods parents should still exert control over adolescent behaviors, respond to negotiable and nonnegotiable limits, and otherwise closely supervise the process of assuming increasing autonomy. Parents who don't encourage autonomy (e.g., authoritarian parents) during these crucial periods miss an important opportunity to closely supervise the necessary process of acquiring independence.

Supporting autonomy involves not only granting more permission for adolescents to do things on their own (e.g., go to the movies with friends) but also encouraging adolescents to express their own choices and opinions, even if these sometimes lead to disagreement. Adolescents appear to do best when they grow up in an atmosphere of close family ties that permits the development of individuality (Steinberg 1999).

■ *Development support* is the degree to which parents foster and enhance the adolescent's underlying developmental capacities for emotional and logical thinking. Effective parents are more likely to engage their children in verbal give-and-take, which plays an important part in the development of reasoning abilities, role-taking, emotional thinking, empathy, and moral judgment. In these families, verbal give-and-take is the norm, emphasizing at the same time the importance of maintaining close relationships and considering how actions may affect other family members (Steinberg 1999, Rueter and Conger 1995). Hauser, Powers, and Noam (1991) describe these characteristics as *enabling interactions* and promoters of healthy adolescent development, in contrast to *constraining interactions*, which are judgmental or devaluating of a family member's opinion.

Enabling interactions, or verbal give-and-take, should not only foster reasoning abilities and problem-solving, but also emotional thinking. Parents have a unique opportunity to help pre- and early adolescents recognize their emotions and express them verbally, thereby discouraging the need for them to be "acted out" in more indirect ways. By exercising empathy, parents can guide their adolescents in the discovery of healthier strategies to regulate intense feelings of sadness, fear, envy, jealousy, anger, and even uncontrolled excitement, while at the same time providing the adolescent with a strong role model for individualized empathy development.

By the time young people reach middle adolescence (ages 15–16) their autonomy is growing, while at the same time their developmental capacity to confront and resist peer pressure is tested on a daily basis. Therefore, it is crucial that adolescent health promotion and prevention programs start earlier (preadolescence and early adolescence) and coordinate efforts with programs directed toward younger children to gradually strengthen adolescents' capacities to develop their own healthy choices as they achieve more autonomy.

It is also important to keep in mind that socialization is a two-way process, in the sense that adolescent behavior also affects parental behavior. Some adolescents are less challenging to raise than others, due to different interactive styles (Greenspan 1995). Secondly, parents naturally tend to have different parenting styles, perhaps as a product of their own upbringing, childhood experiences, and social and cultural values. Thus, it is not uncommon to see opposing parenting styles in the same household (e.g., authoritarian and permissive), which results in confusion and the child or adolescent receiving mixed messages. Lastly, parenting styles can also be affected by environmental constraints, such as economic stress and poverty. Studies show that parents under economic strain are less involved, less nurturing, less vigilant, harsher in their treatment, more inclined toward depression, more enmeshed in marital conflict, and less consistent in their disciplinary methods than their more economically stable counterparts (Steinberg 1999, McLoyd 1990). Under these circumstances, adolescents present more anxiety, depression, conduct problems, and diminished school performance (Steinberg 1999; Conger, Patterson, and Ge 1995). Conger et al. (1993) developed the Family Process Model linking economic stress and adolescent adjustment to explain how economic stress and poverty can adversely affect adolescent development and behaviors by affecting parents' emotional tone and parenting skills. Several studies (Kim et al. 2001, Sheeber et al. 2000) support aspects of this model by linking parents' angry, irritable, and/or depressive emotional tone and poor parenting with health-compromising behaviors. The interaction of these factors and how they contribute to unhealthy adolescent behavior is shown in Figure 18-2.

Studies of families living in poverty also provide insight into what parents living in poor neighborhoods can do to help protect their children from the adverse consequences of growing up in poor inner-city or rural areas. In general, families fare better when they have adequate sources of social support (Taylor 1996) and when they have strong ties to religious institutions (Brody, Stoneman, and Flor 1996). In addition, two specific sets of family management strategies employed by parents in poor neighborhoods seem to work: *promotive strategies*, which attempt to strengthen the adolescent's competence through effective child-rearing within the home environment and/or through involving the child in positive activities outside the home; and *restrictive strategies*, which attempt to minimize the child's exposure to dangers in the neighborhood.

Figure 18-2. **The Effects of Economic Strain on Parenting and Adolescent Adjustment**

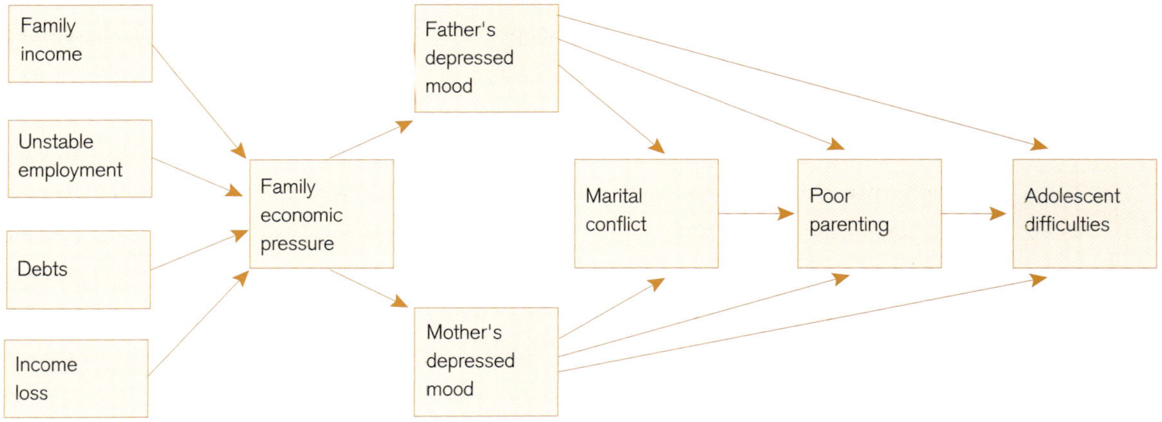

Source: adapted with permission from *Developmental Psychology*, 1993; Conger et al., "Family Economic Stress and Adjustment of Early Adolescent Girls," Vol. 29, pp. 206–219. Copyright © 1993 by the American Psychological Association.

Concentrated poverty has negative effects on the adolescent's transition to adulthood; these effects are above and beyond those attributable to growing up in a poor family. Adolescents growing up in impoverished communities are more likely than their peers from equally poor households—but those nestled within, or closer to, more affluent neighborhoods—to bear children as teenagers and to drop out of high school (Brooks-Gunn et al. 1993). Interestingly, it seems to be the absence of more affluent neighbors, rather than the presence of poor neighbors, that places adolescents in impoverished communities at greatest risk (Ensminger, Lamkin, and Jacobson 1996).

In Latin America and the Caribbean, adolescents are surrounded by economic stress and poverty. In 1997, 32.5 million adolescents between the ages of 13 and 19, or 47% of this age group, were living in poverty (Schutt-Aine and Maddaleno 2003). In Haiti, more than 70% of the population lives below the absolute poverty level. Adolescents who grow up in poor neighborhoods are far more likely than other youth to be exposed to chronic community violence.

Family structure is also changing in many Latin American and Caribbean countries. The percentage of adolescents raised in households headed by women ranges between 21% and 35% (Schutt-Aine and Maddaleno 2003). It is also estimated that 80% of adolescent mothers in urban areas and 70% in rural areas belong to the poorest 50% of Latin American and Caribbean households (Comisión Económica para América Latina y el Caribe 1997). Many adolescent mothers raise their children while living in households headed by their mothers (United Nations Children's Fund 1998). A recently published Swedish research study found increased risks of psychiatric disease, suicide or suicide attempt, injury, and substance addiction in children in single-parent households, compared with those in two-parent households (Ringbäck Weitoff et al. 2003). A recent study in nine English-speaking Caribbean countries indicates that 24% of youth feel that their mother "understands little about their problems," and 32% of adolescents feel the same lack of understanding from their fathers (Pan American Health Organization 2000a). Adolescent boys from nine countries in the Region of the Americas indicate that sexual information received from parents is often provided too late and is laden with myths and taboos (Aguirre and Güell 2002).

Research and Evidence of Practical Applications of the Authoritative Parenting Model to Adolescent Lifestyles

Substantial research supports the relationship between the authoritative or effective parenting style and the adoption of health-promoting lifestyles. Authoritative parenting has been positively associated with self-control, conflict resolution, and peer resistance in ethnically diverse samples of adolescents from fourth to 10th grades (Carlson, Uppal, and Prosser 2000; Jackson, Henriksen, and Fosheen 1998). Authoritative parenting is associated inversely with tobacco, alcohol, and drug use in adolescents, in contrast to authoritarian, uninvolved, and permissive parenting styles, which have been positively related to these adolescent behaviors (Pierce et al. 2002, Simons-Morton and Hartos 2002).

Pierce and colleagues (2002) decided to further test this evidence, examining whether tobacco industry marketing practices towards young people undermine the protective effect of recommended authoritative parenting against adolescent smoking in a representative sample of 1,641 U.S. adolescents aged 12 to 14 years living in California. The study measured the level of receptivity to tobacco industry advertising and promotion among these adolescents. Those who named a brand but did not have a favorite cigarette advertisement were considered as having a low level of receptivity. A high level of receptivity required the adolescent to be willing to use an item with a brand image or to have obtained the product. Although the study results confirmed that adolescents in families with more authoritatively inclined parents were half as likely to smoke by follow-up (between 1996 and 1999) as adolescents in families with less authoritative parents (20% vs. 41%, $p < .0001$), the promotion of smoking by the tobacco industry was found to undermine these effects among adolescents who were highly receptive to tobacco industry advertising and promotions. In families with more authoritative parents, these adolescents were 3 times more likely to smoke compared to those who were minimally receptive. The average California retail outlet has 17 tobacco ads, with half of these placed at the eye level of young children (3 feet high or lower), and a quarter of all retail outlets offer cigarette products right next to candy displays (Pierce et al. 2002, Feighery et al. 2001). This evidence highlights the key role that authoritative parents can have in helping pre- and early adolescents, who are highly receptive to tobacco industry advertising and promotions, to develop media literacy skills so they may become more resilient to those marketing strategies.

The single most studied component of the Authoritative Parenting Model is parental monitoring. Low parental monitoring has been directly related to increased risk behaviors (Borawski et al. 2003; Stanton et al. 2002; DiClemente et al. 2001; Raboteg-Saric, Rijavec, and Brajsa-Zganec 2001; Griffin et al. 2000b). These behaviors include cigarette smoking and alcohol consumption (Raboteg-Saric, Rijavec, and Brajsa-Zganec 2001; Baker et al. 1999; Jackson, Henrikson, and Dickenson 1999), substance use (Stanton et al. 2002, DiClemente et al. 2001), sexual involvement and intercourse (Borawski et al. 2003, Henderson et al. 2002, Stanton et al. 2002), unsafe sexual practices (Huebner and Howell 2003, Short et al. 2003, DiClemente et al. 2001), teen pregnancy (Crosby et al. 2002; Unger, Molina, and Teran 2000), sexually transmitted infections (Crosby et al. 2003; DiClemente, Crosby, and Wingood 2002; Crosby et al. 2001), and violent and delinquent behaviors (DiClemente et al. 2001, Pettit et al. 2001, Stattin 2001, Griffin et al. 2000b).

These studies unanimously support the value of involved parents and stress the important role that effective parental monitoring and parenting styles serve as a protective factor to promote the adoption of healthy lifestyles and prevent risky behaviors among adolescents.

Of the above studies, of particular note is the research by Borawski and colleagues (2003). The authors recognize that often the role of parental practices in preventing health risk-taking behaviors in adolescence is examined in a limited manner that focuses solely on the dimension of parental monitoring. The Borawski et al. study introduces a developmental analysis by suggesting that parents need to adjust their supervisory practices as adolescents mature and require more independence for their own decision-making. Based on this evidence, the authors compare in their study two different parenting practices, parental monitoring and negotiated unsupervised time, and ascertain perceived parental trust in the reporting of health risk behaviors among 692 adolescents from six urban high schools (mean age 15.7 years) in the Midwestern United States. The results confirmed that higher levels of parental monitoring are significantly associated with less sexual activity, lower intentions to have sex in the future, and lower rates of alcohol, tobacco, and marijuana use, as well as higher rates of consistent condom use. Although reports of higher levels of negotiated unsupervised time were significantly associated with more sexual activity and alcohol, tobacco, and marijuana consumption, this second parenting style was also associated with the health-promoting behaviors of carrying condoms for protection and choosing not to have sex when condoms were not available.

Another striking finding of this study was that students who reported having more unsupervised time were no more likely to initiate sex early, intend to have sex, engage in unprotected sex, or report having sexually transmitted infections (STI) than those reporting permission for fewer unsupervised opportunities. Furthermore, reports of higher perceived parental trust were associated with lower prevalence of sexual activity, intentions to have sex, and reports of STI; higher rates of consistent condom use; and lower use of tobacco, alcohol, and marijuana. Thus, as the authors of this study suggest, there appears to be more to effective parenting than merely knowing the adolescent's whereabouts in order to promote the adoption of healthy behaviors and the prevention of health-compromising ones. Kerr, Stattin, and Trost (1999) found that parental knowledge of adolescent daily activities that came from the latter's own spontaneous disclosure was most closely linked to parental trust. Based on these findings, the authors propose a reinterpretation of parental monitoring as one that emanates from parental knowledge based principally on the adolescent's spontaneous disclosure rather than parental questioning of their adolescents regarding where they will be and with whom. Effective parental practices, then, will need to adjust and evolve to acknowledge and accommodate the numerous changes and emerging needs that characterize the adolescent's passage from one developmental stage to the next.

Authoritative or effective parenting—in contrast to authoritarian, permissive, and uninvolved parenting—has also been inversely related to anger, alienation, aggression, psychological distress, delinquency, and school misconduct in adolescents. The role of different parenting practices predicting later antisocial behaviors and violence, including dating violence, among adolescents has been widely studied (Chapple 2003; Conger et al. 2003; Howard, Qui, and Boekeloo 2003; Lavoie et al. 2002; Scaramella et al. 2002; Orpinas et al. 1999). Lavoie and colleagues (2002) followed up 717 Canadian boys living in low income families, beginning at age 10 through age 18, and found a direct relationship between harsh parenting styles (insulting, rejecting, constant quarreling, and/or hitting), antisocial behavior, and later dating violence. Scaramella and colleagues (2002) also found that a lack of nurturing and involved parenting indirectly predicted delinquency, and the adolescent's antisocial behavior over time predicted similar decreases in nurturing parenting. Conger and colleagues (2003) examined intergenerational continuities in both angry, aggressive parenting and also the angry, aggressive behavior of children and adolescents among three generations: 22-year-old young parents (G2), their mothers (G1), and the children of G2 (G3). The authors found in this prospective, longitudinal study a direct connection between observed G1 aggressive parenting and observed G2 aggressive parenting from 5 to 7 years later.

Adolescent attitudes towards violence are strongly associated with witnessing inter-parental violence, as well as with lower parental attachment, and this association appears to intensify with the simultaneous presence and interaction of these two factors. Furthermore, dating violence is significantly associated with having witnessed inter-parental violence, high dating frequency, and low parental monitoring (Chapple 2003). Champion (1999) had also previously found, in a study conducted among rural Mexican-American adolescents in the southwestern United States, that histories of family violence are predictors of adolescent acceptance of interpersonal violence within intimate relationships.

The perception of parents' attitudes toward fighting has been also identified as the strongest predictor of aggression in a study conducted among 8,865 12–15-year-old ethnically diverse U.S. adolescents living in Texas. The study found an inverse relationship between aggression scores, fighting, injuries due to fighting, and weapon-carrying and the following family variables: parental monitoring, positive relationship with parents, and the lack of parental support for fighting (Orpinas et al. 1999). In another study, Simons-Morton and Hartos (2002) similarly found that weapon-carrying and interpersonal violence among middle adolescents were inversely correlated to effective parenting and positively associated with permissive, authoritarian, and uninvolved parenting.

The role of parenting practices in promoting the adoption and maintenance of physical activity and healthy nutrition among adolescents has been less studied than other typical adolescent risk-behavior concerns. Schmitz and colleagues (2002) conducted a study to examine associations between demographic and psychosocial factors and self-reported physical activity and sedentary leisure habits among 3,798 U.S. adolescents ages 11–15 (mean 12.8 years). One of the important findings was that girls who reported that their mothers had an authoritative parenting style also reported higher physical activity and lower sedentary leisure habits. Kremers and colleagues (2003) found in another study that fruit consumption and fruit-specific knowledge were higher among adolescents (mean age 16.5) who were being raised with an authoritative parenting style. Adolescents raised by permissive parents consumed more fruit than adolescents from authoritarian or neglectful homes. Mellin and colleagues (2002) found that overweight teenagers who reported having a close relationship with their parents (feelings of being understood, sharing activities and problems) were more likely to be involved in healthy behaviors. They also found that extremes in parental monitoring (high and low) were associated with lower breakfast consumption among boys and higher rates of extreme dieting behaviors among girls.

Simons-Morton and Hartos (2002) propose adoption of the Authoritative Parenting Model, as described earlier in this chapter, to guide the design of health promotion programs seeking to improve parenting and adolescent health. The model recommends specifying adolescent outcomes of interest and defining aspects of an authoritative parenting style and the practices that will affect adolescent outcomes, and then planning interventions based on these findings. Currently, the authors are conducting a Young Drivers Intervention Study, which seeks to improve teen driving through the application of this Authoritative Parenting Model.

Foxcroft et al. (2001) consider "Strengthening Families," discussed in Chapter Seven, to be one of the most effective U.S. alcohol and drug prevention programs developed to date for adolescents. It also has demonstrated effectiveness in violence prevention. The theoretical framework that helped to design the program's interventions included the Family Process Model (Conger et al. 1993), which describes the relationship between economic stress and adolescent adjustment and is described earlier in this chapter, and concepts from the Resiliency Theory, which will be discussed in Chapter Nineteen.

The acquisition of effective parenting skills is not formally taught at any point or place in life. Yet there is a growing body of evidence regarding parenting best practices and the positive effects these practices can have on adolescent behaviors and lifestyle choices. The Authoritative Parenting Model has been presented in this chapter with the hope that professionals involved in the design and implementation of health promotion and prevention programs for adolescents will seek to actively involve parents as part of a multicomponent health promotion and prevention program that can impart to parents the knowledge and skills necessary to become more effective parents whose attitude and approach to raising adolescents increase the likelihood that their sons and daughters will adopt and maintain healthy lifestyles.

In many communities throughout the world, parents—as we saw earlier in this chapter—are additionally burdened with the tremendous economic strain of poverty and the accompanying emotional stress this situation brings into the family nucleus. Economic stress indirectly influences adolescents through disruptions in parental mood and behavior and its tendency to exacerbate existing problems in marital interactions (Conger et al. 1993), which in turn decrease the likelihood of exercising authoritative or effective parenting practices and increase the chance of adopting more permissive or authoritarian parenting styles. It is crucial that health promotion and prevention programs for adolescents which include a parenting component take into account the economic stress in which the particular family at hand might be immersed. These programs would need to include interventions directed toward helping parents develop or regain authoritative or effective parenting practices, particularly the necessary balance between nurturance and demandingness, and to consciously distance themselves from less effective parenting styles (uninvolved, permissive, authoritarian, even harsh and abusive) when confronted with stress.

Table 18-1. presents a breakdown of the number of studies found using the Authoritative Parenting Model according to health behaviors.

It is important to note, however, that fully two-thirds (i.e., 53 out of 80) of these published research articles focus primarily on the effect of only one component of the Authoritative Parenting Model, that of parental monitoring (or demandingness), as illustrated in Table 18-2.

The significant number of articles found reviewing parenting styles and their impact on adolescent health behaviors also reveals that this area is of great interest to researchers. Along with the Social Networks and Social Support Theories (Chapter Seventeen) and the Social Cognitive Theory (Chapter Sixteen), the Authoritative Parenting Model is among the most studied of all theoretical framework components. The area of parenting and its influence on the development of violent adolescent behaviors appears to elicit the most interest of all in the social sciences research community, as the table further indicates.

Table 18-1. **Most Commonly Researched Adolescent Behaviors Using the Authoritative Parenting Model (APM)**

ADOLESCENT BEHAVIORS	NUMBER OF ARTICLES USING THE APM	NUMBER OF ARTICLES BY KEYWORDS	
Sexual and Reproductive Health	19	Teen Pregnancy	3
		HIV/AIDS	2
		STIs	1
		Condom Use	5
Tobacco, Alcohol, and Drug Use	29	Tobacco	15
		Alcohol	20
		Drugs	10
Physical Activity and Nutrition	3	Obesity	1
		Physical Activity	1
		Nutrition	1
Violence	29		
TOTAL	**80**		

Table 18-2. **A Comparison of the Authoritative Parenting Model (APM) and Parental Monitoring for Adolescent Behavioral Change**

ADOLESCENT BEHAVIORS	NUMBER OF ARTICLES USING THE APM	NUMBER OF ARTICLES FOCUSING ON PARENTAL MONITORING ONLY
Sexual and Reproductive Health	7	22
Tobacco, Alcohol, and Drug Use	1	18
Physical Activity and Nutrition	2	1
Violence	17	12
TOTAL	**27**	**53**

Table 18-3. **A Comparison of the Authoritative Parenting Model, the Social Network and Social Support Theories, the Social Cognitive Theory, and the Individual Level Theories for Adolescent Behavioral Change**

Number of Articles on Adolescence and Individual Behavior Change Theories and Models	Total	Sexual and Reproductive Health	Tobacco, Alcohol, and Drug Use	Physical Activity and Nutrition	Violence
Authoritative Parenting Model	**80**	19	29	3	29
Social Networks and Social Support Theories	**105**	21	45	19	20
Social Cognitive Theory	**85**	19	48	9	9
Health Belief Model	**66**	37	18	9	2
Sensation-Seeking Theory	**65**	6	52	2	5
Transtheoretical Model and Stages of Change	**51**	9	27	15	0
Self-Regulation Theory	**42**	4	31	3	4
Theory of Reasoned Action	**31**	13	14	3	1
Theory of Planned Behavior	**29**	13	12	4	0
Goal-Setting Theory	**23**	10	5	8	0

Box 18-1. Summary of the Authoritative Parenting Model and Adolescent Lifestyles

- Authoritative parenting is associated inversely with tobacco, alcohol, and drug use in adolescents, in contrast to authoritarian, uninvolved, and permissive parenting styles, which have been positively related to these adolescent behaviors.
- Low parental monitoring has been directly related to increased adolescent risk behavior including cigarette, alcohol, and substance use; sexual involvement and intercourse; unsafe sex practices; teen pregnancy; sexually transmitted infections; and violent and delinquent behaviors.
- Although higher reports of negotiated unsupervised time are significantly associated with more sexual activity and alcohol, tobacco, and marijuana consumption, this parenting style is also associated with the health-promoting behaviors of carrying condoms for protection and choosing not to have sex when condoms are not available.
- Adolescents who report greater unsupervised time are no more likely to initiate sex early, intend to have sex, engage in unprotected sex, or report having sexually transmitted infections than those reporting permission for fewer unsupervised opportunities.
- Reports by adolescents of higher perceived parental trust are associated with a lower prevalence of sexual activity and intentions to have sex, fewer reports of sexually transmitted infections, higher rates of consistent condom use, and lower use of tobacco, alcohol, and marijuana.
- Parental practices, in order to be optimally effective, will need to adjust and evolve as adolescents transition from one developmental stage into the next, as parents acknowledge and accommodate the numerous changes and emerging needs that characterize this passage and natural growth process.
- There is a direct relationship between harsh parenting (insulting, rejecting, constant quarreling, and/or hitting) and antisocial behavior, including dating violence.
- Lack of nurturing and involved parenting indirectly predicts delinquency, and the adolescent's antisocial behavior over time predicts similar decreases in nurturing parenting.
- Adolescent attitudes towards violence are strongly associated with witnessing interparental violence, as well as to lower parental attachment, and this association appears to intensify with the simultaneous presence and interaction of these two factors.
- The perception of parents' attitudes toward fighting has also been identified as a strong predictor of aggression among adolescents.
- Weapon-carrying and interpersonal violence among middle adolescents have been inversely correlated to effective parenting and positively associated with permissive, authoritarian, and uninvolved parenting.
- Girls who report that their mothers have an authoritative parenting style also report higher physical activity and lower sedentary leisure habits.
- Fruit consumption and fruit-specific knowledge are higher among adolescents who are being raised with an authoritative parenting style.
- It is crucial that health promotion and prevention programs for adolescents which include a parenting component take into account the economic stress in which the targeted families might be immersed. Such programs would need to include interventions directed toward helping parents develop or regain authoritative or effective parenting practices, particularly the necessary balance between nurturance and demandingness, and to consciously distance themselves from less effective parenting styles (uninvolved, permissive, authoritarian, even harsh and abusive) when confronted with stress.

[Chapter Nineteen]

The Resiliency Theory

The Resiliency Theory seeks to understand how children, adolescents, and adults thrive despite adverse conditions such as extreme poverty, parental mental illness, abuse, and/or catastrophic events (Infante 2001). Much of resilience research focuses on the personality traits, coping skills, and support systems that help individuals endure, survive, and even thrive in challenging environments.

For more than two decades, a number of educational researchers have been probing the issues surrounding youth and resiliency. One of the most influential works is a classic study conducted by Werner and Smith (1992). Over a 32-year period, they studied 505 at-risk children born in Hawaii under adverse circumstances, including chronic poverty. By the time the study participants reached their mid-30s, almost all had become constructively motivated and responsible adults. Only a small percentage of the original group did not effectively "bounce back" from their adverse conditions. A distinguishing factor shared by each resilient child was a long-term, close relationship with a caring, responsible parent or other adult.

The International Resilience Project defines resilience as a universal capacity, which allows a person, group, or community to prevent, minimize, and overcome the damaging affects of adversity (Grothberg 1995). The Project, sponsored by the Civitan International Research Center at the University of Alabama, was developed to examine resilience-promoting behavior in many nations around the world. Its scope of work includes gaining a better understanding of the specific actions taken by parents or other caregivers and children themselves that seem to promote resilience, with a focus on children up to age 12, as well as how the promotion of resilience may vary according to the child's age and gender, and what are the cultural and ethnic similarities and differences in the promotion of resilience in children. The Project's Advisory Committee is supported by an international community which includes the United Nations Educational, Scientific, and Cultural Organization; Pan American Health Organization; World Health Organization; International Children's Center; International Catholic Child Bureau; and Bernard van Leer Foundation.

Resiliency theory proposes that although resilience is an emergent capacity present to some degree in most people, its full development depends on the presence of protective factors during childhood. According to Stanley Greenspan in his book *The Growth of the Mind and the Endangered Origins of Intelligence*, the mind's most important faculties are rooted in emotional experiences from very early in life, where affect, behavior, and thought must be seen as inextricable components of intelligence (Greenspan 1997a). Specific protective factors have been identified repeatedly by different studies of resilient children. These protective factors seem to fall into three general categories: qualities of the child, characteristics of the family, and support from outside the family involving relationships with friends and other members of the community (teachers, mentors, family social network). Grothberg (1995) describes three sources of resilience, labeled as: "I Have," "I Am," and "I Can." The "I Have" source refers to children having parents and other caregivers who promote resilience through their words, actions, and the supportive environment they provide. The "I Am" source refers to the inner qualities of the child (e.g., likeable, pleasing, witty, optimistic, respectful). The "I Can" source refers to skills or behavioral capabilities that help the child overcome adversity (e.g., verbalizing emotions, solving problems, self-control, asking for help). Grothberg underscores that resilience results from a combination of these three sources. Combining Greenspan's and Grothberg's postulates, children who *have* parents and other caregivers who help them to process *early emotional experiences* and promote their *intelligence* so they *can* later integrate *affect*, *behavior*, and *thought* to overcome future adverse emotional experiences with their *inner personal qualities* develop resiliency.

In her literature review, Infante proposes that resilience is not only a personal trait but rather a *process* of positive adaptation despite adversity, which requires the participation of a variety of actors in order to be optimally achieved. This process occurs as a result of the characteristics and dynamic transactions among the individual, the family, the community, and the culture. Greenspan, like Infante, also considers that resiliency is not an attribute of the child alone but a product of the relationships the child has with his or her caregivers and how well these relationships can mesh with the child's unique developmental profile. He argues that merely looking at poverty and children who survive these precarious conditions, or looking at disruptive families and children who survive in those settings, fails to reveal the true essence of resiliency. "This," he writes, "comes only from a closer understanding of the nature of the particular relationships children have in these different settings" (Greenspan 2002). Infante includes among these not only the child-caregiver relationships, but also the ongoing interactions with neighbors, the community, and surrounding culture. She proposes that the most effective strategies will be those that foster resilience at different levels: political, institutional, community, family, and individual (Infante 2001). Chapter Four of this book reviews these multiple levels of influence and their impact on health-related behaviors and conditions.

Greenspan also proposes that true resilience means much more than succeeding in family life, academically, or career-wise in the face of adversity. He argues that positive adaptation includes the ability to enter fully into life's opportunities and meet its challenges without compromising any essential aspects of our humanity, particularly the capacity to empathize and experience intimate, warm relationships with a partner and/or children. He considers that an individual is fully resilient when he or she is able to retain a full range of feelings and abilities in the midst of hardship. "Genuine resilience allows a person to grow and use the sorrows or frustrations to become a fuller, deeper, and more humane person in the future" (Greenspan 2002).

Research and Evidence of Practical Applications of the Resiliency Theory to Adolescent Lifestyles

Between September 1993 and August 1996, the International Resilience Research Project collected data from parents and children up to age 12, including a group of preadolescents 9–12 years old, from 27 sites in 22 countries around the world. The data analysis indicated that about one-third of the parents studied are promoting the development of resilience in their preadolescents. An unexpected finding was that socioeconomic status did not have a significant impact on parental efforts to promote resilience. Resilience was promoted with equal frequency among preadolescents living in lower income families as in those living in higher income families. The only difference was that parents of preadolescents from higher income families provided a greater number of protective factors, a finding that is consistent with results from a developmental assets study conducted by the Search Institute, which will be described in the next paragraph. The International Resilience Research Project also found that resilience was promoted in preadolescents who were considered less intelligent or even intellectually impaired, particularly when their parents helped them to learn how to reach out for help when faced with difficulties or when in need of help (International Resilience Research Project 2004).

The Search Institute is an independent nonprofit organization based in Minneapolis, Minnesota, whose mission is to provide leadership, knowledge, and resources to promote healthy children, adolescents, and communities. Guided by the Resiliency Theory, it has surveyed over 2,000,000 young people in Canada and the United States since 1989 and has identified the presence of a series of powerful developmental assets that positively affect adolescent behavior by protecting young people from harmful and unhealthy behaviors, on the one hand, and by promoting positive attitudes and behaviors on the other. To illustrate the power of these assets, the Institute surveyed 217,277 sixth-to-twelfth-grade adolescents in 33 states and 318 communities across the United States during the 1999–2000 school year. The results showed that youth with the most assets were least likely to engage in four different patterns of high-risk behavior: problematic alcohol use, illicit drug use, sexual activity, and violence. A similar impact was noted with other problem behaviors, including tobacco use, depression and attempted suicide, antisocial behavior, school problems, driving and alcohol, and gambling (Search Institute 2004). Table 19-1. illustrates the inverse correlation between the number of assets possessed by students and the likelihood of their participation in high-risk behaviors.

In this same study, it was found that in addition to protecting youth from negative behaviors, having more assets increases the chances that young people will have positive attitudes and behaviors. A positive correlation between the number of assets and success in school, good health, and ability to delay gratification was also found. The need to develop and nurture these assets during the critical adolescent years clearly suggests a number of important roles families, schools, congregations, neighborhoods, youth organizations, and others in the community may play in shaping young people's lives.

Table 19-1. **The Relationship between Assets and High-Risk Behaviors**

	0–10 Assets	11–20 Assets	21–30 Assets	31–40 Assets
Alcohol Use	49%	27%	11%	3%
Illicit Drug Use	39%	18%	6%	1%
Tobacco	31%	14%	4%	1%
Driving and Alcohol	35%	19%	9%	3%
Sexual Intercourse	32%	21%	11%	3%
Violence	61%	38%	19%	7%
Depression/Suicide	42%	27%	14%	5%

Source: reprinted with permission from *The Asset Approach: 40 Elements of Healthy Development* (Minneapolis, MN: Search Institute). Copyright © Search Institute, 2002. www.search-institute.org. All rights reserved.

Based on the results of a decade of developmental research, the Search Institute formulated the Developmental Assets Framework (Scales and Leffert 1999). This framework identifies 40 critical factors for young people's growth and development, which are divided into 20 external assets and 20 internal assets.[1]

The *external assets* focus on positive experiences that young people receive from people and institutions in their lives. Four categories of external assets are included in the framework:

- *support* (six assets): includes family support and love, positive family communication, three or more nonparental adult relationships, a caring neighborhood, a caring school climate, and parental involvement in schooling.
- *empowerment* (four assets): includes the young person's perception that adults in the community value youth; provide them with useful roles to play in the community; make adolescents feel safe at home, at school, and in the neighborhood; and encourage youth to participate in community service initiatives for one or more hours per week.
- *boundaries and expectations* (six assets): includes family, school, and neighborhood rules, monitoring, and consequences (three assets); parental and other adult role models for positive, responsible behavior; positive peer influence from best friends; and high expectations from parents and teachers to do well.
- *constructive use of time* (four assets): includes spending three or more hours per week on lessons or practice in music, theater, and/or other creative activities; an equal number of hours participating in sports, clubs, school, or community organizations; one or more hours per week in activities in a religious institution; and two or fewer nights per week "hanging out" with friends with no set plans.

The Developmental Assets Framework considers that a community's responsibility towards its adolescents does not end with the provision of external assets, but rather emphasizes the need for a similar commitment to nurturing internal qualities that guide choices and create a sense of centeredness, purpose, and focus. Four categories of *internal assets* are included in the framework:

- *commitment to learning* (five assets): includes the motivation to achieve, active school engagement, doing at least one hour of homework every school day, caring about one's school, and reading for pleasure three or more hours per week.
- *positive values* (six assets): includes placing high value on caring about and helping others and on promoting equal-

---

[1] Framework category descriptions adapted by Cecilia Breinbauer and Matilde Maddaleno with permission from the Search Institute, Minneapolis, Minnesota. The original list of Developmental Asset™ categories may be found at www.search-institute.org. Copyright © Search Institute, 2002. All rights reserved.

ity and reducing hunger and poverty (two assets), choosing to be honest and tell the truth even when circumstances make this more difficult, acting on convictions and standing up for one's beliefs, accepting and taking personal responsibility for actions, and restraining oneself from becoming sexually active and using alcohol or other drugs.

- *social competencies* (five assets): includes abilities for planning ahead and making decisions; empathy, sensitivity, and friendship skills; solving conflicts nonviolently; resisting negative peer pressure and dangerous situations; and having knowledge of and feeling comfortable around people of different cultural, racial, and ethnic backgrounds.
- *positive identity* (four assets): includes feelings of being in control over things that happen, and possessing high self-esteem, a sense of purpose in life, and an optimistic view regarding one's personal future.

The Search Institute suggests that while there is no "magic number" of assets young people should possess, the data indicate that achieving 31 out of 40 "is a worthy, though challenging, benchmark for experiencing their positive effects most strongly." Yet, according to the 1999–2000 study, only 9% of U.S. youth experienced this level of assets, and more than half have 20 or fewer assets, as seen in Table 19-2.

These statistics, as well as the role assets play in predicting both positive and nega-

Table 19-2. **Number of Assets among 217,277 Sixth-to-Twelfth-Grade Youth in 318 U.S. Communities during the 1999–2000 School Year**

	Total Sample (%)
0–10 Assets	15
11–20 Assets	41
21–30 Assets	35
31–40 Assets	9

Source: reprinted with permission from *The Asset Approach: 40 Elements of Healthy Development* (Minneapolis, MN: Search Institute). Copyright © Search Institute, 2002. www.search-institute.org. All rights reserved.

tive outcomes for youth, underscore the importance of the Developmental Assets Framework and the application of its principles in families, schools, and other key community settings for the purpose of "asset-building," the Search Institute's term for purposefully helping youth acquire more assets in their daily lives.

The powerful and positive influence of asset-building has been demonstrated across cultural and socioeconomic groups of youth. A number of promising programs have helped Mexican adolescent immigrants living in the United States to increase their resiliency (Chavkin and González 2000). One example is the Advancement via Individual Determination (AVID) in San Diego, California, which placed students from low-income, ethnic, and linguistic minority backgrounds in college preparation classes along with high-achieving peers. The project resulted in higher college enrollment compared with the school district and national averages (Mehan, Villanueva, and Lintz 1996). In Houston, Texas, Project GRAD (Graduation Really Achieves Dreams) has resulted in higher attendance rates, reductions in teenage pregnancies, fewer disciplinary problems, and better test scores (McAdoo 1998). Zimmerman et al. (2002), using the Resiliency Theory framework, explored the presence and role of natural mentors in the lives of 770 U.S. adolescents. Fifty-two percent reported having a natural mentor. Those with natural mentors were less likely to smoke marijuana or be involved in nonviolent delinquency and had more positive attitudes toward school.

Stronski and colleagues (2000), utilizing the Resiliency Theory, identified protective factors that discouraged Swiss adolescents from progressing from marijuana use to that of other illicit drugs. The statistically significant factors included communicating well with parents, academic achievement, being able to confide in a family member, and regular participation in a sports facility. In the United States, Resnick et al. (1997) had previously found among 12,118 middle and late adolescents that parent-family connectedness and perceived school connectedness were protective measures against every health risk behavior except teen pregnancy.

"Conceptually, the work on resilience suggests that we need to move positive goals front and center," observes Ann S. Masten, Director of the University of Minnesota's Institute of Child Development. "Promoting healthy development and competence is as important, if not more important, than preventing problems, and will serve the same end. As a society, we will do well to nurture human capital—to invest in the competence of our children. This means understanding how the capacity for academic achievement, rule-abiding behavior, and good citizenship develops. It is important to identify risks and prevent them whenever possible, but it is also important to identify assets and protective systems, and support these to the best of our knowledge" (Masten 2000).

Table 19-3. summarizes the number of studies found using the Resiliency Theory according to health behaviors.

Table 19-3. **Most Commonly Researched Adolescent Behaviors Using the Resiliency Theory (RT)**

ADOLESCENT BEHAVIORS	NUMBER OF ARTICLES USING THE RT	NUMBER OF ARTICLES BY KEYWORDS	
Sexual and Reproductive Health	8	Teen Pregnancy	5
		HIV/AIDS	4
		STIs	0
		Condom Use	4
Tobacco, Alcohol, and Drug Use	29	Tobacco	13
		Alcohol	13
		Drugs	17
Physical Activity and Nutrition	0	Obesity	0
		Physical Activity	0
		Nutrition	0
Violence	16		
TOTAL	53		

Box 19-1. **Summary of the Resiliency Theory and Adolescent Lifestyles**

- International analysis indicates that approximately one-third of parents promote resilience in their preadolescent children.
- Socioeconomic status does not appear to have a significant impact on the promotion of resilience among preadolescents. Instead, it is promoted with the same frequency in lower income families as in those with higher income levels.
- However, parents of preadolescents from higher income families provide a greater number of protective factors.
- The Search Institute has identified the presence of a series of powerful developmental assets (40) that positively affect adolescent behavior by protecting young people from harmful and unhealthy behaviors, on the one hand, and by promoting positive attitudes and behaviors on the other.
- Youth with the most assets are least likely to engage in four different patterns of high-risk behavior: problematic alcohol use, illicit drug use, sexual activity, and violence.
- Having more assets increases the chances that young people will have positive attitudes and behaviors.
- External developmental assets (20) are divided into four main categories:
  - support
  - empowerment
  - boundaries and expectations
  - constructive use of time
- Internal developmental assets (20) are divided into four main categories as well:
  - commitment to learning
  - positive values
  - social competencies
  - positive identity
- The powerful and positive influence of asset-building has been demonstrated across cultural and socioeconomic groups of youth.
- Having a natural mentor, communicating well with parents, being able to confide in a family member, parent-family connectedness, and perceived school connectedness are all protective measures against the adoption by youth of risky health behaviors.

[Chapter Twenty]

The Stress and Coping Theories

Stress is a part of everyday emotional life, and the adolescence period is among the most stressful in life. An understanding of the origins of stress and coping is essential to health promotion, in the sense that the presence of stress can trigger health-compromising behaviors (e.g., poor eating habits, insufficient sleep, depression, smoking, alcohol abuse), and the development of healthy coping mechanisms can prevent the initiation of these behaviors or counteract or reverse their harmful effects.

Stress is an unpleasant state of arousal that occurs when people *perceive* that an event or condition threatens their ability to effectively and comfortably cope with the situation (Smith and Carlson 1997, Lazarus and Folkman 1984). A moderate level of stress may be beneficial and is to be expected in many situations in life. But as people begin to feel overwhelmed by the demands placed on them, their moods become negative and they experience more stress than they can handle, which threatens their mental, physical, and emotional well-being. The variation of the effect that the same stressor can have on different people depends on a variety of factors, including how the person *perceives* the stressful event, if the stressor is accompanied by other stressors, the individual's tolerance for stress, and his or her personal beliefs about the resources he or she possesses to cope with the stressor.

Adolescence is a particularly stressful period of life for several reasons (Kaplan 2004). Adolescents are required to adapt to a series of normative changes and increased expectations to act in a more mature manner. They also develop more self-consciousness and devote more time to judging themselves and evaluating how others see them. This process is usually based on the verbal and nonverbal reinforcements they perceive from others (peers, parents, teachers), in which girls are particularly alert to facial expressions that communicate emotions (e.g., angry look from friend or teacher). It also marks the first time for several experiences related to changes in the body (e.g., wearing a bra, using deodorant, menstruation, wet dreams), social changes (e.g., first flirting experiences and first dates), and increased behavioral autonomy (e.g., staying at home alone, using public transportation on one's own).

A *stressor*, the source of stress, is an environmental event or stimulus that threatens an organism and that leads to a coping response, which is any response made by an organism to avoid, escape from, or minimize an aversive stimulus (Gazzaniga and Heatherton 2003). Stressors usually are divided into two categories:

- *major life stressors*: changes or disruptions that affect aspects of great importance in one's life (e.g., severe illness or death of someone close; moving to a new school, neighborhood, city, or country; parental divorce; chronically stressful conditions such as poverty, disabling illness, family conflict, physical and/or sexual abuse); and
- *daily hassles*: small day-to-day frustrations and irritations (e.g., dealing with unfair or unpleasant teachers, school examinations, being teased by friends, arguments with siblings and parents).

Research shows that unpredictable and uncontrollable catastrophic events (e.g., earthquake, hurricane, fire, flood, civil unrest, urban crime and violence, terrorist attack) are especially stressful. Life changes of any type are stressful in and of themselves, and the greater the number of changes, the more intensely the individual will likely feel stress. The effect of day-to-day hassles, if a large number of them present themselves simultaneously, can be comparable to those of major life changes. Although people seem to adjust to daily problems over time, interpersonal difficulties appear to have a cumulative effect on health (Gazzaniga and Heatherton 2003).

Adolescents most often report daily hassles as their most stressful event, particularly those involving parents and teachers. Nearly half of all U.S. adolescents report difficulty in coping with stressful situations at home and/or at school (Gans 1990). School-related stressors include examinations, grades, and feeling rushed (Burnett and Fanshawe 1997; Puskar, Lamb, and Bartolovic 1993). Home- and family-related stressors include parental or sibling health problems, general conflict with parents, conflict between parents, and parental divorce, which are all reported as being very stressful (Forehand, Biggar, and Kotchic 1998).

As early as 1932, Walter Cannon described the *fight-or-flight* response as both an animal and a human reaction to stress, which causes the person to either confront and combat danger or flee rapidly from it (Cannon 1932). Shelley Taylor and her colleagues (2000) have suggested, however, that the fight-or-flight response is more typical for men, whereas females often respond to stress in a *tend-and-befriend* pattern, by protecting and caring for their offspring, as well as by forming alliances with social groups to reduce individual risk. Taylor and colleagues further note that women under stress seek out social support, particularly from other women, and that they remain more connected to their social networks than men do under similar circumstances.

How the stressor is perceived and interpreted (*cognitive appraisal*) affects the process of coping with the stimulus or event. Lazarus (1993) described a two-step appraisal process when a person is confronted with a stressful situation:

- *primary appraisal*: The person evaluates how stressful the situation is and the potential threat or harm of the event. If the person considers the stimulus stressful enough, the next step is a
- *secondary appraisal*: The person evaluates his or her ability to alter the situation, manage negative emotional reactions, evaluate response options, and choose coping behaviors.

In the Transactional Model of Stress and Coping (Folkman and Moskowitz 2000, Lazarus and Folkman 1984), stressful experiences are construed as person-environment *transactions* wherein the impact of an external stressor, or demand, is mediated by the person's appraisal of the stressor and the psychological, social, and cultural resources at his or her disposal. Two basic primary appraisals are *perceptions of susceptibility* to the threat and *perceptions of severity* of the threat.

According to the Transactional Model of Stress and Coping, appraisals of personal risk and threat severity prompt efforts to cope with the stressor. However, heightened perceptions of risk can also generate distress and prompt escape-avoidance behaviors to minimize the significance of the threat. Beliefs of invulnerability, on the other hand, enhance perceived control and active coping, as well as reduce distress. This is often the case for many adolescents. Minimizing appraisals may diminish motivation to adopt recommended preventive health behaviors. Smokers, for example, are significantly more likely than nonsmokers to perceive themselves as less personally susceptible to the health effects of smoking (Chapman, Wong, and Smith 1993).

Other primary appraisals that have been described (Smith and Lazarus 1993, Smith et al. 1993) are *motivational relevance* of the stressor (i.e., when the stressor is considered to have a major impact on a person's goal or concerns, that person is likely to experience anxiety and situation-specific stress) and *causal focus* of the stressor (e.g., when perceiving oneself as being responsible for the stressor).

The primary appraisal, in the life of a typical adolescent, is heavily influenced by emotions. Emotion (or *affect*) refers to feelings that involve subjective evaluation, physiological processes, and cognitive beliefs. Emotions are immediate responses to environmental events, such as receiving a poor grade or having a family argument (Gazzaniga and Heatherton 2003). Emotions also provide information about the importance of stimuli to personal goals and then prepare the individual to take actions aimed at achieving those goals (Frijda 1994). Adolescents are more affected by their own emotional reactions in the presence of daily stressors (e.g., feelings of hurt when teased, anger when insulted) than by the perceived susceptibility or severity of a health threat or risky situation. Emotions are part of the daily interpersonal dynamics in which adolescents are immersed, and emotional expressions are powerful nonverbal communications. For example, Gazzaniga and Heatherton (2003) found that, in terms of facial expressions, the lower half of the face, and particularly the mouth (e.g., smile), has been identified as more important than the upper half of the face (eyes) in communicating emotion, especially for positive affect. This finding could be of significant relevance to parents and teachers as a mechanism they can use (e.g., a daily smile) to help adolescents buffer daily hassles at school and home, in full awareness of the positive impact this gesture in particular has on young people.

Secondary appraisal is an assessment of a person's coping resources and options. In contrast to primary appraisals that focus on the features of the stressful situation, secondary appraisals address what one can do about the situation. Key examples of secondary appraisals are:

- *perceived ability to change the situation* (perceived control over the threat)
- *perceived ability to manage one's emotional reactions* to the threat (perceived control over feelings)
- *expectations about the effectiveness of one's coping resources* (coping self-efficacy)

Sturges and Rogers (1996) found that among adolescents and youth, the threat appeals of some health education interventions worked only if the people believed they could cope effectively with the danger; if they believed they could not cope, higher levels of the threat resulted in decreased intentions to refrain from, in this case, tobacco use. Although adolescents elaborated and integrated the information about threat severity, personal vulnerability, and response efficacy, the fragility and malleability of the adolescents' beliefs in self-efficacy demonstrated the importance of adding a developmental perspective to theories of preventive health psychology.

The secondary appraisal, in the life of an adolescent, is also heavily influenced by emotions. According to Slovic and colleagues (2002), emotions serve as heuristic guides providing feedback for making quick decisions when confronted with complex, multifaceted situations. The judgment concerning risky situations is significantly affected by the emotions experienced at the moment of decision-making, given that emotions usually have more impact than cognitions on rapidly made decisions (Loewenstein et al. 2001).

Folkman and Lazarus (1980) suggested that there are two general categories of *coping efforts* or *coping strategies*:

- *emotion-focused coping*: These are strategies of coping with stress that focus on reducing the discomfort associated with stress (Kaplan 2004). This category includes efforts to prevent having an emotional response to the stressor or changing the way one feels about the stressful situation. Emotion-focused coping involves strategies such as seeking social support, the venting of feelings, use of avoidance techniques, attempting to minimize the problem's significance, efforts to distance oneself from the problem's outcomes, overeating and/or overdrinking, to even complete denial of the situation at hand (Gazzaniga and Heatherton 2003). Emotion-focused strategies will be most adaptive when the stressor is unchangeable or when all problem-focused coping attempts have been made. The adoption of one or more of these strategies allows people to continue performing in the face of stressors that are out of their control.
- *problem-focused coping*: These are strategies of coping with stress that involve actively confronting the problem in an effort to solve it (Kaplan 2004). This form of coping is directed at changing the stressful situation by taking steps to solve the problem (e.g., seeking information, generating alternative solutions, evaluating costs and benefits for each possible solution, and choosing a response). Problem-focused strategies will be most adaptive for stressors that are perceived as controllable and changeable.

People usually use either one or the other of the above categories of coping responses, depending on the situation. Emotion-based strategies, such as choosing to ignore a problem, are effective only in the short term (e.g., ignoring sibling rivalry issues may work on individual occasions, but it will not improve relations over time), whereas problem-focused coping is often effective in the long term. Some strategies, such as denial, are considered to be maladaptive in both types of situations; Herman-Stahl and Petersen (1996) found that teens who respond to problems with denial have worse outcomes (e.g., depression) than those who do not adopt this response.

Although some emotion-focused strategies are proactive in terms of helping the person to process the emotion that he or she feels when confronted with the stressor, (e.g., seeking social support, venting feelings with a friend) other emotion-focused strategies (e.g., avoidance, minimizing the problem's importance, efforts to distance oneself from the problem's outcomes, denial) discourage the processing of emotions and have been described by Carver and colleagues (1993) as *disengaging coping strategies*. In contrast, problem-focused coping strategies may be considered *engaging coping strategies*, since these involve consciously facing the problem and adopting active coping (e.g., developing a plan for solving the stress-causing problem, seeking information and social support).

Moos's model (Moos 1993), employed extensively in health psychology, is particularly useful because it combines measurements of the focus of coping (emotion vs. problem) with the method of coping (cognitive vs. behavioral) in a relatively brief instrument. Moos's division of coping into "approach" and "avoidance" categories classifies behaviors and cognitions into those which are used by the subject to face the problem squarely (approach), and those which divert the individual's attention away from the problem (avoidance) (Steiner et al. 2002).

Additional coping strategies have been described by Folkman and Moskowitz (2000) and Folkman (1997):

- *meaning-based coping*: the interpretation of a stressful event in a personally meaningful way (e.g., the use of spirituality and religious beliefs)
- *positive reappraisal*: a cognitive process that includes a positive reinterpretation and acceptance of a stressful event the individual is facing by viewing its positive aspects (e.g., comparing one's own situation with that of others in less fortunate circumstances)
- *creation of positive events*: a strategy in which the individual infuses ordinary events with positive meaning, allowing him or her to focus on the positive aspects of life (e.g., enjoying a beautiful sunset, quality family time in the presence of a serious injury or illness)

In contrast to coping strategies or efforts, which will vary according to different situations, *coping styles* are considered dispositional; i.e., a stable, unchanging characteristic of each person, despite the presence of a stressor. There has been interest in analyzing individual differences in coping, particularly in studying people who remain healthy even while enduring stressful life experiences. In this line of research, two coping styles have been described:

- *hardiness* (Kobasa 1979): a stress-resistant coping style characterized by three main components
    - a strong sense of *meaningfulness* and *commitment* to self and one's daily activities
    - a vigorous attitude toward life in which *threats are viewed as challenges or opportunities for growth*

- an *internal locus of control*, in which individuals see themselves as being in control of their lives
- *dispositional optimism*: an innate tendency to expect positive, rather than negative, outcomes from stressful situations. The description of dispositional optimism emerges from a new line of research referred to as *positive psychology*, which studies how people develop and sustain positive features such as hope, courage, perseverance, and future-mindedness despite levels of significant stress in their lives. Several studies have found positive associations between possessing a sense of purpose in life and life satisfaction, positive mood states, and well-being (Kwan et al. 2003, Ryff and Keyes 1995, Ryff et al. 1994).

Regardless of the existence of different coping strategies and styles, one of the most important factors enabling individuals to deal effectively with stress is the level of *social support* they receive. According to Cohen and Wills (1985), social support can have a stress-buffering effect on well-being, in the sense that this support will have a consistently stronger positive impact on adjustment as the stressors become more intense or persistent. Gazzaniga and Heatherton (2003) note that "social support needs to imply that people care about the recipient of the support," and emphasize that receiving emotional support is much more important than the simple provision of information to buffer stressful events. *Coping outcomes*, a person's adaptation to a stressor, may be observed through the person's emotional well-being, functional status, and health-related behaviors.

Research and Practical Applications of the Theories of Stress and Coping to Adolescent Lifestyles

Levels of stress tend to increase from preadolescence into later adolescence, the time at which gender differences become more obvious. There is also evidence indicating that the transition into adolescence represents a period of particular vulnerability for girls (Rudolph 2002). In a variety of studies, coping has been shown to make significant contributions to adolescent adjustment (Steiner et al. 2002). Prospectively, it has been related to good or poor health outcomes in depressed and chronically ill youths (Moos 1993).

According to Ann Masten (2001), adolescents develop and maintain skills that help them to deal with stress through having warm, nurturing relationships with others. Within this context, an interesting question for future research might be to analyze to what degree adolescents develop resiliency by growing up with parents or caregivers who themselves present healthy coping styles, such as hardiness and dispositional optimism, in addition to having a nurturing relationship with their children.

Forehand, Biggar, and Kotchic (1998) examined the relationship between the number of familial stressors and psychological

> **Box 20-1. The Stress and Coping Theories: Key Theoretical Concepts in the Adoption of Healthy Behaviors**
>
> **stress**: an unpleasant state of arousal that occurs when people perceive that an event or condition threatens their ability to effectively and comfortably cope with the situation
>
> **stressor**: a source of stress; an environmental event or stimulus that threatens an organism
> - **major life stressors**: changes or disruptions that affect aspects of great importance in one's life
> - **daily hassles**: small day-to-day frustrations and irritations
>
> **fight-or-flight response**: a reaction to stress in which the organism either directly confronts and combats danger or flees rapidly from it
>
> **tend-and-befriend response**: a reaction to stress in which the organism protects and cares for its offspring and forms alliances with social groups to reduce individual risk
>
> **cognitive appraisal**: the perception and interpretation of a stressor
>
>   **primary appraisal**: The person evaluates how stressful the situation is and the potential threat or harm of the event. Primary appraisals include:
> - *perceptions of susceptibility* to the threat
> - *perceptions of severity* of the threat
> - *motivational relevance* of the stressor
> - *causal focus* of the stressor
> - *role of emotion in evaluating how stressful the situation is*
>
>   **secondary appraisal**: The person evaluates his or her ability to alter the situation, manage negative emotional reactions, evaluate response options, and choose coping behaviors. Secondary appraisals include:
> - *perceived ability to change the situation*
> - *perceived ability to manage one's emotional reactions* to the threat
> - *expectations about the effectiveness of one's coping resources*
> - *role of emotions in rapid decision-making*
>
> **emotion (or *affect*)**: feelings that involve subjective evaluation, physiological processes, and cognitive beliefs
>
> **coping efforts or strategies**: actual strategies used to adapt to stressful circumstances
> - **emotion-focused coping**: strategies of coping with stress that focus on reducing the discomfort associated with stress
> - **problem-focused coping**: strategies of coping with stress that involve actively confronting the problem in an effort to solve it
> - **meaning-based coping**: the interpretation of a stressful event in a personally meaningful way
> - **positive reappraisal**: a positive reinterpretation and acceptance of a difficult situation the person is facing by viewing its positive aspects
> - **creation of positive events**: infusing ordinary events with positive meaning, allowing the person to focus on the positive aspects of his/her life
>
> **coping styles**: dispositional (i.e., stable and unchanging) characteristics of each person, even in the presence of a stressor
> - **hardiness:** a stress-resistant coping style characterized by a strong sense of *meaningfulness* and *commitment,* viewing stress as a *challenge* to be overcome, and feeling *in control* of one's life
> - **dispositional optimism**: a tendency to expect positive, rather than negative, outcomes from stressful situations
>
> **coping outcomes**: a person's adaptation to a stressor, observable through the individual's emotional well-being, functional status, and health-related behaviors

adjustment over time. They measured five stressors in a sample of adolescents 11 to 15 years old: parental marital status, parental depressive mood, maternal physical health problems, maternal depressive mood, and mother-adolescent relationship problems. The adolescents in the study were followed for six years, and then measures of depression, conduct disorders, and academic progress were obtained. The researchers found that as the number of stressors increased, so did the adolescent's vulnerability to internalizing problems (e.g., depression) and/or externalizing them (e.g., conduct disorders) later on. An increase from three to four stressors led to a significant increase in problems six years later. The authors conclude that although some adolescents may initially handle stress effectively, as the number of stressors increase, over time their resources begin to become depleted and the adolescents are less able to cope than they were earlier.

Steiner et al. (2002) examined 1,769 nonclinical high school students (48% of whom were girls, mean age 16 years) to establish a link between coping styles, health problems, and health risk behaviors. The findings showed that approach coping correlated negatively with indicators of health problems and health risk behaviors, while avoidance coping correlated positively with these domains. When both forms of coping (approach coping and avoidance coping) were used on different occasions, the presence of approach coping served to mitigate the negative effects of using avoidance coping alone. The authors highlight the importance of giving special attention to youth who present a high preponderance of avoidance coping. They describe these adolescents as quite elusive, as evidence suggests they do not come to the attention of surveys, studies, or health care personnel readily and willingly. The authors also found that a certain type of coping (i.e., high avoidance in the presence of low approach coping) seems to be associated with the highest health risks and risk-taking behaviors. Steiner et al. propose that this association of avoidance coping in the face of adversity and a high tendency to take risks is compatible with a psychodynamic formulation of risk-taking as a form of acting out (i.e., action taken to avoid confronting painful realities and emotions).

Studies of adolescent populations have found that smoking is positively related to indices of negative affect and life stress (Lloyd and Lucas 1998, Sussman et al. 1993). Prospective studies have found stress measures to be predictive of smoking onset and escalation (Sussman and Dent 2000; Dugan, Lloyd, and Lucas 1999). In a 1999 journal article, Parrot proposed conversely that cigarette smoking causes increases in stress.

Wills, Sandy, and Yaeger (2002b) conducted a comparative test of both hypotheses: stress as an etiological factor for smoking and cigarette smoking as a cause of increases in stress. Participants were a sample of 1,364 adolescents who were initially surveyed at mean age 12.4 years and received three yearly follow-ups. Measures of negative affect, negative life events, and cigarette smoking were obtained at all four assessments. Latent growth modeling showed negative affect was related to an increase in smoking over time. There was no path from initial smoking to change in negative affect. Comparable results were found for negative life events, with no evidence for reverse causation. Relations between stress and smoking were comparable for boys and girls. The authors suggest that a primary aim for prevention programs should be to strengthen efforts toward the development of coping mechanisms and to build engagement in alternative sources of reinforcement.

Stress might explain also why low-income pregnant adolescent girls smoke. Lawson (1994) found that this population group smoked to cope with anxiety and depression, particularly when rejected by their families and/or boyfriends. They also reported smoking to cope with weight gain during pregnancy. Furthermore, the girls reported fearing the pain of delivery and knew that smoking would help them to deliver smaller infants, which in turn would decrease the duration of labor.

Siqueira, Rolnitsky, and Rickert (2001) examined the relationship of nicotine dependence, stress, and coping methods between U.S. inner-city adolescent smokers and quitters and, using the Transtheoretical Model and Stages of Change, among adjacent smoking cessation stages. Smokers were significantly more likely to report smoking additional cigarettes per day as well as have higher levels of physical addiction, greater levels of perceived stress, and less use of cognitive coping methods than quitters. Comparison of consecutive stages revealed a significant difference only between pre-contemplation and contemplation in cognitive coping methods. Three out of 20 withdrawal symptoms (cravings, difficulty dealing with stress, and anger) were reported more frequently among current smokers who had attempted to quit in the last six months than among former smokers. The authors suggest that interventions for inner-city adolescents who smoke should be designed to target those with the highest levels of nicotine dependence, stress, and decreased use of cognitive coping methods, since the members of this group are the least likely to quit on their own.

Sussman et al. (1999) reviewed the effects of 34 adolescent tobacco use cessation and prevention trials on regular users of tobacco products. The authors found that among cessation studies, an emphasis on the immediate consequences of use and instruction in the development and strengthening of coping strategies led to relatively successful programs.

Wills et al. (2001b) tested the relation of seven coping dimensions to substance use (tobacco, alcohol, marijuana) with a sample of 1,668 U.S. early adolescents who were assessed at a mean age of 12.5 years and received two annual follow-ups. An associative latent-growth model showed one index of engagement (*behavioral coping*) to be inversely related to the initial level of adolescent use and growth over time in peer use. Behavioral coping was defined as taking action to try to solve the problem (getting information, thinking about the choices before making a decision, considering which steps to take). Three indices of disengagement (*anger coping*, *helpless coping*, and *hangout coping*) were positively related to initial levels of peer use and adolescent use and to growth in adolescent use. Anger coping was defined as becoming angry at and criticizing other people because of the problem; helpless coping as giving up on trying to solve the problem; and hangout coping as choosing to socialize with friends instead of confronting the problem. Life stress was positively related to initial levels for peer use and adolescent use and to growth in adolescent use. Moderation tests indicated that the effects of coping were significantly greater at a higher level of stress, while behavioral coping buffered the effects of disengagement. The effects of life stress were greater for girls than for boys.

Wills and Cleary (1996) examined how the effect of parental emotional and instrumental support on substance use (tobacco, alcohol, and marijuana) in adolescents is mediated. Data were from a sample of 1,702 adolescents in the United States who were surveyed between the seventh and ninth grades. Structural modeling analyses indicated the effect of support was mediated through more behavioral coping and academic competence and less tolerance for deviance and behavioral lack of control. Multiple-group analyses suggested buffering effects occurred because high support reduced the effect of risk factors and increased the effect of protective factors.

Laniado-Laborin, Molgaard, and Elder (1993) demonstrated that a program emphasizing training to cope with the social pressures of cigarette smoking was effective in preventing initial experimentation among sixth graders in Tijuana, Mexico. Although not intended for this purpose, the program was also effective in helping adolescent smokers to quit smoking. The proportion of adolescents in the intervention group that quit smoking was significantly higher (72% vs. 35%) compared to the control group that was not affected by the coping skills training intervention.

Shimai et al. (2000) studied the relationship between snacking behavior and stress coping among elementary and junior high school students in Japan and found a close relationship. The authors suggest that behavioral interventions to encourage healthy eating habits should be included in the development of stress-coping skills against various kinds of life demands. Norris, Carrol, and Cochrane (1992) examined the effects of physical activity on psychological stress and well-being in an adolescent population. The analysis revealed that those who reported greater physical activity also reported less stress and lower levels of depression.

The process of moving to a new country, adapting to a new culture, and learning to integrate one's own culture with a new one can be a major stressor in the lives of an increasing number of adolescents migrating for better opportunities. Infante (2003) describes the resilience factors that help Latino adolescents to cope successfully when immigrating to the United States. These include having parents with a strong sense of responsibility, optimism, autonomy, and the confidence that they can create positive change by giving hope and opportunities to their sons and daughters; adolescents with strong social skills enabling them to express their feelings, to have others find them likeable, and to establish strong relationships with service providers; a strong relationship within the family; and maintaining a strong cultural attachment and identification with the Latino community even as the adolescent learns more about the values of the dominant culture.

Stress and coping has been vastly researched for adolescent behaviors related to tobacco, alcohol, and drug use, but very poorly linked to violent and sexual health-related behaviors and physical activity and nutrition in adolescents. Literature reviews indicate that stress and coping theories seem to be among the most crucial theories to utilize when planning, implementing, and monitoring health promotion interventions for adolescents. The theoretical framework helps to foster an important developmental task of pre- and early adolescence, which is the development of healthy coping styles to deal with life's minor day-to-day stressful events. The evidence also shows that most of the adolescent lifestyle decisions (tobacco, alcohol, and drug use; physical activity and nutrition; sexual practices; anger expression) are at least partly influenced by the anxieties surrounding male-female interactions and masculine-feminine expectations, although not always significantly.

Table 20-1. presents the number of studies found using Stress and Coping Theories to research adolescent health behaviors.

Table 20-1. **Most Commonly Researched Adolescent Behaviors Using the Stress and Coping Theories (SCT)**

ADOLESCENT BEHAVIORS	NUMBER OF ARTICLES USING THE SCT	NUMBER OF ARTICLES BY KEYWORDS	
Sexual and Reproductive Health	15	Teen Pregnancy	4
		HIV/AIDS	2
		STIs	0
		Contraceptives	0
Tobacco, Alcohol, and Drug Use	56	Tobacco	30
		Alcohol	43
		Drugs	43
Physical Activity and Nutrition	10	Obesity	5
		Physical Activity	2
		Nutrition	2
Violence	5		
TOTAL	**86**		

Box 20-2. **Summary of Stress and Coping Theories and Adolescent Lifestyles**

- Levels of stress tend to increase from pre-adolescence into the later periods of adolescence, particularly among girls.
- Nearly half of all U.S. adolescents report difficulty in coping with stressful situations at home or at school (daily hassles).
- School-related stressors include being teased by friends, examinations and grades, dealing with unfair or unpleasant teachers, and feeling rushed.
- Home-related stressors include parental or sibling health problems, general conflict with parents, conflict between parents, parental divorce, and arguments with siblings.
- *Primary appraisal* (evaluating how stressful a situation is) is heavily influenced by emotions among adolescents.
- Adolescents are more affected by their own emotional reactions in the presence of daily stressors (e.g., feeling hurt when teased, angry when insulted) than by the perceived susceptibility or severity of a health threat or risky situation.
- Emotions are part of the daily interpersonal dynamics in which adolescents are immersed, and emotional expressions are powerful nonverbal communications.
- *Secondary appraisal* (deciding what to do in the presence of a stressful event) is also heavily influenced by emotions among adolescents.
- The judgment concerning risky situations is significantly affected by the emotions experienced at the moment of decision-making, given that emotions usually have more impact than cognitions on rapidly made decisions.
- Adolescents who use denial to respond to problems have worse outcomes (e.g., depression) than those who do not respond this way.
- Adolescents develop and maintain skills that help them to deal with stress through having warm, nurturing relationships with others.
- As the number of stressors increase, so does the adolescent's vulnerability to internalizing problems (e.g., depression) and/or externalizing them (e.g., conduct disorders).
- High avoidance in the presence of low approach coping seems to be associated with the highest health risks and risk-taking behaviors among adolescents.
- Smoking among adolescents is positively related to indices of negative affect and life stress. Stress measures are predictive of smoking onset and escalation among this group.
- Low-income pregnant adolescent girls smoke to cope with anxiety and depression, particularly when rejected by their families and/or boyfriends, and to cope with weight gain during pregnancy.
- Adolescent smokers are significantly more likely to report smoking additional cigarettes per day as well as have higher levels of physical addiction, greater levels of perceived stress, and less use of cognitive coping methods than quitters.
- Life stress is positively related to initial levels for peer and adolescent use of tobacco, alcohol, and marijuana and to growth in use over time.
- Training to cope with the social pressures of cigarette smoking has been shown to be effective in preventing initial experimentation among Mexican adolescents.
- A close relationship between snacking behavior and stress coping has been shown for elementary and junior high school students.
- Physical activity is associated with lower levels of stress and depression among adolescents.

[Chapter Twenty-one]

At a Glance: The Interpersonal Level Theories and Models for Behavior Change

Of all the theories and models reviewed in Chapters Sixteen through Twenty to promote change at the interpersonal level, the Social Networks and Social Support Theories (Chapter Seventeen) have been the most utilized to address adolescent behaviors, particularly those involving sexual and reproductive health, as well as the promotion of physical activity and healthy nutrition. Interestingly, tobacco, alcohol, and drug prevention efforts have relied more on the Stress and Coping Theories to explain underlying factors and have used the Social Cognitive Theory to promote healthy behaviors. On the other hand, comparatively little research has been conducted on adolescent sexual and reproductive health utilizing the Stress and Coping Theories, compared to their application to studies of tobacco, alcohol, and drug use, even though the two classifications are intimately related as risky behaviors, particularly the link between alcohol use and unprotected sexual activity. Finally, while there have been a few efforts to understand aggressive behaviors at the individual level, violence among adolescents, either as perpetrators or as victims, has been much more studied at the interpersonal level, particularly within the framework of different parenting practices and the influence of social networks and social support, as well as from the resiliency perspective.

Table 21-1. illustrates these ideas and summarizes the number of studies using the theories and models discussed in Chapters Sixteen through Twenty according to health behaviors.

Table 21-2. presents a comparison of the total number of research articles on adolescent behaviors utilizing individual and interpersonal level theories and models. An interesting observation that emerges from this comparison is that tobacco, alcohol, and drug use behaviors have been by far more researched than the other reviewed behaviors, both at the individual level as well as at the interpersonal level.

Table 21-3. provides a summary of the behavior change theories and models discussed in Chapters Sixteen through Twenty and the most salient characteristics of each.

Table 21-1. **Summary of Most Commonly Researched Interpersonal Level Theories and Models for Changing Adolescent Behaviors**

Number of Articles on Adolescence and Interpersonal Level Behavior Change Theories and Models	Sexual and Reproductive Health	Tobacco, Alcohol, and Drug Use	Physical Activity and Nutrition	Violence	Total
Social Cognitive Theory	19	48	9	9	85
Social Networks and Social Support Theories	21	45	19	20	105
Authoritative Parenting Model	19	29	3	29	80
Resiliency Theory	8	29	0	16	53
Stress and Coping Theories	15	56	10	5	86
Total	82	207	41	79	319

Table 21-2. **A Comparison of the Individual Level and the Interpersonal Level Theories and Models for Adolescent Behavioral Change**

Number of Articles on Adolescence and Behavior Change Theories and Models	Sexual and Reproductive Health	Tobacco, Alcohol, and Drug Use	Physical Activity and Nutrition	Violence	Total
Total Individual Level Behavior Change Theories and Models	92	159	44	12	307
Total Interpersonal Level Behavior Change Theories and Models	82	207	41	79	319

Table 21-3. **Interpersonal Level Theories and Models and Their Application to Adolescent Behavioral Change: A Comparison of Conceptual Frameworks, Applications, and Benefits**

Theory/Model	Conceptual Framework	Application	Benefits
Social Cognitive Theory (Chapter Sixteen)	This theory encompasses both determinants of behavior and the methods of promoting behavior change. The theory explains behavior as a triadic, dynamic, and reciprocal model in which socio-environmental, personal or cognitive, and behavioral factors all interact. Its three main principles are that: (1) behavior is influenced by both socio-environmental and personal factors; (2) socio-environmental factors play a significant role in the onset of behaviors, but their influence is mediated via personal cognitions; and (3) behavior is not only influenced by socio-environmental and personal factors, but also, in turn, influences these factors (called *reciprocal determinism*). The theory also describes key constructs that help in promoting the adoption of a new behavior, including observational learning, reinforcements, outcome expectations and expectancies, self-efficacy, behavioral capability, mastery learning, and self-control of performance.	The Social Cognitive Theory has been identified as the underlying theoretical framework for many adolescent health promotion and prevention programs, probably because of its consideration of socio-environmental factors affecting individual behaviors. However, one of the drawbacks of such a broad theoretical formulation (environmental, personal, and behavioral factors) is that program designers might feel pressured to explain almost any phenomenon using one or more of the constructs without a complete understanding of how they operate separately and together. At the same time, there is considerable conceptual confusion about how to apply, measure, and analyze these constructs. Keeping this precaution in mind, the application of this theory to promote the adoption of health behaviors and the prevention of risk behaviors among adolescents has been successful, particularly among behaviors related to tobacco, alcohol, and drug use, and, more recently, to increased condom use.	This theory provides a particularly useful framework for understanding and describing the potential impact of the social environment on health behaviors among adolescents. The theory is also helping health promotion planners and project developers to move away from the mere provision of information to adolescents. This theory emphasizes the importance of teaching adolescents the necessary skills to perform new behaviors through effective role models and increasing their self-efficacy and behavioral capability. It additionally has raised awareness regarding the significant impact that negative role models and messages in the media can have, through observational learning, on the adoption by adolescents of health-compromising behaviors (e.g., violence; unsafe sex practices; tobacco, alcohol, and drug use). It is important, however, to combine this theory with others at the interpersonal and community levels, since evidence shows that skills training alone is likely to not have sustainable positive results in the long term if interventions only target adolescents and not their surroundings (e.g., peers, parents, community at large).
Social Networks and Social Support Theories (Chapter Seventeen)	Personal social networks are essential for receiving social support, which ranges from emotional support (love, caring, empathy) to the provision of aid or a service; information, advice, or suggestions; and input that is useful for self-evaluation purposes (constructive feedback,	The Social Networks and Social Support Theories have been applied to guide the design of health promotion and prevention programs for adolescents. However, most of the research has been related specifically to parental support or the influence that peers can have on adoles-	The beneficial and protective health effects of supportive social networks may be cultivated in any community, where a variety of human resources most likely already exist. Understanding peer networks within a community can be very helpful in the design and implementation of health promo-

Table 21-3. **Interpersonal Level Theories and Models and Their Application to Adolescent Behavioral Change: A Comparison of Conceptual Frameworks, Applications, and Benefits**–*(continued)*

Theory/Model	Conceptual Framework	Application	Benefits
Social Networks and Social Support Theories *(continued)*	affirmation of beliefs, social comparison). Social networks and social support are critical to the health and well-being of adolescents within the community where they live.	cent behaviors, and much less attention has been focused on creating and strengthening protective social networks for adolescents and tailoring these to the adolescent's changing developmental needs and wants and including a gender perspective.	tion and prevention programs for adolescents of different ages and gender. Strengthening adult supportive networks in the community can also play a major role, not only for adolescents but also for their parents during the process of accommodating their parenting skills to new and constantly changing developmental needs of their sons and daughters and the challenges these changes bring.
Authoritative Parenting Model (Chapter Eighteen)	Parenting approaches have been classified as authoritative, authoritarian, permissive, and uninvolved, and analyzed along the dimension of each's demandingness and responsiveness. A model which enables the quantification of these two dimensions has been developed (Maccoby and Martin 1983), and studies have demonstrated a positive relationship between parental demandingness and adolescent behavioral adjustment, as well as between parental responsiveness and adolescent psychosocial development. The main components of authoritative parenting are warmth, structure, and autonomy and development support. Growing evidence shows inverse relationships between effective (authoritative) parenting and health-risk behaviors among children and adolescents.	Research using this model has been conducted with ethnically diverse adolescent populations and to study the effects of poverty on adolescent adjustment and development. The relationship between authoritative parenting and tobacco, alcohol, and drug use; violence and HIV/STI prevention; school delinquency; and teen driving are among the specific adolescent behaviors that have been studied to date.	This model holds particular relevance for health promotion and prevention program designers in Latin America and the Caribbean, where nearly half of the adolescent population lives at or below the poverty line. A model has been developed (Conger et al. 1994, 1993) to explain how economic stress and poverty may adversely affect adolescent development and behaviors by affecting parental emotional tone and parenting skills. The results of numerous studies related to adolescent health, parenting styles, and poverty are providing insight into how the design of protective interventions can facilitate the adoption and maintenance of healthy behaviors and lifestyles despite the difficult socio-environmental circumstances and challenges these young people face.
Resiliency Theory (Chapter Nineteen)	This theory seeks to understand how children and adolescents thrive despite adverse conditions such as extreme poverty, parental mental illness, abuse, and/or catastrophic events. Much of resilience research	Studies of resilient children have identified specific protective factors falling under three general categories: qualities of the child, characteristics of the family, and support from outside the family. Resilience appears to result from	This theory utilizes a strengths-based (vs. deficits-based) approach to identify protective factors and focuses on youths' potential contribution to society instead of viewing this group as a social problem and burden.

Table 21-3. **Interpersonal Level Theories and Models and Their Application to Adolescent Behavioral Change: A Comparison of Conceptual Frameworks, Applications, and Benefits**–(continued)

Theory/Model	Conceptual Framework	Application	Benefits
Resiliency Theory (*continued*)	focuses on the personality traits, coping skills, and support systems that help individuals endure, survive in, and overcome challenging circumstances. The theory proposes that although resilience is an emergent capacity present to some degree in most people, its full development depends on the presence of protective factors during childhood and adolescence.	a combination of these three sources, reflecting the different levels of influence (individual, interpersonal, institutional, community) that may mutually reinforce one another and cause positive impact on health-related behaviors and conditions. Based on the results of a decade of developmental research, the Search Institute has identified 40 developmental assets for young people's growth and development, which are divided into 20 external assets and 20 internal assets. Research results show that youth with most assets are least likely to engage in four different patterns of high-risk behavior: problematic alcohol use, illicit drug use, sexual activity, and violence.	There is a growing body of evidence to indicate that taking a strengths-based approach by promoting skills and assets as an alternative to preventing deficits is more effective in engaging and motivating adolescents to develop healthy attitudes and behaviors and grow into responsible, caring adults. The powerful and positive influence of asset-building has been demonstrated across cultural and socioeconomic groups of youth.
Stress and Coping Theories (Chapter Twenty)	An understanding of the origins of stress and coping is essential to health promotion, in the sense that the presence of stress can trigger health-compromising behaviors, and the development of coping mechanisms can prevent the initiation of these behaviors or counteract or reverse their harmful effects. Coping may be classified by the focus of the coping strategy (emotion vs. problem) or the method of coping (cognitive vs. behavioral). Coping mechanisms may further be divided into *approach* and *avoidance* categories, with coping behaviors and cognitions being classified into those which are used by the subject to face the problem squarely (approach), and those which divert the individual's attention away from the problem (avoidance).	Stress and coping has been vastly researched for adolescent behaviors related to tobacco, alcohol, and drug use, but very poorly linked to sexual health-related behaviors and physical activity and nutrition in adolescents. The evidence shows that the majority of adolescent lifestyle decisions regarding the above-mentioned behaviors are at least partly influenced by the anxieties surrounding male-female interactions and masculine-feminine expectations.	The Stress and Coping Theories are among the most crucial theories to use when planning, implementing, and monitoring health interventions for adolescents. The theoretical framework helps to foster an important developmental task of pre- and early adolescence, which is to gain practice and skill in the use of healthy coping mechanisms to deal with life's minor day-to-day stressful events.

Theories and Models that Promote Change at the Community Level

Community level theories and models are essential for comprehensive health promotion efforts. Social norms, regulations, and policies are key factors to support the adoption of health-promoting behaviors and to reduce or eliminate health-compromising reinforcements in the social and physical environments. Community level theories and models help us to better understand how social groups organize themselves to identify their needs and wants, to pinpoint the variety of possible and appropriate solutions to the identified community problems, and to decide how best to promote social and environmental changes that make healthier choices easier choices to make. Community level theories and models are a meeting point for health education approaches and policy, economic, regulatory, and other environmental interventions. As Green and Kreuter (1999) note, "health education provides the consciousness-raising, concern-arousing, action-stimulating impetus for public involvement and commitment to social reform essential to its success in a democracy. Without health education, health promotion would be a manipulative social engineering enterprise. Without the policy support for social change, on the other hand, health education is often powerless to help people reach their health goals even with successful individual efforts." Health services, schools, recreational and sports facilities, community organizations, government agencies, and business and political leaders are all part of the community where the adolescent develops, grows, studies, plays, works, and seeks health advice and services. These entities and individuals are essential stakeholders that can play a pivotal role in promoting healthy lifestyles among adolescents.

Chapters Twenty-two and Twenty-three will review the following constructs for community level change in adolescent health promotion:

- the Community Organization Models
- the Diffusion of Innovations Theory, Behavior Change Models, and Social Marketing

[Chapter Twenty-two]

The Community Organization Models

Community organization has its roots in the Theories of Social Networks and Social Support described in Chapter Seventeen through the use of the ecological perspective (see Chapters Four and Seven). *Community organization* is defined as the process by which community groups come together to identify common needs, problems, and goals; mobilize resources; and develop and implement strategies for reaching the collective goals they have set (Minkler and Wallerstein 2002).

Minkler and Wallerstein (2002) emphasize that the definition of community organization clearly suggests that the needs or problems around which community groups are organized must, by necessity, be identified by the community itself. On the other hand, the authors warn about the growing tendency in recent years for community needs or problems to be identified by an outside organization or agent of change. According to Nyswander (1956), community organization captures one of health promotion's most fundamental principles, which is to "start where the people are." Therefore, health promotion program designers and health education professionals whose departure point reflects the specific needs determined by the target community will be far more likely to experience success in the change process and to promote true community ownership of programs and actions than will their counterparts who follow and/or impose a personal or institutionally dictated agenda developed outside the community and without its input.

This is an important challenge for health intervention planners and developers, who have traditionally relied upon behavioral theories as powerful tools with rigorous methodologies for analyzing and changing behaviors as well as measuring those changes, but whose work calls for them to follow the dictates of a particular institutional agenda or interest originating outside the community. Furthermore, externally funded projects usually come with preset health and/or behavioral objectives that might tempt health promotion program developers to bypass the social assessment phase when using the PRECEDE-PROCEED model discussed in Chapter Four of this book.

Yet Green and Kreuter (1999) encourage community health promotion planners to use an expansionist approach and include this initial phase assessment, regardless of the nature of the particular community project's structure or type of funding, because of its usefulness in determining community members' perceptions of their own needs and quality of life and because of the valuable input this information provides for the additional assessment phases to follow. They reason that this initial social assessment phase is essential because people value their health to the degree that being healthy allows them to achieve other personal goals.

In this sense, community organization is an excellent framework within which to carry out this social assessment. In the case of adolescent target groups, the assessment would yield essential information regarding their needs and wants, by gender and age group, that could be used as the backdrop for a well-designed intervention or program that would be responsive to their specific problems and goals at the particular point where they are now in their lives. In this sense, positive community change and empowerment are most optimally achieved when the design of health promotion programs embodies not only the appropriate mix of behavioral change theories, but successfully integrates them with developmental and ecological perspectives that prioritize the needs and goals of the community or community group desiring change.

In his book *An Ethic for Health Promotion: Rethinking the Sources of Human Well-Being*, David R. Buchanan argues that well-being is achieved by cultivating certain virtues, or dispositions of character, in which case the virtue of mindfulness is essential to the attainment of human well-being. According to Buchanan, "mindfulness is gaining greater self-knowledge, or becoming more aware of felt desires and putting them into perspective, in terms of the kind of person (or community) one aspires to be" (Buchanan 2000). As noted in this book's Introduction, an understanding of behavior change theories includes the awareness that they are health promotion strategies chosen by people and communities for the adoption of health-promoting lifestyles and positive, sustainable behavior change. These strategies, lifestyles, and long-term behavior change are, in this framework, the means to the final goal of human self-realization and optimal well-being. Within this context,

Buchanan's "mindfulness" may be viewed as a consciousness-raising and goal-setting construct leading to self-determined human well-being, as well as to the creation of stable, self-sustaining, and prosperous communities.

In the public health field, a growing emphasis on community participation, begun in the 1970s, culminated in the adoption of the Ottawa Charter for Health Promotion by the member governments of the World Health Organization in 1986. Support of the Charter's precepts signaled a new approach that encouraged governmental and nongovernmental sectors to work together in partnership, to seek universal participation, to create health-promoting public policies and sustainable environments, and, ultimately, to reduce inequities and disparities between groups in community-driven projects (World Health Organization 1986). The concept of *community-building* has also emerged, in which people who identify themselves as members of a shared community engage together in the process of community change. The definition of *community* may be based solely on geographical boundaries and related considerations, or it may refer to people living widely dispersed over large geographical areas who nonetheless view themselves as united through shared interests, ethnicity, profession, sexual orientation, or other similarities.

Rothman (2001) describes community organization as being composed of three alternative change models that sometimes overlap and may also be combined:

- *Locality* or *community development* utilizes a broad cross-section of people in the community to identify and solve its own problems. It stresses consensus-development, capacity-building, and a strong task orientation. Outside consultants or specialists may help to coordinate and enable the community to successfully address its particular concerns.
- *Social planning* uses task goals and addresses substantive problem-solving, with technical consultants providing expertise to benefit community members.
- *Social action* aims to increase the problem-solving capacity of the community and to achieve concrete changes to redress social injustice issues affecting the community's most disadvantaged and/or underserved groups.

The main differences between these models are that the *locality* or *community development* model is seen as being more process-oriented, the *social planning* model is viewed as more task-oriented, and the *social action* model is considered to be both task- and process-oriented (Minkler and Wallerstein 2002).

Community-building (Walter 1997, Gardner 1991) is a newer type of community organization model whose approach is considered to be more strengths-based and community-centered. In contrast to the other models just described, whose approaches are more needs-based and which often rely heavily on input supplied by external consultants, community-building focuses on increasing the community's own capacity to solve current and future problems.

The *Community Coalition Action Theory* (Butterfoss and Kegler 2002; Butterfoss, Goodman, and Wandersman 1993) has also gained recognition during the last decade. Community coalitions are formal, multi-purpose, and long-lasting alliances of individuals representing diverse organizations, factions, or constituencies within a community who agree to work together to achieve a common goal (Feighery and Rogers 1990). As an action-oriented partnership, a coalition usually performs a variety of functions: it analyzes the community problem to be prevented or addressed, gathers data and assesses the needs, develops a plan of action, and implements identified solutions, aiming to achieve community-level outcomes through social and behavioral changes (Whitt 1993).

The *Community Organization and Development* Model (Braithwaite, Bianchi, and Taylor 1994) involves the development of a community coalition board, which then undertakes its own community assessment, facilitates leadership development, sets policy, and designs culturally relevant interventions through a community problem-solving approach.

Several key concepts are shared by these various approaches and are central to effect and measure change at the community level:

- *Empowerment* is a social action process through which individuals, organizations, and communities gain mastery over their lives in the context of changing their social and political environment to improve equity and quality of life. In this regard, Minkler and Wallerstein (2002) pose an interesting question that must be addressed when considering empowerment: "Can people in positions of dominance or privilege derived from culture, gender, race, or class (and with funding attributions), empower others? Or must people empower themselves?" In the case of adolescents, Kim and colleagues (1998) emphasize the need to promote positive development through *youth empowerment*, by shifting the paradigm of considering youth as a community problem to one that views them as community resources and assets. Key components to the empowerment process—active participation, awareness of the surrounding world, and identification of strengths—are all essential aspects of youth development (Holden, Pendergast, and Austin 2000).
- *Critical consciousness* is developing an understanding of the root causes of problems. This concept is directly related to the empowerment concept. According to the Brazilian educator Paulo

Freire (1970), real education enables people to engage in active dialogue and develop a critical consciousness, which in turn allows them to challenge the conditions that keep them powerless.

- *Community capacity* is the approximate community-level equivalent of self-efficacy plus behavioral capability—terms, as we saw in Chapter Sixteen, that are integral components of the Social Cognitive Theory—that is, the confidence and skills to solve problems effectively. Seven dimensions have been described as critical to the development of community capacity (Norton et al. 2002):
  - *level of skills, knowledge, and resources* (e.g., skills for strategic planning and interpersonal communication);
  - *nature of social relationships* (e.g., social connectedness, sense of community);
  - *structures, mechanisms, and spaces for community dialogue and collective action* (e.g., social networks, community spaces);
  - *quality of leadership and its development* (e.g., communication, analysis and judgment, coaching, visioning, trust-building, teamwork);
  - *extent of civic participation* (e.g., volunteerism, voting behavior, public concern with governance);
  - *value system* (i.e., norms, standards, expectations, and desires of the community); and
  - *learning culture* (i.e., the community's ability to reflect on the outcomes of their actions and on new available options).

- *Participation and relevance* presuppose that citizens become actively involved and possess a collective sense of readiness for change based on their own felt needs, shared power, and awareness of resources.
- *Issue selection* is the identification of the problem(s) the community feels most strongly about. According to Minkler and Wallerstein (2002), a good issue selection must meet several important criteria:
  - *It must be winnable* (i.e., contribute to an achievable goal).
  - It must be *simple and specific*.
  - It must *unite* members of the group.
  - It must involve members in a *meaningful* way in resolving the community's problems.
  - It should deal with a problem that *affects a large number of people*.
  - It should *strengthen the community or organization*.
  - It should be part of *a larger plan or strategy*.

Social action approaches to community organizing can go beyond geographical and political boundaries and are able to coalesce action around common health problems. These types of approaches (e.g., HIV/AIDS prevention) have used *media advocacy* as a powerful tool in their efforts. Media advocacy is the strategic use of mass media as a resource for advancing a social or public policy initiative. Groups such as HIV/AIDS and tobacco control coalitions have made major advances in public support, funding, and policies in a remarkably short time.

The *Communication for Social Change* Model describes a reinforcing process of community dialogue and collective action working in tandem to produce social change in the community that improves the health and well-being of all of its members (Figueroa et al. 2002). This model proposes that usually communities do not initiate dialogue and action on their own. Instead, the catalyst or stimulus for these—which may be external or internal to the community—might take any variety of forms (e.g., mass media messages, new available technologies, a policy proposal, a change agent) and leads to a dialogue about a specific issue of concern or interest to the community. The model describes 10 steps in the community dialogue: (1) recognition of a problem; (2) identification and involvement of leaders and stakeholders; (3) clarification of community's perceptions regarding the issue; (4) expression of individual and shared needs; (5) development of a vision of the future; (6) assessment of current status; (7) setting of objectives; (8) identification of options for action; (9) securing consensus on the proposed action; and (10) creation of an action plan.

This model further proposes that since the community dialogue and collective-action processes are mutually reinforcing, they have the effect of increasing the community's capacity to cooperate effectively each successive time it goes through these processes. The model also postulates seven outcome indicators of social change: (1) leadership; (2) degree and equity of participation; (3) information equity; (4) collective self-efficacy; (5) sense of ownership; (6) social cohesion; and (7) social norms.

As community members and stakeholders in their community's overall health and well-being, adolescents and youth should be considered by planners and promoters of social change as valuable community assets and resources. This group is additionally ideally suited to provide innovative perspectives and other types of input into the development of a vision for the future and should therefore be encouraged to play an active role in community dialogues, coalitions, and all other forms of community organization.

Research and Evidence of Practical Applications of the Community Organization Models to Adolescent Lifestyles

Various initiatives launched in recent years indicate that the strategy of youth empowerment represents a potentially powerful tool in community efforts to encourage health-promoting behaviors among young people.

In an effort to address prevention in a more comprehensive manner, the American Legacy Foundation (2000) developed and implemented a statewide tobacco prevention program in Florida that included a focus on youth empowerment

> **Box 22-1. The Community Organization Models: Key Theoretical Concepts in the Adoption of Healthy Behaviors**
>
> **Community:** a group of people living within defined boundaries of the same geographical area; or alternatively, a group of people living widely dispersed over a large geographical area who view themselves as united through shared interests, ethnicity, profession, sexual orientation, or other similarities
>
> **Community organization:** the process by which members of a community come together to identify common needs, problems, and goals; mobilize resources; and develop and implement strategies to address these concerns and to achieve collectively set expected results
>
> **Community Development Model (Locality):** a process-oriented model that utilizes a broad cross-section of people in the community to identify and solve its own problems, and stresses consensus development, capacity-building, and task orientation
>
> **Social Planning Model:** a task-oriented model used to address substantive problem-solving, in which consultants provide technical expertise to benefit community members
>
> **Social Action Model:** both a task- and process-oriented model whose aim is to increase the community's problem-solving capacity and to achieve concrete changes to redress social injustice issues affecting the community's most disadvantaged and/or underserved groups
>
> **Community-Building Model:** a strengths-based and community-centered model focused on increasing the community's own capacity to solve problems
>
> **Community coalition:** a formal, multipurpose, and long-lasting alliance of individuals representing diverse organizations, factions, or constituencies within a community who agree to work together to achieve a common goal
>
> **Community Organization and Development Model:** involves the development of a community coalition board, which then undertakes its own community assessment, facilitates leadership development, sets policy, and designs culturally relevant interventions through a community problem-solving approach
>
> **Empowerment:** a social action process through which individuals, organizations, and communities take control over their lives in the context of changing their social and political environment to improve equity and quality of life
>
> **Community capacity:** refers to the community-level equivalent of self-efficacy and behavioral capability (i.e., the confidence and skills of a community to solve its problems effectively)
>
> **Communication for Social Change Model:** based on a mutually reinforcing process of community dialogue and collective action that produces social change, at the same time that it increases community capacity to cooperate effectively each time similar issues or problems are faced in the future

through the initiation of youth-led and youth-driven coalitions. The Foundation's goals were to engage youth in community actions against tobacco use by developing a broad-based coalition that reflected the state's ethnic and social diversity, building or extending statewide youth movements against tobacco use, and fostering meaningful youth-led tobacco prevention activities or programs that encouraged and increased youth empowerment, positive development, civic involvement, and leadership and decision-making responsibilities.

Another teen empowerment movement to prevent tobacco use aspires to be a model for the rest of the United States in overcoming barriers related to tobacco use prevention. Martin and colleagues (2001) describe the North Carolina-based program in a recently published journal article and emphasize that "youth speak with a fresh voice, bringing energy and conviction, as well as nontraditional ideas and strategies, to the achievement of their goals."

The use of cigarettes among U.S. teens has been dropping steadily and substantially since the peak rates seen in 1996 and 1997. Between 2001 and 2002, the proportion of teens saying that they had tried smoking fell by 4 or 5 percentage points in each grade surveyed (8, 10, and 12), more than in any other recent year (Monitoring the Future 2002). One of the factors mentioned as facilitating the achievement of these results is the major anti-smoking campaign aimed at youth launched by the American Legacy Foundation. The Monitoring the Future organization attributes part of the success to the important role played by the American Legacy Foundation's "Truth" campaign in increasing the perceived risk of smoking among teens.

While youth empowerment has proven to be a successful strategy in decreasing adolescent tobacco use in the United States (Monitoring the Future 2002, Martin et al. 2001, American Legacy Foundation 2000), it has not been widely explored as an alternative option to promote delay in sexual initiation and the adoption of safer sex practices among adolescents. The authors of this book found only two successful experiences, both directed towards African youth: the Kenyan Youth Initiatives Project and the Promotion of Youth Responsibility Project-Zimbabwe (Johns Hopkins University Center for Communications Program 1999). The first one aimed to empower young people with information on their reproductive health through a radio variety show targeted to this group in which young people also developed and oversaw the presentation of the show's contents. The second experience involved young people in the development of an extensive six-month communication campaign and in the identification of "youth-friendly" health centers.

These experiences point to the possibility that HIV and teen pregnancy prevention programs could benefit from fresh, nontraditional ideas and strategies, created by youth themselves through the initiation of youth-led and youth-driven coalitions. These would foster meaningful youth-inspired and -directed HIV and teen pregnancy prevention interventions, activities, and programs. Most of the interventions to date involving youth in sexual and reproductive health prevention programs use them as peer educators, with some successful experiences (Pearlman et al. 2002, Feudo et al. 1998). However, the role of adolescents typically is limited to that of serving as outreach agents to provide the prevention services, and their participation is excluded from the programs' assessment and planning phases. A model for a youth-based approach to HIV/AIDS services is being implemented in San Francisco, California. Bay Positives is a peer-run, peer-based organization funded by and for youth living with HIV. Among its executive directorship, board of directors, staff, and cadre of volunteers, the oldest member is only 26 years old (Bettencourt et al. 1998).

A literature review by this book's authors of publications describing community coalitions to prevent teen pregnancy revealed that very rarely do these incorporate youth as active participants in the project development and implementation stages. Kegler and Wyatt (2003) have identified a series of factors associated with successful neighborhood mobilization to prevent adolescent pregnancy. These include a strong sense of community, consensus on the perceived need for the initiative, support by key organizations, shared leadership, effective group action processes, and a competent staff contingent. An innovative approach to increase male involvement in teen pregnancy prevention was initiated in the United States by the Teen Pregnancy Task Force of Bucks County, Pennsylvania. Through two local gatherings open only to men, the Task Force promoted community dialogue among adolescent and adult men around such issues as male responsibility in preventing pregnancy and sexually transmitted infections, feelings about sexual abstinence, and providing advice to younger siblings about teen pregnancy prevention (Boyer and Yanoff 1995).

The evaluation of youth-targeted community organization interventions has also presented challenges of its own, particularly when substantial financial resources have been invested in the intervention and the expected results elude program sponsors. Hallfors et al. (2002) highlight one such example of this in a research paper presenting evidence on the effectiveness of community antidrug coalitions in reducing substance abuse in 12 U.S. communities participating in the Fighting Back program. The federal government, through the Center for Substance Abuse Prevention's Community Coalition Program, had supported local coalitions by investing almost half a billion dollars during the 1990s. Based on this precedent, and following several large-scale community trials for chronic disease prevention that had had significant influence in developing community-based, comprehensive health promotion programs, the Robert Wood Johnson Foundation launched the Fighting Back program. The program promoted the development of community coalitions that would assess substance abuse problems in their local areas and respond with a comprehensive and coordinated action plan. Communities were encouraged to develop their own programs based on local needs and to include separate components on public awareness, prevention interventions for children and youth, early identification, treatment, and relapse prevention. Despite the planning and organization that had preceded the program's launching, the results of the Fighting Back evaluation showed no effects in reducing substance abuse among youth. Furthermore, strategies aimed at improving adult-focused outcomes showed significant negative effects over time, compared to matched controls.

Hallfors and colleagues also describe some lessons learned from this experience. First, they note, the Fighting Back program had extremely broad goals. It was expected that the process would stimulate a reduction in demand for all drugs and alcohol among all target groups, which in effect forced the coalitions to work on too many fronts and to juggle competing programmatic priorities. Based on the evaluation's disappointing results, the authors recommend that communities keep their goals focused and manageable, with well-defined expected results and appropriate corresponding data for the evaluation process. Secondly, leaders in the 12 communities chose, developed, and implemented strategies without proper supervision that could have ensured that the chosen strategies were supported by scientific evidence. Thirdly, the Fighting Back coalitions were expensive to maintain, and policymakers assumed the effectiveness of the strategies at the same time that key elements had not been given due consideration. These included encouraging communities to choose research-based programs and to acquire the necessary technical expertise to effectively carry them out, and incorporating appropriate environmental level interventions (e.g., reducing youth access to alcohol and tobacco), in addition to strategies focused at the individual level.

Green and Kreuter (2002) offer a series of possible strategies to help communities bridge the gap between scientific evidence and the desire to develop their own local interventions. One of these is for communities to partner with the nearest and most interested university-based research teams or schools of public health, in order to ensure the community's access to best practices and adequate support in monitoring and evaluating the intervention. Another alternative would be to encourage the engaging of researchers, community program developers, and local policymakers in the joint research, planning, and evaluation process. This collaborative effort would assure the use of evidence-based interventions adapted to local circumstances and adequate levels of monitoring and evaluation supervision.

The Communities Mobilizing for Change on Alcohol (CMCA) initiative is an example of a successful U.S. community-based effort to change community policies and practices and reduce youth access to alcohol. CMCA was a group-randomized trial that included seven Midwestern communities assigned to the intervention condition and eight communities assigned to the control condition. The intervention consisted of a 2.5-year process in which a part-time community organizer worked with local government officials, enforcement agencies, alcohol retailers, the media, schools, and other community groups to reduce youth access to alcohol. The target group was youth ages 18–20 years old. The evaluation of this process showed that the CMCA intervention had a significant effect in reducing alcohol consumption among the target group, as well as in reducing the propensity to sell alcohol to minors. The intervention also had a significant effect in reducing the number of arrests of 18–20-year-olds driving while under the influence of alcohol (Wagenaar et al. 2000a, 2000b).

New Zealand is currently carrying out a project focused on youth and drug use that consists of a partnership with six communities in rural and urban areas, many of whose residents are predominantly of the Polynesian-speaking Maori cultural group. This project illustrates a model that aims to bridge the gap between research and practice and to improve human health and well-being by working with communities to increase their capacity to deal with alcohol and drug issues and to introduce sustainable initiatives (Conway et al. 2000).

Rudd, Goldberg, and Dietz (1999) have written one of the few articles to date which describes community organization efforts to increase physical activity and healthy nutrition among adolescents. They suggest that:

(1) Community members themselves should take the initiative to identify the strongest needs among the various population groups they serve and suggest where new resources could be most strategically utilized.
(2) Community experts who are familiar with or belong to the culture of the target population should become members of the pilot program planning and implementation team.
(3) In order to actively engage members of the targeted population, there must be a strong foundation for community linkages and for community-building.

These basic principles are indeed key to the success of any community health promotion program. They help to ensure that the initiatives will be able to increase their effectiveness over time and thus become self-sustaining in the long term.

Table 22-1. presents a breakdown of the number of studies found using Community Organization Models according to adolescent health behaviors.

As seen in Table 22-1., community organization models have been vastly researched for adolescent behaviors related to tobacco, alcohol, and drug use, but very poorly linked to physical activity and nutrition in adolescents. Although there are various publications describing community interventions to improve adolescent sexual and reproductive health, and to reduce teen pregnancy and youth violence, the effectiveness of these interventions alone is less evident unless they are part of comprehensive programs that include interventions at multiple levels (individual, interpersonal, community, and policy).

Table 22-1. **Most Commonly Researched Adolescent Behaviors Using the Community Organization Models (COM)**

ADOLESCENT BEHAVIORS	NUMBER OF ARTICLES USING THE COM	NUMBER OF ARTICLES BY KEYWORDS	
Sexual and Reproductive Health	39	Teen Pregnancy	22
		HIV/AIDS	17
		STIs	1
		Condom Use	1
Tobacco, Alcohol, and Drug Use	76	Tobacco	30
		Alcohol	28
		Drugs	18
Physical Activity and Nutrition	6	Obesity	1
		Physical Activity	4
		Nutrition	3
Violence	22		
TOTAL	**143**		

Box 22-2. **Summary of Community Organization Models and Adolescent Lifestyles**

- Youth empowerment has been a successful strategy in decreasing adolescent tobacco use in the United States through youth-led coalitions that have fostered meaningful tobacco prevention activities and programs and increased youth civic involvement and leadership and decision-making responsibilities.

- Despite its demonstrated success in reducing adolescent tobacco use, youth empowerment has not been widely explored as a potential strategy to promote delay in sexual initiation, the adoption of safer sex practices, adequate physical activity, and healthier eating patterns among this age group.

- While adolescents may be used as peer educators or outreach agents in the provision of prevention services in sexual and reproductive health promotion programs, they typically are not involved in the assessment and planning phases of these programs.

- Factors that have been associated with successful neighborhood mobilization to prevent adolescent pregnancy include a strong sense of community, consensus on the perceived need for the initiative, support by key organizations, shared leadership, effective group action processes, and a competent staff contingent.

- The evaluation of youth-targeted community organization interventions has been problematic and challenging. Some lessons learned are:

- Communities should keep their goals focused and manageable, with well-defined expected results and appropriate corresponding data for the evaluation process.

- Communities should choose research-based programs and acquire the necessary technical expertise to effectively carry them out.

- Communities may wish to partner with the nearest or most interested university-based research teams or schools of public health, in order to ensure the community's access to best practices and appropriate support in monitoring and evaluating the intervention.

- Communities should also explore the possibility of engaging researchers, community program developers, and local policymakers in the joint research, planning, and evaluation process. This collaborative effort would assure the use of evidence-based interventions adapted to local circumstances and appropriate levels of monitoring and evaluation supervision.

- Community organizing efforts involving local government officials, enforcement agencies, alcohol retailers, the media, schools, and other community groups can be an effective strategy to reduce youth access to alcohol products.

[Chapter Twenty-three]

The Diffusion of Innovations Theory, Behavior Change Communication Models, and Social Marketing

An innovation is the introduction of an idea, practice, method, device, or object that is perceived as being new by an individual, family, organization, community, or even larger group of people. Diffusion is defined as "the process by which an innovation is communicated through certain channels over time among members of a social system" (Rogers 1983). The Diffusion of Innovations Theory addresses how new ideas and practices spread within and between communities.

Within the context of health promotion, innovation presents special challenges, since first the need for it must be demonstrated; then the innovation must be developed and proven to be effective; and finally, ways must be found to widely disseminate information about it and encourage the adoption of its use among the population. Thus, the theory focuses on both the characteristics of the particular innovation and how the innovation will be communicated to its intended audience.

Within the framework of adolescent health and positive behavior change, this chapter will highlight the theory's background and applications, principally within the school and educational environment. It also contains a special section on a representative selection of social marketing techniques and behavior change communication models used to diffuse innovative health messages and promote positive behavior change among young people, both at the individual and community levels.

Following is a summary of key characteristics of innovations, based on the work of Rogers (1995, 1983), which determine if the given innovation will be adopted by new individuals and groups and how quickly this adoption will occur.

- **Characteristics of innovations:**
    - *relative advantages*: the degree to which an innovation is perceived as an improvement over the idea, practice, program, or product it proposes to replace
    - *compatibility*: how consistent the innovation is with the values, habits, experiences, and needs of those to whom it is targeted and who will potentially adopt it
    - *complexity*: how difficult the innovation is to understand and/or adopt
    - *communicability*: the degree of ease with which the proposed innovation may be described to potential adopters so that they may clearly understand the benefits it offers
    - *trialability*: the extent to which the innovation may be experimented with before a commitment to adopt it is required
    - *observability*: the extent to which the innovation provides tangible or visible results readily observable in others who have already adopted it
    - *risk and uncertainty level*: the extent to which the innovation may be adopted with minimal risk and uncertainty
    - *reversibility*: the degree to which the innovation may be reversed or discontinued easily
    - *time required*: an expression of the minimal time investment required to adopt the innovation
    - *commitment*: an expression of the minimal level of commitment required to adopt the innovation
    - *modifiability*: the extent to which the innovation may be modified and/or updated over time
    - *impact on social relations*: an expression of the degree to which adoption of the innovation may have a negative effect on the individual's surrounding social environment
    - *cost-effectiveness*: Although this characteristic is not explicitly mentioned by Rogers, it is nonetheless a key consideration in developing countries wherever and whenever economic resources are relatively scarce.

- **Communication channels**: Diffusion theorists view communication as a two-way process, in which opinion leaders (e.g., public figures well known to the community) mediate the impact of radio, television, newspapers, and other public information sources by emphasizing the value of social networks or interpersonal channels, over and above mass media, when making decisions. The basic premise of this theory, confirmed by empirical research, is that new ideas and practices spread through interpersonal contacts largely consisting of interpersonal communication. These interpersonal networks, then, act as an informal vehicle to accelerate the diffusion of innovations originally presented through the mass media, with the result that the work of the networks and media becomes complementary and mutually reinforcing. One example of this synergy would be the use by public health specialists of both the mass media and community leaders to support and diffuse messages relating to a new smoking cessation program being offered in the community.

The work of Valente and Davis (1999) sheds further light on the use of communication channels in innovations diffusion. The authors propose that using opinion leaders that have been selected by all community members, instead of having them recruited by non-community members or nominated by a few individuals within the community, can accelerate the diffusion of innovations. This selection system ensures the credibility and trustworthiness of the opinion leaders and facilitates more efficient learning because the individuals receive the messages of innovation from community members whom they have chosen as their role models.

The implementation of a structured, well-thought-out program is an essential part of the health promotion process. School programs for the prevention of smoking are ineffective, for example, if teachers do not understand the intrinsic benefit of this innovation and do not properly apply it with their students. On the other hand, underestimating the barriers to diffusion and adoption is one of the principal reasons why innovations are sometimes ineffective. While the need for information about the determinants of individual behavior is commonly accepted, it is hardly recognized that information about the determinants of institutional "behavior" (such as the adoption of a prevention program by organizations) is also needed for the development of successful implementation strategies.

The focus of contemporary research on the diffusion of school health promotion interventions has gradually shifted from the attributes of a particular innovation and the characteristics of the target audience to the planning behavior, thought processes, and actions of the schoolteacher, with regard to the proposed innovation process. This process, as it refers to the educational representative and his/her responsibility of sharing the innovation with the students, involves four subsequent stages: dissemination, adoption, implementation, and continuation. *Dissemination* refers to the transfer of information about the innovation from its developers to its potential users (in this case, teachers). *Adoption* refers to the potential users' intentions to adopt the innovation. *Implementation* refers to the actual use of the innovation. *Continuation* refers to the final stage in which the innovation has become current practice. Patterns of adoption have been described as having a normal, bell-shaped distribution, divided in five categories: innovators, early adopters, early majority adopters, late majority adopters, and laggards (Rogers 1995). As Green, Gottlieb, and Parcel (1987) have noted, special efforts to identify barriers for late adopters would be particularly useful as research continues to unfold in the field of innovations diffusion.

According to Orlandi et al. (1990), many health promotion innovations have failed because of the gap that is frequently left unfilled between the point where innovation development ends and diffusion begins. To bridge this gap, Orlandi and colleagues stress the need for linkage between the *resource system* that develops and promotes the intervention (e.g., the ministry of health's adolescence program) and the *user system* that is supposed to adopt the intervention (e.g., schools, community health centers, sports clubs). Such a liaison group should include representatives of the user system (e.g., school principal, teachers, health professionals, sports coaches, town mayor) and of the resource system (experts who developed the intervention), and a *linkage agent*, or diffusion coordinator, who facilitates the collaboration between user system and resource system. This person or group plays a critical role in providing training, answering questions, and solving problems that may occur during the implementation phase. The essential point is that the diffusion planning process has been developed through cooperation among diverse players, with the goal of improving the fit between innovation and user, of fine-tuning intervention innovations to local realities, of identifying and working to overcome barriers, and of facilitating widespread implementation. In this sense, a strategy to stimulate implementation should be based on a careful analysis of the determinants of implementation behavior, at both the individual and organizational levels.

Box 23-1. The Diffusion of Innovations Theory: Key Theoretical Concepts in the Diffusion of Adolescent Health Promotion and Prevention Programs

characteristics of innovations
- relative advantages
- compatibility with target group
- complexity in adopting
- communicability of features
- trialability before adoption
- observability in others prior to adoption
- risk and uncertainty level
- reversibility
- time required to adopt
- commitment level required
- modifiability
- impact on social relations
- cost-effectiveness

communication channels
- media
- opinion (community) leaders

diffusion stages
- dissemination
- adoption
- implementation
- continuation

patterns of adoption
- innovators
- early adopters
- early majority adopters
- late majority adopters
- laggards

linkage system (liaison group)
- resource system: those who developed the intervention
- user system: those who will adopt the intervention
- linkage agent: person or group which facilitates the partnership between resource system and user system

Diffusion of Innovations through Behavior Change Communication and Social Marketing

During the last decade, particular attention has been placed on the role that social marketing and mass media can have in diffusing innovative health promotion messages among adolescents and youth. Within this context, the concept of *behavior change communication* (BCC) has gained visibility as a particularly appealing and cost-effective vehicle for disseminating innovative ideas and practices to large audiences. According to Family Health International (1996), behavior change communication is "a multi-level tool for promoting and sustaining risk-reducing behavior change in individuals and communities by distributing tailored health messages in a variety of communication channels." This strategy has been used by a variety of agencies (international, national, nongovernmental) as a tool for combating HIV/AIDS in developing countries. A variety of multi-level activities has been implemented across Africa under the rubric of BCC, ranging from HIV/AIDS media campaigns, promoting general awareness through community mobilization activities, and interpersonal/small-group communications, to social marketing of condoms and HIV/STI-related services and supplies. Media advocacy and policy advocacy approaches have also been used. BCC constituted a major component of the global AIDS Control and Prevention (AIDSCAP) Project, funded by the U.S. Agency for International Development from 1991 to 1997. AIDSCAP supported such activities as radio call-in shows, peer education activities, and the production of musical revues and comic book and television serial dramas.

BCC is also included among the technical strategies recommended by the Global AIDS Program (GAP) of the U.S. Centers for Disease Control and Prevention (U.S. Department of Health and Human Services 2001e). For the GAP program, the CDC analyzed the techniques employed by successful BCC campaigns and health behavior change literature and then proposed a series of "best practice" features of BCC:

- The communication should be *personalized*. Successful public health projects, even when applied on a large scale (and perhaps especially so), work best when the public message is reinforced interpersonally and in concert with other services and sectors. Members of target populations will almost always require individualized attention in obtaining general information and attempting to relate it to their unique situations and concerns.
- The messages should be *emotionally compelling*. Communication campaigns and programs that succeed in modifying behaviors appear to do so because they create an emotional stake that motivates the population to act, instead of relying upon a purely cognitive approach.
- The strategy includes a *role models component*. The use of role models is at the heart of many interpersonal communi-

cations and community mobilization activities. From testimonials by persons living with AIDS to peer education strategies, real-life models in the form of peers, friends, family members, and opinion leaders are extremely powerful. Role models are a particularly effective way to motivate individuals to change behavior by increasing their confidence in their ability to change, by persuading them of the positive benefits of change, and by showing them how to change. Thus, the use of role models not only contributes to creating the sort of emotional commitment that can lead to change, but also demonstrates concrete examples of behavior that can be emulated.

- The messages must be *embedded in existing social and cultural norms and expectations*. For information to make sense and be useful to members of the target population, it must be easily integrated into their social expectations, norms, and values, as well as be a part of their popular culture and relevant to their socioeconomic milieu. It must be applicable to people's everyday lives and presented in a narrative form (i.e., storytelling) that is familiar to the target audience.

- There must be *recognition of impediments to and facilitators of new behaviors*. Successful BCC activities recognize the variables in the environment that either impede or facilitate the implementation of desired behaviors. Programs that have the greatest impact are usually linked to specific services or supplies (e.g., provision of condoms, birth control pills) in the community. Where the infrastructure and/or supplies are limited, these conditions should be accurately reflected and compensated for in the program.

The CDC's GAP report (U.S. Department of Health and Human Services 2001e) proposes that the BCC approach that combines these elements most effectively is the "entertainment-education" modalities. These may range from professional to amateur street theater, and from film and popular music to radio and television soap operas. One reason that "entertainment-as-education" is both popular and effective is because it focuses on the emotional as well as cognitive factors that influence behavior, and it is closely aligned with the customs, norms, and narrative forms that are familiar to the target audiences.

One entertainment-education approach that is highlighted in this report as promising, due to its recently demonstrated behavioral impact in Africa, is the use of long-running serialized dramas on radio using a methodology first developed in the 1970s by Mexican theater and television producer Miguel Sabido. An evaluation of a Sabido-based program was conducted in Tanzania (1993–1997), where part of the country did not receive the radio drama *Twer Na Wakati* for the first two years of the program. This two-year period permitted a quasi-controlled study. Listeners in areas receiving the Radio Tanzania broadcast reported increased commitment to use family planning methods and to adopt sexual and reproductive health practices to prevent HIV infection. There was a 153% increase in condom distribution (compared to a 16% increase in the control area) and a 33% increase in new clients at family planning clinics (Vaughan et al. 2000, Rogers et al. 1999). Research has also shown that entertainment-education programming with social change messages is a cost-effective method for reaching large audiences (Singhal and Rogers 1999, Westoff and Bankole 1997).

Social marketing techniques have also been employed, through a variety of media channels, to diffuse new messages and/or programs to adolescents and youth. Social marketing theory predicts that target market members (e.g., adolescents) will voluntarily exchange their resources (e.g., money, time) for a product when they become aware that the innovation offers them attractive benefits at a reasonable cost or price and that it is available at the right place and at the right time.

Despite its demonstrated effectiveness, the use of social marketing techniques, as well as behavior change communication, has at times drawn the attention of critics (Buchanan 2000), principally due to the ethical dilemma they present of imposing or selling an innovation without the voluntary participation of the targeted group. Maibach, Rothschild, and Novelli (2002), for example, argue that several public health specialists, confusing its definition with commercial marketing, have poorly understood the concept of social marketing. In an attempt to rescue social marketing from these criticisms and elevate its role in public health, Maibach and colleagues have extracted from different authors (Rothschild 1999, Andreasen 1995, Kotler and Roberto 1989) a series of concepts considered key in defining social marketing:

- Social marketing's primary objective is to influence the voluntary behavior of target market members (e.g., adolescents and youth).
- Social marketing offers to target market members an attractive package of benefits and reduced barriers to behavior change, in order to enhance the possibilities for the adoption of new and healthier behaviors.
- Social marketing's primary beneficiaries are members of the target market, whereas commercial marketing's primary beneficiaries are those who decide

---

Box 23-2. **Behavior Change Communication: Best Practice Features**
- The communication should be *personalized*.
- The messages should be *emotionally compelling*.
- The strategy includes a *role models component*.
- The messages must be *embedded in existing social and cultural norms and expectations*.
- There must be *recognition of impediments to and facilitators of new behaviors*.

to market the innovation (e.g., product or service).

- Social marketing activities seek to create a voluntary exchange between the marketing organization and members of the target market through mutual fulfillment of self-interest (e.g., participation in campaigns promoting safer sex practices that contain appealing messages and offer youth opportunities to participate in interesting campaign activities with their friends).

Research and Evidence of Practical Applications of the Diffusion of Innovations Theory, Behavior Change Communication Models, and Social Marketing to Adolescent Lifestyles

The Diffusion of Innovations Theory holds great potential in helping to scale up effective interventions that promote the adoption of healthy behaviors or change of risk behaviors among adolescents in a variety of settings, including schools, community organizations, and sports clubs.

One of the best examples found of research projects in the diffusion of innovations is the implementation of "Smart Choices," a smoking prevention program for adolescents in which more than 100 Texas school districts participated (Parcel et al. 1989). The Smart Choices local implementation strategies followed these four phases:

Dissemination: The objectives were for teachers and administrators to indicate their awareness of the program, to view the program favorably, and to discuss the program with other colleagues participating in the innovation process.

Adoption: The objectives were that school districts would see the advantages of the program in terms of outcomes, expectancies, and social reinforcements. The determinants study showed that the most powerful incentives were making a difference in the lives of students and complying with the essential instructional elements mandated by the Texas educational system.

Implementation: The objectives were that the participating teachers possessed the necessary skills and self-efficacy to use the program with acceptable proficiency, completeness, and fidelity.

Continuation: The objectives were that teachers and administrators would have experienced positive feedback and reinforcement on the use of the program after one year and would continue using it.

An evaluation of the adoption phase (Parcel et al. 1995b) showed the expected results. In the intervention group, 56.3% of the districts adopted the Smart Choices program, while in the comparison group only 10.5% adopted the program. Stepwise logistic regression indicated that the variables most closely related to adoption among intervention districts were teacher attitudes towards the innovation and organizational considerations of administrators. In the evaluation of the implementation phase, two strategies were compared: live workshop training and video training.

The results showed that a lower proportion of video-trained teachers implemented the program (video training: 78.9%; live workshop training: 97.4%).

The Diffusion of Innovations Theory was also employed in Texas to plan the dissemination and adoption phases of the Child and Adolescent Trial for Cardiovascular Health (CATCH) health promotion project among elementary schools (Hoelscher et al. 2001). The project was designed to decrease saturated fat and sodium levels, increase physical activity, and prevent tobacco use among preadolescent-age children. Its effectiveness had been previously demonstrated among 5,106 elementary schoolchildren ages 9–11 in California, Louisiana, Minnesota, and Texas (Luepker et al. 1996), and the behavioral changes resulting from the project were shown to persist three years later into the study group's early and middle adolescent years (Nader et al. 1999).

During the CATCH dissemination stage in Texas, the project's earlier successes and its state-of-the-art design were highlighted in order to emphasize the innovation's relative advantage over other initiatives that had been tested in the past. Developing teacher-friendly materials minimized the complexity involved in adopting the program. Networking and the forming of partnerships were crucial to project implementation, as were the participation and support of local decision-makers. Yet the scaling up of projects of this nature takes time, careful planning, and persistence, as was shown in this particular case, where only 24% of schools in Texas had adopted the intervention during its first two years of dissemination.

The El Paso del Norte Health Foundation also chose CATCH as its first community-wide preventive health initiative for the El Paso, Texas/Juárez, Mexico border area. This predominantly Hispanic, low-income border community has actively embraced the El Paso CATCH program, with 108 elementary schools from New Mexico to West Central Texas (Heath and Coleman 2003) agreeing to participate in the initiative, illustrating the potential of diffusion projects of this type to scale up over time.

One research study conducted in Europe has yielded important results regarding the role of teacher attitudes and behavior in the diffusion of new health promotion curricula. Paulussen and colleagues (1995, 1994) have described the steps involved in the diffusion and implementation of AIDS prevention programs in Dutch schools. They identified the steps leading from the initial development of the innovation to an increase in teachers' awareness and knowledge and to the uptake and implementation of four nationally disseminated AIDS curricula. An extended model of planned behavior (see Chapter Eleven), the *attitude/social influence/self-efficacy* model, was used as an organizing schema for a questionnaire addressing teachers' social and psychological disposition towards the AIDS curricula innovation and decision-making. When the extent of diffusion of classroom AIDS education was examined, the rates were similar to those reported for most externally developed curricula, indicating that around 50% of teachers generally receive the curricula, while only 25% actively take notice of the curricula content, and only 5%–10% use the curricula in one way or another (Paulussen 1994).

The different steps involved in the diffusion and implementation of the AIDS prevention programs in Dutch schools were determined by two principal factors. First of all, the diffusion of the curricula through teachers' networks within the participating schools mainly determined the extent of knowledge acquisition by the individual teachers about the programs. Secondly, the teachers' intentions to provide AIDS education in general were mainly determined by:

- subjective norms (i.e., the teachers' perceptions of how others felt about the program, especially students, other colleagues, and the school's principal);
- self-efficacy;
- personal moral beliefs about sexuality issues in general;
- sense of professional responsibility;
- frequency of interaction with other colleagues about HIV instruction; and
- the presence of a formal school policy concerning AIDS education.

In another study based on the Diffusion of Innovations Theory framework, Hallfors and Godette (2002) examined the adoption and implementation of the U.S. Department of Education's new policy, the "Principles of Effectiveness," regarding the governmental requirement to select research-based programs for school health prevention initiatives. Results from a sample of 104 school districts in 12 states indicated that only 19% of the schools were implementing a research-based curriculum with fidelity. Common problems identified included the lack of teacher training and of the requisite materials; use of some, but not all, of the required lessons and teaching strategies; and failure to deliver lessons to age-appropriate student groups. The authors concluded that low levels of funding, inadequate infrastructure, decentralized decision-making, and the lack of adequate program guidance contributed to the slow progress in improving school-based prevention practices.

A study by Buston and colleagues (2002) also concluded that interventions are unlikely to achieve their desired aims unless they are implemented as intended. These authors analyzed the factors that impeded and facilitated the implementation of a specially designed sexual education program in Scotland. The analysis revealed that program implementation was negatively affected by competition for curriculum time; brevity of lessons; the assignation of low priority to implementation by school managers, particularly in relation to time-tabling; and teachers' limited experience and ability in the use of role-playing. The nature of the adoption process, staff absence and turnover, lack of theoretical understanding of the package, and commitment to the research were also factors influencing the extent of implementation within and across schools. The authors recommend that health promotion program managers take these lessons learned into account when designing and implementing teacher-delivered, school-based health promotion initiatives.

Behavior Change Communication, Social Marketing, and Adolescent Lifestyles

To date, one of the most innovative behavior change communication initiatives targeting young people is *loveLife*, a multimedia communications strategy developed in South Africa which includes advertising on the Internet, television, radio, billboards, taxis, and in print materials and uses behavior change as the cornerstone of HIV prevention. Launched in September 1999, *loveLife*'s design responds to the fact that risky sexual behavior among teenagers is currently driving the HIV epidemic in this country. Since the highest rates of new infection occur in late adolescence and early adulthood, the initiative targets principally youth ages 12 to 17. Major predictors of high-risk sexual behavior in this age group are coercion, peer pressure, transactional sex, and abdication of sexual responsibility by boys.

loveLife combines its high-profile multimedia approach with institutional support from government authorities, health services delivery, and community outreach with the goal of creating a new vision for youth in which they come to associate the lifestyles depicted in *loveLife*'s messages with healthy and positive behavioral changes they can achieve in their own lives. The content of communication is framed by three values: informed choice, shared responsibility, and safe sexual practices. Since its launch, *loveLife* "branding" has positioned itself as part of South African popular youth culture by focusing on sensitive issues related to sex, sexuality, and gender inequities, while at the same time rapidly transcending the boundaries that would narrowly define it as an HIV prevention initiative (*loveLife* 2002).

loveLife has significant public and political support. Public approval ratings are around 85–90%. Political support is expressed through a formal public-private financing partnership between the South African Government and the Henry J. Kaiser Family Foundation. In addition to the above, considerable funding has been received from the Bill and Melinda Gates Foundation and UNICEF. *loveLife*'s current budget is estimated at US$ 3.33 per capita in the country's 12- to 17-year-old population segment.

Although young people in South Africa exposed to *loveLife* programming reported significant behavior change by the end of year two (*loveLife* 2002), the multimedia initiative has not been able to reach young people living in extreme poverty with the same positive results.

A number of initiatives are currently underway to address this obstacle, such as the expansion of *loveLife* Y-Centres in poor peri-urban and rural communities that are supported by mobile outreach programs with regular radio broadcasts. The Y-Centres combine educational skills development, such as computer literacy, personal motivation and leadership training, and communications and broadcast skills, with popular sports such as basketball and volleyball. All Y-Centres include a fully equipped sexual health clinic providing clinical and counseling services in a nonclinical setting.

Another innovative BCC project in South Africa targeting young adolescents is Soul Buddyz (The Communication Initiative 2003). The project was launched in 1999 as a way to build on the success of the Soul City multimedia series, which debuted in 1992 and targeted its health and development issues to the general public. Soul Buddyz is best described as an "edutainment" vehicle conceived to promote good health among children ages 8–12. Its developers note that all the issues dealt with in the series (e.g., HIV/AIDS, sexuality, nutrition, road safety, disability, gender equality, bullying, and conflict resolution) are framed within the U.N. Convention on the Rights of the Child (see Chapter Five of this book). At the same time, the series highlights a number of underlying issues, including children's rights and responsibilities, respect for and sensitivity toward cultural differences, role-modeling good behavior towards others, and the need for children to view themselves as proactive, valuable, and productive members of the community. The communications media employed include a 26-part television drama series representing "children from all walks of life ... who form a bond" and depicting "issues that children are facing every day of their lives" and a half-hour-long radio program consisting of 10-minute dramas with young actors, a five-minute documentary insert for adults and children, and 15 minutes of interactive talk with the audience hosted by a young person. In addition, a life skills booklet has been designed for use by seventh-grade students, a parenting booklet has been distributed as a newspaper supplement, and children have taken the initiative to form their own Soul Buddyz clubs. Based in schools and libraries across South Africa, these clubs have served as a platform where the children may acquire additional knowledge and skills related to health issues and "be empowered to realize and voice their rights, needs, and interests and interact with peers on an educational and recreational level" (The Communication Initiative 2003).

While behavior change communication initiatives geared toward adolescents have primarily taken place in Africa, social marketing has led to several media campaigns in Europe and the United States. Kennedy and colleagues (2000) evaluated a multimodal social marketing intervention aimed at reducing HIV infection among adolescents in California. Condom use at last sex with a principal partner was associated with the number of channels through which an adolescent had been exposed to the intervention, with a significant increase in the proportion of adolescents using condoms (4.3%) during a one-year intervention. Penfold and Kirkman (2002) also used the social marketing of condoms to develop an innovative national pilot project in the United Kingdom. The design of the intervention involved selling packets of three condoms each at an affordable price through strategically placed vending machines throughout Manchester. In marketing these condoms, the intervention designers decided to partner with Galaxy 102, Manchester's leading youth-focused commercial radio station, and branded the condoms as a Galaxy product. Evaluation of the Manchester intervention's success is currently underway.

Media campaigns have also focused on improving anti-smoking advertising directed toward young people. Florida's "truth" campaign is an excellent example of a counter-marketing, anti-tobacco youth-driven media campaign. Zucker et al. (2000) describe that the campaign has been associated with a 92% brand awareness rate among teens, a 15% rise in adolescents who agree with key attitudinal statements about smoking, a 19.4% decline in smoking among middle adolescents, and an 8% decline among late adolescents. Wakefield and colleagues (2003), after conducting a comprehensive review of the published literature on the effects of anti-smoking advertising on youth smoking, concluded that these campaigns appear to have more reliable positive effects among pre- and early adolescents by preventing smoking initiation. These authors highlight, however, that family and peer interactions can play a crucial role in reinforcing, denying, or neutralizing the potential effects of anti-smoking campaigns, and they warn against isolated anti-smoking campaigns that are not enhanced by the use of other tobacco control strategies.

Diffusion of innovations, behavior change communication, and social marketing are complementary theories and models which serve as instruments to reach different population levels, through various channels, with the unifying goal of scaling up effective adolescent health promotion and prevention interventions. Table 23-1. presents a breakdown of the number of studies found using the Diffusion of Innovations Theory, behavior change communication, and social marketing according to adolescent health behaviors.

As seen in Table 23-1., the diffusion of health messages has mainly focused on the prevention of tobacco, alcohol, and drug use, followed by the promotion of safer sex practices among adolescents. Table 23-2. presents a further breakdown of the results in Table 23-1. by comparing the research and evidence published using the Diffusion of Innovations Theory with that available utilizing behavior change com-

Table 23-1. **Most Commonly Researched Adolescent Behaviors Using the Diffusion of Innovations Theory (DIT), Behavior Change Communication Models (BCC), and Social Marketing Techniques (SM)**

ADOLESCENT BEHAVIORS	NUMBER OF ARTICLES USING THE DIT, BCC, AND SM	NUMBER OF ARTICLES BY KEYWORDS	
Sexual and Reproductive Health	39	Teen Pregnancy	3
		HIV/AIDS	24
		STIs	5
		Condom Use	17
Tobacco, Alcohol, and Drug Use	54	Tobacco	39
		Alcohol	11
		Drugs	8
Physical Activity and Nutrition	10	Obesity	2
		Physical Activity	7
		Nutrition	7
Violence	2		
TOTAL	**105**		

munication models and social marketing techniques.

The Diffusion of Innovations Theory has primarily been used to date to introduce and scale up adolescent health promotion and prevention programs as part of a school health curriculum. Initially this strategy showed great promise within the context of adolescent health and the promotion of positive behavior change, because its design allows for large populations of adolescents to be reached simultaneously and interventions to be delivered in a setting where this group spends a significant amount of time—the

Table 23-2. **Most Commonly Researched Adolescent Behaviors Using Diffusion of Innovations Theory Compared to Social Marketing and Behavior Change Communication**

ADOLESCENT BEHAVIORS	NUMBER OF ARTICLES USING DIT	NUMBER OF ARTICLES USING SM AND BCC	TOTAL
Sexual and Reproductive Health	8	31	39
Tobacco, Alcohol, and Drug Use	13	41	54
Physical Activity and Nutrition	4	6	10
Violence	0	2	2
TOTAL	**25**	**80**	**105**

school classroom. Yet as we have seen in this chapter, the adoption and implementation of health promotion curricula by schoolteachers have presented challenges of their own. This is particularly the case for sexual education, where personal beliefs may interfere with the fidelity of the curricula implementation.

In contrast to this approach, behavior change communication and social marketing have been widely used to diffuse health messages through multimedia channels that young people find appealing and to which they often turn as a source for reliable information and entertainment. As seen in Table 23-2., BCC- and social marketing-based adolescent health initiatives have also generated more interest in the research community and have been far more studied than their primarily school-based innovations diffusion counterparts.

Although BCC and social marketing might appear to be more attractive strategies to use in scaling up health behavior messages directed toward adolescents, it is important to not confuse these strategies with the channels (e.g., media) or settings (e.g., schools) that are used most commonly to introduce the innovative messages. As noted in this chapter, the Diffusion of Innovations Theory, behavior change communication models, and social marketing techniques are all complementary constructs used to reach large populations of adolescents, with a variety of channels and settings options available to program developers.

It is interesting to further note that some of the key characteristics of innovations in the Diffusion of Innovations Theory, such as the innovation's relative advantages, compatibility, complexity, trialability, and observability, have been successfully applied to social marketing strategies. On the other hand, while entertainment-education interventions with social change messages have been shown to be effective, this approach has yet to be introduced in any significant way in the school setting, even though adolescents often tend to complain about the lack of novelty and creativity in traditional educational approaches.

To date, no magic bullet has emerged that clearly demonstrates its effectiveness in reaching a wide range of adolescents, which may consist of different age groups, genders, and cultures, through the use of only one strategy applied in one setting. There are indications, however, based on the research findings discussed in this chapter, that a more synergistic approach—one which integrates effective multimedia social campaigns with the scaling up of evidence-based interventions in the school environment and at the community level—holds promise as a possible best practice for the future.

Models that Promote Change at the Policy Level

The World Health Organization defines *policy* as a written "expression of goals for improving the health situation, the priorities among these goals, and the main directions for attaining them" (World Health Organization 1986). Widely defined, policy is a statement of aims and ideals or a guide for the achievement of goals (Rodríguez-García et al. 1999). Health care policy, then, may be seen as a network of interrelated decisions, which together form an approach or strategy in response to practical issues concerning the provision of quality health care to all members of the community. Policies are expressed in a body of practices, statements, regulations, and laws (Barker 1996). A policy statement only acquires true significance, however, if it is put into action. Policies are a way of addressing the broader social, economic, and environmental determinants of health.

Health policy may be approached from different perspectives. For an economist, health policy will be seen as actions to optimize the allocation of scarce resources. From a clinical physician's point of view, improving the quality of health services will be of vital importance. From a public health perspective, the development of health promotion strategies—to *prevent* poor health to the greatest degree possible—will be paramount. And in the specific case of adolescents, the focus will be to forge health-promoting lifestyle policies that include opportunities for adopting health-promoting behaviors and that ensure protections against adopting health-compromising behaviors, utilizing a comprehensive approach that goes beyond the health sector to include public and private partners, such as schools, churches, commercial advertisers and services, the mass media, and families. In an ideal scenario, mutually reinforcing policies of this type will be in place at all levels—institutional, community, national, and even international.

As has already been pointed out in this book, adolescence is a singularly pivotal period of life in which increasing autonomy and exposure to risk are approaching the crossroads of discovery, opportunity, and decision-making. On the one hand, the adolescent enjoys decreasing adult supervision, while on the other, he/she may still possess insufficient instruments (social, emotional, and cognitive skills and economic resources) to effectively manage and overcome the numerous risks faced.

The World Bank's Social Risk Management framework for social protection (Holzmann and Jorgensen 2000) proposes that all individuals, households, and communities are vulnerable to multiple risks from different sources, whether they are natural (e.g., earthquakes, hurricanes, floods) or man-made (e.g., those related to industrialization, urbanization, social unrest, civil war, etc.). The framework also states that poverty relates to vulnerability since the poor are typically more exposed to risk, and they have a more limited access to appropriate risk management instruments than less disadvantaged groups. This framework considers that the best social risk management is to take the needed steps to ensure that the risk does not occur at all. One of the roles of international governments in the Social Risk Management framework, then, is to implement appropriate policy actions for risk prevention (Holzmann and Jorgensen 2000). The framework also identifies empowerment, capacity-building, and increased opportunities for socioeconomic stability as crucial for poverty reduction.

Adolescents who are still growing and developing are in particular need of social protection, in the form of public interventions designed to assist them to better manage risk, take advantage of opportunities for self-improvement, master the necessary skills and assets to achieve their self-set goals, and express their needs and wants through positive and healthy channels.

The next chapter will present various models for policy and legislation development that can guide program developers in designing more effective policies for promoting healthy lifestyles among adolescents.

[Chapter Twenty-four]

Models of Policy and Legislation Development

A policy is a framework that guides decision-making in an organization or government and is usually expressed in a statement of intended actions. Policies may be general statements regarding national or organizational priorities, written regulations, guidelines, procedures, and/or standards to be achieved. Alternatively, they may be informal (i.e., unwritten) but widely recognized practices (Family Health International 1996). Usually, the creation of new policies (e.g., regarding community health) does not occur in a vacuum, but instead within established networks of interrelated decisions that together form an integral approach or strategy in relation to practical issues regarding health care delivery (Barker 1996).

Carol Barker, along with numerous other colleagues, has described the process of policy-making as a specific sequence of events. The stages of this process are shown in Figure 24-1.

However, Barker's work presents a caveat about such a stylized and vertical configuration, because it gives the false impression that policy-making is always within the full control of the policymaker, involving no outside interests or agendas. She emphasizes that public policies address complex realities, and, on the one hand, the process needs to be conducted in a style that emphasizes flexibility, responsiveness, accountability, transparency, and broad participation. On the other hand, by virtue of the presence of these elements, a policymaker's freedom to act will be constrained at various different stages

Figure 24-1. **Stages in the Policy-Making Process**

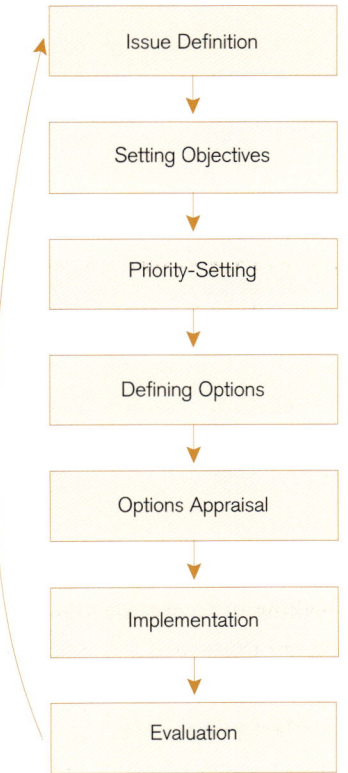

Source: *The Health Care Policy Process*, by C. Barker. Reprinted by permission of Sage Publications, Ltd. ©1996.

during the policy-making process. It is also a fact that policies are made by politicians and people who hold positions of authority. Gill Walt (1994) declares that although health policy is concerned with *content*, health policy is really about *process* and *power*. She proposes that policy development is ultimately determined by who influences whom in the making of policy, and how this comes about. There are different theories about the roles of power and influence in policy-making:

- *pluralist view*: Power is unequally distributed and shifts between different individuals, interest groups, and pressure groups.
- *elite view*: Power is in the hands of small networks of elites who are powerful because of their economic wealth and social position.
- *Marxist approach*: Power is understood in relationship to the ownership of the means of producing and distributing goods and services.
- *structuralist approach*: Power is understood to be organized into various structural groups in which distinctions are made among dominant interest groups, challenging interest groups, and repressed interest groups. The dominant interest groups are those who are basically content with the status quo and whose interests are being well served by the way in which their sector is currently structured within an organization or government. Challenging interest groups are those who are less content with the status quo and who feel that their interests would be better served by structural change. The repressed interest groups are those who are least content with the current situation and conditions and who feel that their interests are not being well served at all within current structures.

Each of the above approaches may contribute to the process of policy-making, and the power influence will depend upon the type of policy that is being decided upon.

Policy Categories and Levels

Policies may be differentiated between *macro policies* (high political issues) and *micro policies* (low political issues) (Walt 1994, Evans and Newnham 1992).

- *Macro policies* affect everyone; they involve or reflect long-term objectives of the State or of those in power (e.g., major economic decisions, perceived national security crises). These policies are usually formulated by the government and are passed into law through the legislative branch. Government leaders are likely to discuss them only with groups considered important to the nation's economic and political security, and the policy process is likely to be relatively closed. The macro policy process may be considered to be elitist.
- *Micro policies* involve more localized, sectoral interests. These low politics are usually placed in the hands of the department in charge of the sectoral issue (e.g., the ministry of health) and are not considered by the government as a whole. Sectoral policies may be communicated through institutional statements, memoranda, letters, or circulars rather than through formal legislation. The policy process may be much more open to groups with special interests, including nongovernment organizations; professional, community, and advocacy groups; and the church. These groups may have considerable access to government and may be extended opportunities to influence policy. Low political issues can shift and become high political issues over time. The micro policy process may be considered to be more pluralist.

Health policies usually fall into the micro policy category, which does not mean that health policies are always noncontroversial or low political issues. Mass marketing of condoms and sexual education for adolescents, for example, often elicit impassioned public debate and discussion emanating from different sectors of society with varying interests and values. Nevertheless, it is interesting to point out that the Social Risk Management framework for social protection described in the introductory section to this chapter categorizes the AIDS epidemic as a type of high political issue requiring the development of a macro policy, given the level of risk it presents at all levels of society everywhere. The framework calls for the creation of publicly mandated or provided arrangements that would become the principal instruments of risk management strategies.

Policymakers will need to recognize, however, that even seemingly commonplace sectoral policies are very often based on networks of decisions that are interwoven with other high political issues. Frenk (1994) describes four operational levels of health policy:

- *The systemic level* deals with main features that shape the health system over-

all (e.g., the nature of public institutions involved in health care, the public/private mix, and the relationship between health and other sectors).
- *The programmatic level* decides on the priorities for health care, the actual nature of health care programs, and the way in which resources will be allocated.
- *The organizational level* addresses the way in which resources may be used most productively to provide high quality service.
- *The instrumental level* is the one at which various types of technical expertise and instruments of good organization, such as the systems for human resources development and information collection, are managed.

The type of policies developed at the programmatic, organizational, and instrumental levels will depend on the nature of systemic level policy-making, which may also be considered to be of the high political or macro category.

Policy Agenda-Setting Models

Theorists also have examined how an issue is placed on the *policy agenda*. Following is a discussion of several different theoretical models and constructs that explain this process.

- **The Hall Model:** This model (Hall et al. 1975) suggests that an issue becomes part of the policy agenda only when it has high *legitimacy*, *feasibility*, and *support*. Legitimacy refers to those issues in which governments feel most people will accept State intervention. As Walt (1994) explains in her book *Health Policy: An Introduction to Process and Power*, some evidence-based issues have a low-legitimacy public profile because of a protracted ideological debate about the boundaries between individual freedom and the right of the State to restrain that freedom. For example, policies to protect adolescents from certain health-compromising behaviors such as tobacco use have low legitimacy in several Latin American countries, where the prerogative of individual freedom still prevails over public health concerns despite overwhelming scientific evidence in support of the proposed policy.

Feasibility refers to the potential for implementing the policy. This will depend on the technical and theoretical evidence, financial and other resources, availability of skilled personnel, capability of administrative structures, and existence of necessary infrastructure. As we saw in Chapter Twenty-three, research has shown that teacher-delivered, school-based sexual education initiatives have low feasibility of being implemented (Buston et al. 2002, Hallfors and Godette 2002) due to lack of proper teacher training, insufficient funding levels, and inadequate infrastructure, among other factors.

Support refers to public support, in the sense of powerful and highly visible interest groups providing strong support for, or resistance against, a specific policy issue. Governments may successfully challenge important interest groups such as the church, but only if they have secured sufficient support among other high-profile interest groups. Advocacy movements play a key role in supporting health-promoting policies for adolescents (e.g., smoke-free schools, drug-free zones, violence prevention in schools, sexual education, and access to condoms and contraceptives).

- **The Policy Windows Theory:** Kingdon (1995) states that governments pay attention to policies only when a major window of opportunity opens up simultaneously in each of three "streams": the problem, the politics, and the policy. The role of the policy advocate is to create, monitor, and capitalize on these opportunities. This theory is also known as the *Kingdon Model*.

The *problem stream* refers to the issues that capture government officials' attention at a given point in time. This might happen because of a generalized increase in prevalence of a specific social problem (e.g., teen pregnancy), news of high local impact (e.g., children dying from alcohol intoxication), or even a personal experience (e.g., a family member or close relative unexpectedly commits suicide). Policymakers will only identify an existing condition as a problem when they feel (or others convince them to feel) that something needs to be changed.

The *politics stream* refers to the participation of visible organized groups, who highlight a specific problem and manipulate the mass media to focus attention on it, and of much less visible groups of specialists, who work towards proposing alternative options for solving the problem at hand (e.g., academics, researchers, consultants). The politics stream will be affected by political party platforms, elections, changes in administration, and national mood regarding the role of government.

The *policy stream* selects the proposals resulting from the previous streams that have technical feasibility, congruence with existing values, public acceptability, politicians' receptivity, and no significant financial restraints. Kingdon argues that although policies might be developed in stages (such as those described by Barker and shown in Figure 24-1.), the policies might be advocated for long periods before the opportunity appears for their acceptance.

- **The Agenda-Building Theory:** Cobb and Elder (1983) have described three models for agenda-building: the outside-initiative model, in which the public supports an issue that requires action from the government; the inside-initiative model, in which the government takes the lead in supporting an issue; and the mobilization model, in which the government proposes a policy and seeks public support for its successful implementation. According to Cobb and Elder, media attention and the support of opinion and political leaders are essential to place an issue on the policy agenda.

- ***Media advocacy:*** Wallach and colleagues (1993) have proposed a media advocacy framework that may be used by community groups to influence policy. The authors describe three steps of media advocacy: setting the agenda, shaping the debate, and moving forward the policy by suggesting solutions and placing pressure on policymakers.

The Ontario Public Health Association published *Making a Difference in Your Community: A Guide for Policy Change* (Danaher and Kato 1995), which includes a Policy Development Model, an adaptation of which is shown in Figure 24-2. The figure depicts the previously-mentioned stages in Barker's policy-making process but also incorporates aspects such as assessing feasibility, legitimacy, and support from the Hall model.

The Web page of The Health Communication Unit (THCU) of the University of Toronto's Centre for Health Promotion (http://www.thcu.ca/infoandresources.htm) also offers practical materials (publications, workshop slides and workbooks, and other print and electronic resources) that can provide guidance to program developers as they advocate for health-promoting policies. "Policies define and support particular values and behaviors," the THCU emphasizes in the site's policy development section. "If implemented well, policy can profoundly influence the way people live and the choices that they make. In terms of health promotion, policies should make healthier choices easier and unhealthy ones more difficult."

Effective communication within and between social networks is essential for successful legislative and policy formulation and implementation. This ranges from face-to-face or small group level to media-based communication. Short advocacy statements and fact sheets are other tools that program developers may use to guide their public actions in support of policies, laws, and programs that will facilitate the adoption of health-promoting lifestyles among adolescents (Rodríguez-García et al. 1999).

Policy Implementation and Legislation Development

The Pan American Health Organization (PAHO) promotes the use of risk assessment and risk management to guide its technical cooperation activities in the Region of the Americas and works with its Member Governments to increase institutional capacity for the management of health risks. One of the Organization's principal focuses in risk management has been tobacco use prevention. Aware that a policy statement regarding health risks acquires real significance only if it is implemented through legislation, PAHO has published a series of guidelines in which legislation is described as an evolving process that consists of three basic phases: development, implementation, and enforcement (Pan American Health Organiza-

Figure 24-2. **The Policy Development Model**

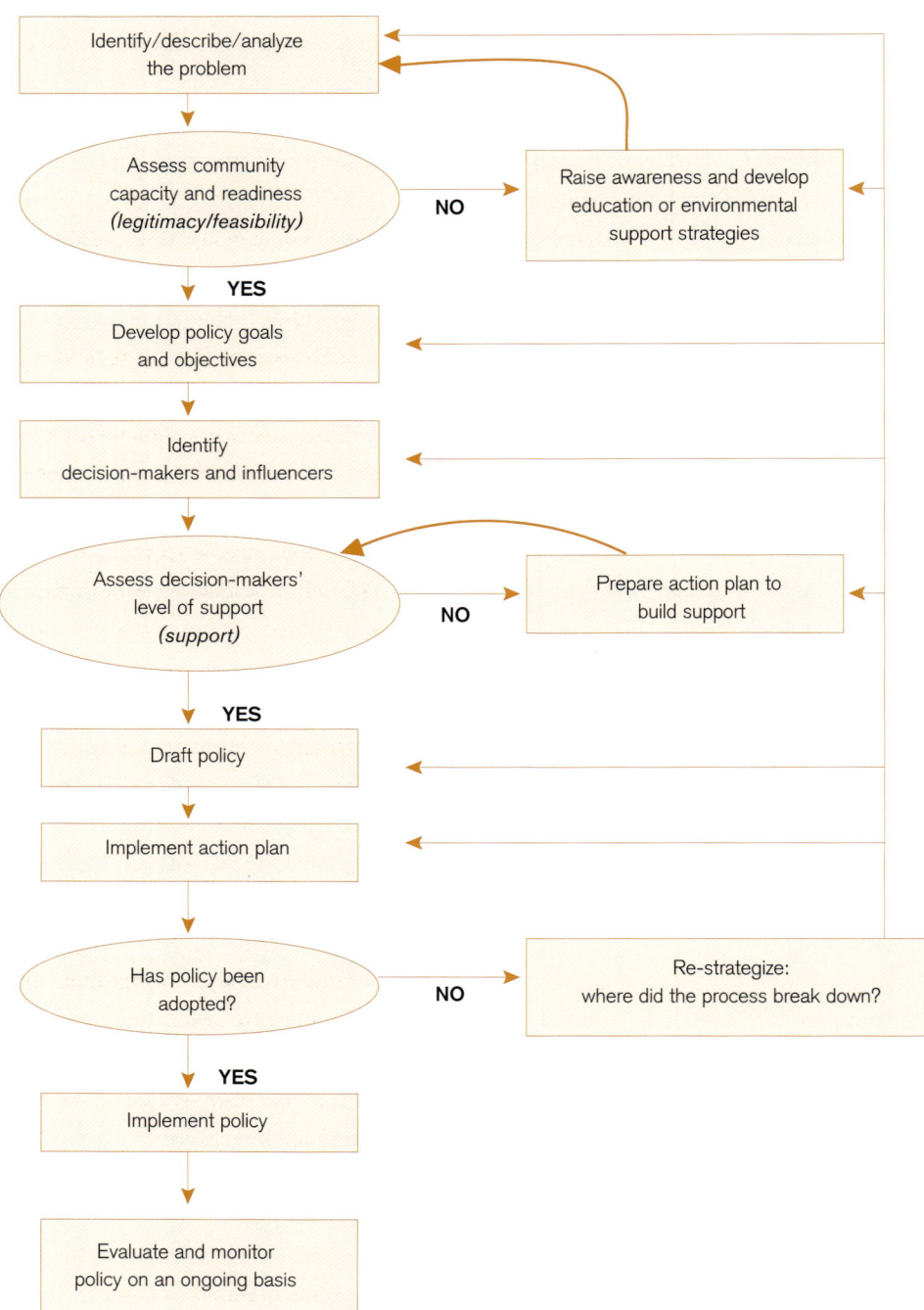

Source: adapted from the THCU Roadmap for Policy Development, The Health Communication Unit, Centre for Health Promotion, University of Toronto, 2004.

tion 2002a). The guidelines describe various factors that need to be considered while preparing the law's specific content:

- *the broader goals of a country's tobacco use reduction strategy*
  This is considered to be the most important of the factors, since it defines the country goals and the role of legislation/regulation in achieving those goals.
- *scientific evidence*
  Focusing on empirical, scientifically validated evidence of "what works" is the most effective way to reduce tobacco use and should guide any tobacco control strategy. This type of foundation will not only ensure effectiveness in achieving the desired results, but also ensures that the law is defensible in the judicial system if the tobacco industry challenges the law on constitutional or other grounds.
- *human or consumer rights perspective*
  Any tobacco control legislation should include provisions to protect human or consumers' rights (e.g., the right to be informed about the ingredients of tobacco products and their harmful effects on health, the right to be protected from second-hand smoke).

Additionally, the PAHO guidelines describe several other steps to be considered during the legislation development phase:

- *consulting experts* to ensure compatibility with constitutional requirements and other relevant national laws;
- *directly addressing the public*, which helps build support, and similarly,
- *creating a communications strategy* with fact-based, positive, and persuasive messages; and
- *anticipating and developing an effective response to industry or other groups' opposition* (e.g., "the proposal won't work," "it will harm the economy/business community/religious community," "implementation is not possible within the proposed time frame").

These factors should be taken into account not only when developing tobacco control legislation, but also when formulating nearly any type of health promotion legislation for adolescents (e.g., marketing and sale of alcohol and tobacco products to minors, treatment of teen driving-while-intoxicated violations, gun control legislation, availability of contraceptives and condoms in youth-friendly health services). Bartholomew and colleagues (2001) describe several legal and economic policy instruments, including direct spending (e.g., grants, contracts, production of goods and services), regulation and monitoring (e.g., minimum age for a behavior, fines), and fiscal incentives (e.g., subsidies, taxation, and tax deductions), that may be incorporated into health promotion legislation.

Research and Evidence of Practical Applications of Policies and Legislation Development to Adolescent Lifestyles

According to research studies conducted in the United States, the two policy and legislative actions that have had the most decisive and immediate effects on preventing youth smoking are the establishment of smoke-free environments and cigarette tax increases (U.S. Department of Health and Human Services 2000). Existing literature suggests that a 10% increase in cigarette taxes leads to approximately a 1%–4% decline in adult smoking and that teenagers are more susceptible than adults to the economic pressures caused by taxation (Glied 2003, Lantz et al. 2000).

There is also research evidence suggesting that higher cigarette taxes decrease the intensity of marijuana use. According to Farrely and colleagues (2001), a 10% increase in cigarette prices would lead to a 5.4% decrease in total marijuana use, and this effect would be greater among males, where a 10% increase in cigarette taxes would lead to a 10% decrease in total marijuana demand. However, Emery, White, and Pierce (2001) found that price is not significantly associated with tobacco experimentation, although it is an important factor for more advanced smoking behavior among adolescents. Experimenters consume only sporadically and very few cigarettes, frequently obtaining them from friends. Price becomes relevant only when teens begin smoking enough to buy their own cigarettes. Sherry Glied (2003), on the other hand, worries that higher taxes only delay smoking initiation without having a significant reduction in prevalence rates through adulthood. She suggests that efforts to reduce smoking among teens need to be continued into adulthood, thereby also promoting adult cessation rather than simply focusing on adolescent initiation.

Levy, Cummings, and Hyland (2000) developed a simulation model that supports Glied's argument. The model predicts that even if tobacco policies eliminate youth initiation, the number of smokers would not be halved for more than 30 years, reinforcing the need for more balanced policies that also increase cessation rates. Lantz and colleagues (2000) conducted a comprehensive review of policies aimed at reducing youth cigarette smoking in the United States. Based on the evidence found, the authors recommend an aggressive approach to changing the social context of smoking, which would include decreasing the number of smoking adult role models by emphasizing adult smoking cessation policies and expanding state and local clean indoor air laws. They also highlight the need to accelerate the development and implementation of adolescent smoking cessation programs.

Policies aimed at reducing youth access to tobacco do not show strong evidence of effectiveness. Fichtenberg and Glantz (2002) conducted a rigorous meta-analysis of nine controlled studies on this topic and found that there was no evidence that an increase in compliance with youth access restrictions was associated with a decrease in youth smoking prevalence. The authors even suggest that this type of policy has had two negative effects: first, that it has created an opportunity for the tobacco industry to build coalitions with local merchants; and secondly, that it has reinforced the tobacco industry's central marketing message that smoking can be attractive to adolescents since it makes them appear to be more adult. Non-retail sources, such as purchasing from older peers or through black markets, borrowing from parents or siblings, and stealing, usually increase as retail access is reduced (Levy and Friend 2000). Furthermore, adolescents are generally familiar with laws and rules about access and possession for minors, but consider them ineffective (Crawford et al. 2002). On the other hand, strong local restaurant smoking regulations have been associated with reduced environmental tobacco smoke exposure among youth (Siegel et al. 2004). While this finding does not address active behavior change on the part of adolescents themselves, it does suggest that the existence of strong smoking restrictions in restaurants and other public places contributes to the subliminal "denormalization" of smoking and of its perception as an accepted and widespread behavioral norm.

Not surprisingly, tobacco advertising increases tobacco consumption (Saffer and Chaloupka 2000). A significant portion of youth experimentation with smoking can be attributed to tobacco marketing campaigns and promotional activities, such as give-aways of free tobacco samples, clothing, sporting equipment, and paraphernalia for outdoor activities (Pierce et al. 1998, Altman et al. 1996). Smoking initiation among adolescent girls has been associated with target advertising towards women (Pierce, Lee, and Gilpin 1994). Saffer and Chaloupka (2000) provided empirical evidence of the effect of tobacco advertising bans in 22 countries. The results showed that comprehensive bans can reduce tobacco consumption by approximately 6%, but a limited set of advertising bans will have little or no effect, only resulting in substitution by the tobacco industry in the remaining non-banned media.

Crawford and colleagues (2002) conducted focus groups among 785 adolescents, ages 12–19, from different ethnic and socioeconomic backgrounds living in 13 different sites across the United States, with the purpose of exploring their responses to potential tobacco control policies. In every focus group in each of the 13 sites, only two policies were identified as being potentially effective in encouraging them to stop smoking: a sudden and large price increase, and listing ingredients with common uses. Most agreed that they would stop buying cigarettes at a price of US$ 6 per pack, which was about twice the current price at the time the study was conducted. The adolescents were familiar with cigarette prices and knew how and where to find the best deals. Participants at all sites felt that warning labels alone are ineffective, vague, ambiguous, and/or meaningless. They were shocked and repulsed, however, to find out the common uses of several potentially harmful substances that are added to cigarettes or that occur as a byproduct of burning tobacco, such as those also used to make pesticide, wood stripper, and nail polish remover. During interviews, the adolescents said they felt that the general public has a right to have this information, and they expressed the need to require tobacco companies to disclose it on every cigarette package and to display it at places where cigarettes are sold. They added that the industry should be further required to provide complete information on all the additives, identifying them not only by their chemical names—with which most of the adolescents were unfamiliar—but also by their more common names and usages in everyday life.

Policies affecting the price of alcohol have a similar effect on youth alcohol consumption. Economists use the concept of *price elasticity of demand* to describe the percentage change in consumption resulting from a 1% increase in price. For adults, the price elasticity of demand for beer, wine, and distilled spirits is −0.3%, −1.0%, and −1.5%, respectively (Leung and Phelps 1993). This means that a 1% increase in price reduces beer consumption only by 0.3%, but wine by more than three times that much and the higher-alcohol-content distilled spirits by five times that amount.

Chaloupka, Grossman, and Saffer (2002) also reviewed the effect of price on alcohol consumption and alcohol-related problems among U.S. youth and young adults. These authors describe two scientifically rigorous studies predicting the effects of price on alcohol use by youths ages 16 to 21. Both studies found an inverse relationship between beer consumption, beer price, and the state's minimum legal drinking age. Price increases had a more pronounced effect on fairly heavy and heavy drinkers than on occasional drinkers. Additionally, increases in beer taxes and/or state minimum legal drinking age were shown to significantly reduce youth motor vehicle fatalities (Saffer and Grossman 1987). Chaloupka and colleagues (1993) additionally demonstrated that increases in the full price of alcohol—whether through tax increases, reduced availability, and/or increases in the expected legal costs of drinking and driving, including more severe drunk driving laws—can reduce drinking and driving and its consequences among all age groups. Grossman and Markowitz (2001) describe a 4% reduction in the number of college students involved in violence each year due to a 10% alcohol price increase. These authors had also previously demonstrated that increases in the beer tax can be an effective policy tool in reducing child and adolescent abuse (Markowitz and Grossman 1998). Policies designed to reduce alcohol consumption by increasing beer taxes are also associated with a reduced number of young adult male suicides (ages 20–24), although female suicides seem not to be affected by this policy (Markowitz, Chatterji, and Kaestner 2003).

Although there is striking evidence that increases in the price of alcoholic beverages seem to be an effective policy for reducing alcohol consumption and its consequences, this policy has been largely ignored in the United States. Real prices of alcoholic beverages, after adjusting for the effects of inflation, have declined significantly over the past 50 years, and particularly in relationship to the prices for other consumer goods and services. The principal policy to decrease youth drinking in the United States has been to increase the states' minimum legal drinking age to 21 years (Chaloupka, Grossman, and Saffer 2002).

Di Nardo and Lemieux (2001) analyzed the impact of increases in the minimum drinking age on the prevalence of alcohol and marijuana consumption among late adolescents from 43 states in the United States over the years 1980–1989. During this period, the minimum drinking age was raised in all the states from 18 to 21. The authors found that the policy of increasing the legal minimum drinking age did reduce to some extent the prevalence of alcohol consumption, but the reduction was also associated with a mild increase in the prevalence of marijuana use in this age period. Furthermore, between 1991 and 2001, the percentage of U.S. youths aged 12 to 17 who had tried marijuana increased by 10.4%, from 11.5% in 1991 to a peak of 21.9% in 2001 (U.S. Department of Health and Human Services 2003b). Farrelly and colleagues (2001) found that higher fines for marijuana possession and increased probability of arrest were effective policies in decreasing the probability of use of marijuana among young adults.

Several Latin American and Caribbean countries have minimum-age drinking laws banning alcohol consumption for adolescents under 16 (Trinidad and Tobago), 18 (Argentina, Brazil, Colombia, Honduras, Panama, Peru), or 21 years of age (Chile), but adolescents in these countries are usually unaware of the legal consequences (if any) of trespassing this law. As noted in Chapter One of this book, one of the obstacles to discouraging alcohol consumption among adolescents is the behavior's widespread cultural acceptance, reinforced by the media and reflected in the actions and attitudes of adult role models emulated by adolescents. The starting point for the development of policies and legislation in this area, then, should be based on consideration of the most appropriate measures to protect young people from the unhealthy effects of drinking, to promote a delay in the starting age for alcohol exploration, and to encourage the adoption of reasonable and responsible drinking behaviors. The particular content of these measures might vary from one geographical area to another, depending on the severity of teenage drinking as a public health problem and the specific nature of its relationship to motor vehicle accidents, suicides, sexual and physical violence, and other social phenomena to which alcohol consumption has been linked.

Another area in which health-promoting policies are needed is that of encouraging adolescents to delay sexual initiation and to adopt safer sex practices. These policies may range from protecting their right to seek and receive information to teaching them skills to develop their sexuality in healthy ways. Policies can help protect them from sexual coercion and abuse and define the range of developmentally appropriate confidentiality to which they are entitled when seeking sexual and reproductive health services. It should be noted, however, that adequate counseling may be severely handicapped if adolescents believe that the information they volunteer during counseling will not kept in confidence (World Health Organization 2002b), and fear that parents may learn of their visit to health services is often cited as a reason for not seeking or using services (especially reproductive health) when needed (Senderowitz 1999).

Policies that regulate the price and availability of contraceptives for adolescents who decide to initiate sexual activity are also crucial in the efforts to encourage youth to adopt safer sex practices. Averett, Rees, and Argys (2002) found that making family planning services more available increased contraceptive behavior among 15–19-year-old U.S. women. Availability was measured by the number of clinics per 10,000 women in the county of residence, and a 1-unit increase was associated with an increase of 0.19 in the probability of using some form of birth control at last intercourse. Denmark has been a pioneer in its effort to reduce abortion among adolescent girls. Although Danish law authorizes abortion free of charge before the 12th week of pregnancy, the government has introduced a series of policies to reduce abortion among adolescents. Since 1970, sex education has been mandatory in Danish schools. All counties are required to have at least one clinic that provides contraceptive counseling to adolescents. Jutland, the county with the lowest teen pregnancy rate, has introduced a program in which all middle adolescents are required to visit the county clinic to learn about contraceptives availability and use, pregnancy avoidance, and abortion reduction. Denmark was able to reduce the number of teen abortions by 20% within one year of introducing these policies (Risor 1989).

The introduction of laws in the United States requiring parental involvement in a minor's decision to abort a pregnancy has had mixed results. Joyce and Kaestner (1996) found that this policy had had no impact except for nonblack minors of 16 years of age in South Carolina and Tennessee, a group in which a 10% decline in the probability of abortion was seen. Levine (2003), on the other hand, found that parental involvement laws resulted in fewer abortions for minors; this, in turn, had resulted from fewer pregnancies, in which the reduction in pregnancy seems to be attributable to increased use of contraception rather than a reduction in sexual activity.

The research evidence on the effectiveness of different policies to reduce youth violence is much more limited than that for reducing tobacco, alcohol, and illegal drug use, and risky sexual behaviors. Most of the policy and legislation literature is related to domestic violence in the general population and to protection of minors. The latest report of the U.S. Surgeon General on youth violence mentions that a number of effective intervention and prevention programs are available in this area. The most successful appear to be those which combine components addressing both individual risks and environmental conditions and which include building individual skills and competencies, parent effectiveness training, improving the social climate of the school, and changes in the type and level of involvement in peer groups. However, the report does not provide any evidence on the effectiveness of policies and legislation for the prevention of youth violence, suggesting instead that more research is needed in this area (U.S. Department of Health and Human Services 2001c). The absence of a policy analysis of the potential impact of gun control on youth violence is particularly noteworthy, since at least one study (Vittes, Sorenson, and Gilbert 2003) has shown that most high school students in the United States favor more restrictive firearms policies.

There is also a gap in the research regarding effective policies to promote physical activity and healthy nutrition among adolescents. Dietz and colleagues (2002) state that the rapid increase in adolescent overweight between 1980 and 1999 can only be explained by environmental factors and that there is a need to expand the science base linking environmental conditions and policies to youth health behaviors.

The Ontario Public Health Association, through the Heart Health Resource Centre (Ontario Heart Health and Nutrition Resources Centres 2002), has recently published *Policies in Action*, a collection of international, national, and local policies that community health policy developers in other parts of the world may wish to use as a template during the writing stage of their own healthy policies. *Policies in Action* describes a series of youth-favoring policies to promote physical activity, including:

- ensuring that communities have accessible and safe opportunities to engage in physical activity, including reducing barriers to and facilitating environmental support for physical activity (e.g., implementing bicycle rack requirements for new buildings, making cities more accessible by foot or bicycle, ensuring proper sidewalk construction/repair, improving street lighting);
- mandating quality daily physical activity (30 minutes a day) for students at the elementary and secondary levels;
- mandating comprehensive health education (i.e., development of healthy lifestyles) for elementary and secondary level students; and
- providing extracurricular physical activity programs that address the needs

and interests of all students, taking into account gender, ethnic, and cultural considerations.

Policies in Action also offers a number of youth-favoring policies to promote healthy eating. Among these are:

- providing dietary guidance;
- increasing healthy food choices/reducing unhealthy food choices in school cafeterias;
- reducing the promotion/advertising of unhealthy food choices to pre- and early adolescents;
- increasing taxes on non-nutritious snacks;
- modifying pricing policies to promote healthy food choices;
- mandating nutrition education in elementary and secondary level schools;
- reimbursing for nutrition counseling; and
- regulating nutrition information (e.g., labeling).

As this chapter has indicated, the responsibility for the development of comprehensive, well-integrated health-promoting policies for adolescents will often need to be shared among various interests and/or sectors. These include health, education, justice, finance, agriculture, sports and recreation, transportation and urban development, commerce and industry, housing, and labor. One example worth noting within this context is the Government of the Netherlands, in which youth policy is part of the portfolio of the Ministry of Health, Welfare, and Sport, and other government departments have worked jointly with the Ministry to create the general policy framework. This Ministry also coordinates youth research and the reorganization of the youth health care system, the promotion of healthy lifestyles, local preventive youth policy, parenting and development support, voluntary youth work/national youth organizations, day care and after-school care, sports and cultural development, and youth civic participation. The Ministry of Education, Cultural Affairs, and Science oversees policies to discourage students from dropping out of school, to provide educational opportunities for disadvantaged youth, and to promote safe school projects. The Ministry of Justice has policies targeting youth crime prevention, youth care/protection, ethnic minorities and youth crime, and metropolitan youth safety. The Ministry of the Interior and Kingdom Relations supports metropolitan youth safety and ethnic minorities and youth crime prevention, and the Ministry of Social Affairs and Employment establishes minimum youth wages, oversees a youth employment guarantee act and laws and regulations on working conditions, and provides other types of incentives for youth employment.

"Youth policy [in the Netherlands]," notes its developers, "does not only deal with the well-being and participation of young people, but also with education, employment opportunities, (mental) health care, pre-school education, safety, sports, and culture. Youth policy forms a horizontal layer across society: all the underlying policy areas contribute . . . to achieve better coherence and collaboration between the various policy areas and the associated administrative layers, so as to arrive at a better youth policy" (NIZW International Centre 2001).

Since 1996, Bolivia and the Dominican Republic have approved comprehensive national policies that incorporate strong adolescent health components, including reproductive health. Bolivia approved a national youth policy in October 1998, and its president issued a decree on youth in February 1999. The Dominican Republic formally approved a national youth policy in January 1998 and enacted a youth law in August 2000. In both countries, strong national leadership was instrumental in moving the policy implementation process forward. Other keys to success were having effective intersectoral coordination, consistent support from international agencies, and the availability of reliable information regarding youth needs and behaviors, as well as being able to take advantage of windows of opportunities, mobilize the youth vote, and forge a strong involvement by youth and civil society in the policy process. Adequate funding for implementation, however, has been a persistent problem in both countries, with the severity of the funding constraint being greater in Bolivia (Rosen 2001).

Table 24-1. presents a breakdown of the number of studies found on the effect of policies and legislation on adolescent health behaviors.

As seen in Table 24-1., much of the evidence on the effectiveness of policies and legislation in changing adolescent behavior lies in the area of tobacco, alcohol, and illegal drug use. Perhaps surprisingly, the areas of physical activity and nutrition and violence are the least researched, despite the fact that the prevalence of obesity and gang violence is on the rise in many parts of the world. The paucity of research literature available on these issues could be an indication that insufficient policy work has been done in these areas, or it could mean that the evidence base for "what works" in terms of existing policies and laws is still too small. In either case, the resulting gap suggests an area for future work by both policymakers and public health researchers, who, buttressed by a cross-section of interested stakeholders, might approach this gap utilizing community organization strategies similar to those described in Chapter Twenty-two of this book.

Box 24-1. presents a summary of evidence on the policy and legislation effects on adolescent lifestyles.

Table 24-1. **Most Commonly Researched Adolescent Behaviors Using Policy and Legislation Analysis**

ADOLESCENT BEHAVIORS	NUMBER OF ARTICLES ON POLICIES AND LEGISLATION	NUMBER OF ARTICLES BY KEYWORDS	
Sexual and Reproductive Health	50	Teen Pregnancy	42
		HIV/AIDS	5
		STIs	1
		Condom Use	7
Tobacco, Alcohol, and Drug Use	153	Tobacco	74
		Alcohol	60
		Drugs	19
Physical Activity and Nutrition	10	Obesity	1
		Physical Activity	6
		Nutrition	3
Violence	20		
TOTAL	**233**		

Box 24-1. Summary of Policy and Legislation Effects on Adolescent Lifestyles

- According to research studies conducted in the United States, the two most effective policy and legislation actions to prevent youth smoking are the establishment of smoke-free environments and cigarette tax increases. There is also evidence to suggest that higher cigarette taxes decrease the intensity of marijuana use.

- Price is not significantly associated with tobacco experimentation, although it is an important factor for more advanced smoking behavior among adolescents.

- Policies aimed at reducing youth access to tobacco do not show strong evidence of effectiveness.

- Tobacco advertising increases tobacco consumption: a significant portion of youth experimentation with smoking can be attributed to tobacco marketing campaigns and promotional activities, particularly the provision of free tobacco samples, clothing, sporting equipment, and paraphernalia for outdoor activities.

- Comprehensive bans on tobacco advertising can reduce tobacco consumption by approximately 6%, but a limited and selective set of bans will have little or no effect at all.

- Adolescents have identified two policies as being potentially effective in encouraging them to stop smoking: a sudden and large price increase, and the listing of chemical additives on cigarette packaging and on displays where tobacco products are sold.

- U.S. studies have shown an inverse relationship between beer consumption, beer price, and the state's minimum legal drinking age among young people.

- Increases in beer taxes and/or state minimum legal drinking age have been shown to significantly reduce youth motor vehicle fatalities.

- Price increases have a more pronounced effect on fairly heavy and heavy drinkers than on light drinkers.

- Increases in the price of alcohol have also been associated with reductions in the number of college students involved in violent acts.

- Policies designed to reduce alcohol consumption by increasing beer taxes have been associated with a reduced number of suicides among males ages 20–24.

- Increasing the legal minimum drinking age has been shown to reduce the prevalence of alcohol consumption among late adolescents, but at the same time it has been associated with a mild increase in the prevalence of marijuana use in this age group.

- Higher fines for marijuana possession and increased probability of arrest have been shown to be effective policies in decreasing the probability of marijuana use among young adults.

- Fear that the information they volunteer during counseling will not be kept confidential and that parents may learn of their visit is often cited by adolescents as a reason why they do not seek health services, especially those related to reproductive health issues.

- Making family planning services more available can increase contraceptive behavior, particularly among girls during middle and late adolescence.

- Most high school students in the United States favor the creation of more restrictive firearms policies.

[Chapter Twenty-five]

At a Glance: The Community and Policy Level Theories and Models for Behavior Change

Of all the theories and models reviewed in Chapters Twenty-two through Twenty-four to promote change at the community and policy levels, the level of policy and legislation development (Chapter Twenty-four) has been the most utilized to address adolescent behaviors, particularly those involving tobacco, alcohol, and drug prevention efforts, as well as unprotected sex behaviors. Interestingly, even though today we are witnessing an emerging epidemic of obesity among children and adolescents in some parts of the world, comparatively little research has been conducted on the promotion of physical activity and healthy nutrition at the community and policy and legislation development levels, despite the fact that studies abound describing the effects of interventions at these two levels designed to achieve the same results among the adult population. Also of interest is the research gap at these two levels regarding youth violence prevention, given the fact that the majority of instances of violence reported in the media occur among adolescents and youth. Once again, research studies to date have tended to focus on the general population, and very few have attempted to address the needs of young people in this area.

The significant variance in the number of articles researching the different adolescent behaviors might hopefully serve to raise eyebrows in the public health and social sciences research communities, given the fact that often alcohol use, unprotected sexual activity, and interpersonal violence cluster together, not only among adults, but also among adolescents and youth. This worrisome situation may be a sign of ongoing and excessively fragmented research, in which experts in the various behavior specializations have failed to interact with colleagues focusing on other behaviors and thereby produce more interdisciplinary research. At the same time, many researchers have primarily focused their behavioral change research on adult subjects, and, as we have seen throughout this book, the approaches that have proven most effective among one age group are not necessarily successful among younger cohorts whose physical, cognitive, and socio-emotional development is still incomplete. Clearly, there is a need to more closely integrate research across behaviors and also heed differences in expected results between adult and adolescent research, including differences distinguishing the various developmental stages within adolescence. This gap presents an important opportunity for adolescent health and development experts throughout the world to assume a leadership role in forming interdisciplinary research teams that can work together to reverse today's current trends of fragmentation and draw attention to the unique developmental needs and wants of each stage of adolescence.

Table 25-1. illustrates the ideas presented above and summarizes the number of studies using the theories and models discussed in Chapters Twenty-two through Twenty-four according to health behaviors.

When the community and policy level results shown in Table 25-1. are compared with their counterparts in Table 21-1. (interpersonal level theories and models) and Table 15-1. (individual level theories and models), it becomes apparent that the disproportionate number of studies based on models of policy and legislation development, most notably in the area of tobacco, alcohol, and drug use, is a reflection of prevention efforts by local and national

Table 25-1. **Summary of Most Commonly Researched Community and Policy Level Theories and Models for Changing Adolescent Behaviors**

Number of Articles on Adolescence and Community and Policy Level Behavior Change Theories and Models	Sexual and Reproductive Health	Tobacco, Alcohol, and Drug Use	Physical Activity and Nutrition	Violence	Total
Community Organization Models	39	76	6	22	143
Diffusion of Innovations Theory, Behavior Change Communication Models, and Social Marketing	39	54	10	2	105
Models of Policy and Legislation Development	50	153	10	20	233
Total	128	283	26	44	481

governments. As we have seen in earlier chapters, these behaviors have also been researched far more than sexual and reproductive health, physical activity and nutrition, and violence at the individual and interpersonal levels, as well. These results are shown in Table 25-2. below.

Figure 25-1. shows the different emphases placed on research at the different ecological levels for the four adolescent behaviors and reveals that most of the research on one of the lesser-studied behavior groups—physical activity and nutrition—has occurred at the individual level. This finding indicates that an increase in physical activity and the adoption of healthier nutrition that adolescents have achieved on an individual basis have received more research attention, and that much less is known and/or has been reported as regards the impact of interactive (i.e., interpersonal) health-promoting interventions, as well as community-wide initiatives, policies, and legislation to change these behaviors.

It is also interesting to note that, as shown in Table 25-2. and Figure 25-1., in the area of sexual and reproductive health, the majority of theories and models studied have been at the community and policy levels, while in the area of violence, much of the research has focused on the interpersonal level, and, as earlier stated, tobacco, alcohol, and drug use by adolescents have received the most attention at the policy and legislation development level.

Table 25-3. provides a summary of the health promotion and behavior change theories and models discussed in Chapters Twenty-two through Twenty-four and the most salient characteristics of each.

Table 25-2. **A Comparison of the Four Levels of Theories and Models for Adolescent Behavioral Change**

Number of Articles on Adolescence and Behavior Change Theories and Models	Sexual and Reproductive Health	Tobacco, Alcohol, and Drug Use	Physical Activity and Nutrition	Violence	Total
Total Individual Level Behavior Change Theories and Models	92	159	44	12	307
Total Interpersonal Level Behavior Change Theories and Models	82	207	41	79	409
Total Community and Policy Level Behavior Change Theories and Models	128	283	26	44	481
Total	302	649	111	135	1197

Figure 25-1. **A Comparison of the Four Levels of Theories and Models for Adolescent Behavioral Change**

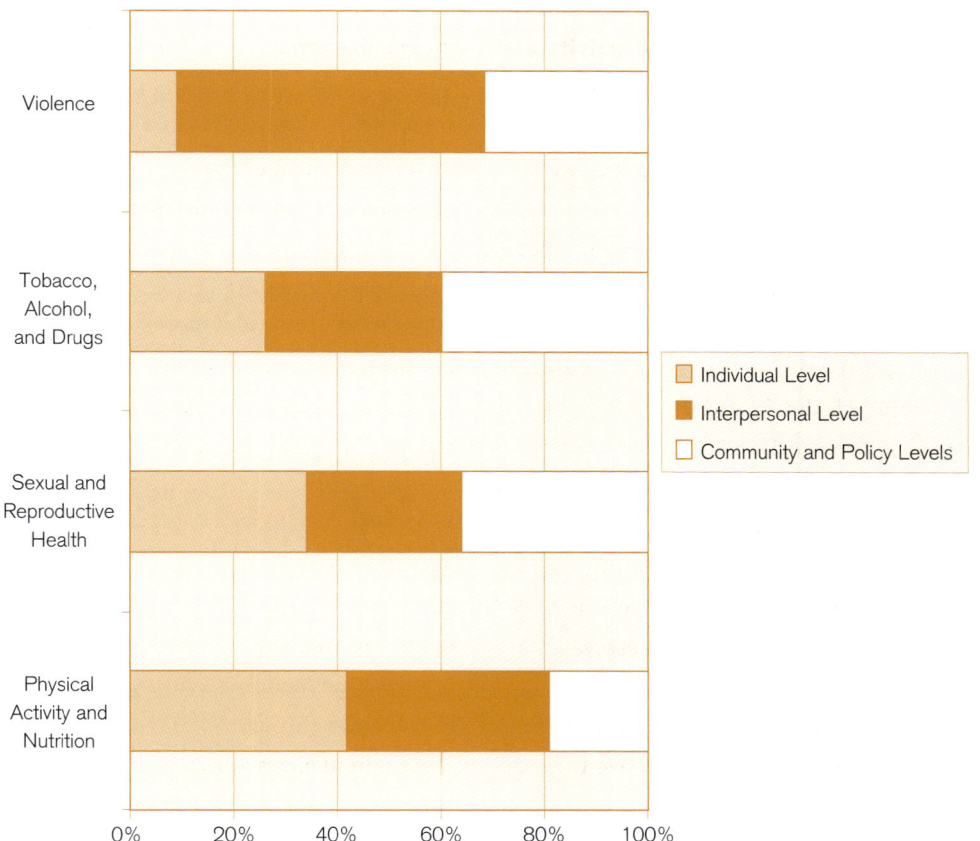

Table 25-3. **Community and Policy Level Theories and Models and Their Application to Adolescent Behavioral Change: A Comparison of Conceptual Frameworks, Applications, and Benefits**

Theory/Model	Conceptual Framework	Application	Benefits
Community Organization Models (Chapter Twenty-two)	Community organization models describe the process by which community members organize themselves to identify common needs, problems, and goals; mobilize resources; and develop and implement strategies for reaching the collective goals they have set. Although some community change models (locality or community development, social	Initiatives launched in recent years indicate that the strategy of youth empowerment represents a potentially powerful tool in community efforts to encourage health-promoting behaviors among young people. Engaging youth in community actions against tobacco has resulted in broad-based coalitions and fostered meaningful youth-led	Community organization is an excellent framework within which to carry out the social assessment phase when using the PRECEDE-PROCEED Model (described in Chapter Four). In the case of adolescent target groups, this assessment would yield essential information regarding their needs and wants, by gender and age group. This

Table 25-3. **Community and Policy Level Theories and Models and Their Application to Adolescent Behavioral Change: A Comparison of Conceptual Frameworks, Applications, and Benefits**—(continued)

Theory/Model	Conceptual Framework	Application	Benefits
Community Organization Models (*continued*)	planning, and social action) emphasize different aspects (process- versus task-oriented) they usually overlap and may also be combined. Community-building is a newer type of community organization model whose approach is considered to be more strengths- than need-based. Community coalitions, also a newer model, describe formal, multipurpose, and long-lasting alliances of individuals representing diverse organizations, factions, or constituencies within a community. Several key concepts are shared by these various approaches and are central to effect and measure community level change: empowerment, critical consciousness, community capacity, community participation, and issue selection. Media advocacy and communication for social change also have emerged as important tools for facilitating community organization towards change.	tobacco prevention activities, which in turn have encouraged and increased youth empowerment, positive development, civic involvement, and leadership and decision-making responsibilities. In contrast, most of the interventions to date involving youth in sexual and reproductive health prevention programs have limited their participation to use as peer educators or as outreach agents to provide the prevention services, while at the same time excluding their involvement in the programs' assessment and planning phases. Similarly, community coalitions to prevent teen pregnancy rarely incorporate youth as active participants in the project development and implementation stages. A series of factors associated with successful neighborhood mobilization in this area, however, include a strong sense of community, consensus on the perceived need for the initiative, support by key organizations, shared leadership, effective group action processes, and a competent staff contingent.	information could, in turn, provide the backdrop for well-designed interventions and programs that would be responsive to their problems and goals at the particular point where they are currently in their lives. Community organization models provide a strategy to involve not only concerned adults in the community in issues of youth development and potential health-compromising behaviors, but also the youth themselves, during the assessment and planning phases. These phases should involve not only motivated youth without risky behaviors, but also those who have already been affected by health-compromising experiences (e.g., gang membership, pregnancy, addictive behaviors). Concepts such as community-building could also be integrated into the work of developmental assets (Chapter Nineteen), in which youth participation would be essential in identifying community networks that could help them strengthen individual capacity to resist health-compromising behaviors and lifestyles.
Diffusion of Innovations Theory, Behavior Change Communication Models, and Social Marketing (Chapter Twenty-three)	The Diffusion of Innovations Theory deals with the introduction of a new idea, practice, method, device, or object and the process by which this innovation is communicated through specific channels over time to its intended target audience. The theory focuses on both the characteristics of the particular innovation (e.g., a new school-based tobacco prevention program) and how the innovation will be communicated to its intended audience (e.g., early adolescents). The timeframe and adoption level	The Diffusion of Innovations Theory has demonstrated its efficacy in scaling up health promotion and prevention programs for adolescents. However, most of its documented applications to date have been in the expansion of tobacco initiation and HIV/AIDS prevention programs as part of a school health curriculum. Yet the adoption and implementation of school health promotion curricula by schoolteachers have presented challenges of their own. This is particularly the case for sexual	The Diffusion of Innovations Theory holds great potential in helping to scale up effective interventions that promote the adoption of healthy behaviors or change of risk behaviors among adolescents in a variety of settings, including not only schools, but also community organizations, sports clubs, and other places where youth frequent and spend their time. As new initiatives of this type are being developed and their effectiveness tested, followed by plans for a scaling up of programs, those

Table 25-3. **Community and Policy Level Theories and Models and Their Application to Adolescent Behavioral Change: A Comparison of Conceptual Frameworks, Applications, and Benefits**–(continued)

Theory/Model	Conceptual Framework	Application	Benefits
Diffusion of Innovations Theory, Behavior Change Communication Models, and Social Marketing (*continued*)	of any given innovation will be affected by the characteristics of the innovation (e.g., its relative advantages over previously used similar strategies, its compatibility with the proposed target group, its complexity in being understood and adopted, its observability in those who have already adopted it, its trialability before final adoption), the communication channels (e.g., opinion leaders, mass media), and how the process of dissemination is carried through. Behavior change communication is a multi-level intervention, using a variety of communication channels, to distribute tailored health messages to individuals and communities. Social marketing theory predicts that target market members (e.g., adolescents) will voluntarily exchange their resources (e.g., money, time) for a product when they become aware that the innovation offers them attractive benefits at a reasonable cost or price and that it is available at the right place and at the right time. Diffusion of innovations, behavior change communication, and social marketing are complementary theories and models which serve as instruments to reach different population levels, through various channels, with the unifying goal of scaling up effective health promotion and prevention interventions.	education, where personal beliefs may interfere with the fidelity of the curricula implementation. In contrast to this approach, behavior change communication and social marketing have been widely used to diffuse health messages through multimedia channels that young people find appealing and to which they often turn as a source for reliable information and entertainment. Entertainment-education has been identified as an effective behavior change communication model. Its effectiveness is attributed to its focus on the emotional as well as cognitive factors that influence behavior, and by being closely aligned with the customs, norms, and narrative forms that are familiar to the target audiences. Research has also shown that entertainment-education programming with social change messages is a cost-effective method for reaching large audiences. There is also evidence that social marketing techniques have contributed to the effectiveness of anti-smoking advertising campaigns. These have been shown to have a reliable positive effect among pre- and early adolescents by preventing smoking initiation. The evidence also points out that family and peer interactions play a crucial role in reinforcing, denying, or neutralizing the potential effects of these anti-smoking campaigns.	involved in this process should keep in mind that the degree of long-term cooperation and cohesion among the team that developed the innovation (e.g., designers of a health promotion intervention targeting preadolescent males through local soccer clubs), the potential user systems (e.g., soccer coaches at local clubs in each neighborhood), and the linkage agent (a designated facilitator who knows in depth the intervention's design and methodology and interacts directly with soccer coaches by training them in the intervention's appropriate implementation) will, to a large extent, determine the initiative's overall effectiveness in achieving the expected results. Although BCC and social marketing might appear to be more attractive strategies to use in scaling up health behavior messages directed toward adolescents, it is important to not confuse these strategies with the channels (e.g., media) or settings (e.g., schools) that are used most commonly to introduce the innovative messages. To date, no magic bullet has emerged that clearly demonstrates its effectiveness in reaching a wide range of adolescents, which may consist of different age groups, genders, and cultures, through the use of only one strategy applied in only one setting. A synergistic approach that integrates effective multimedia social campaigns with the scaling up of evidence-based interventions in the school environment and at the community level holds promise, however, as a possible direction to be explored and tested in the future.

Table 25-3. **Community and Policy Level Theories and Models and Their Application to Adolescent Behavioral Change: A Comparison of Conceptual Frameworks, Applications, and Benefits**–*(continued)*

Theory/Model	Conceptual Framework	Application	Benefits
Models of Policy and Legislation Development (Chapter Twenty-four)	Policies are frameworks that guide decision-making in an organization or government, described in statements of intended action and sometimes constituting an element in a network of interrelated decisions, which together form a comprehensive approach or strategy in relation to practical issues (e.g., health care delivery). The stages in the policy-making process include issue definition, setting objectives and priorities, defining options, options appraisal, policy implementation, and policy evaluation. A policymaker's freedom to act will be constrained at various different stages during the policy-making process, and policy development will be ultimately determined by who influences whom in the making of policy, and how this comes about. Policies may be differentiated between *macro policies* (high political issues) and *micro policies* (low political issues). An issue becomes part of the policy agenda only when it has high *legitimacy, feasibility*, and *support*. Governments pay attention to policies only when a major window of opportunity opens up simultaneously in each of three "streams": the problem, the politics, and the policy. The role of the policy advocate is to create, monitor, and capitalize on these opportunities.	There is significant research evidence regarding how various policies and types of legislation may help to prevent tobacco and alcohol initiation, as well as drug use, among adolescents. In the United States, the two policy and legislative actions that have had the most decisive and immediate effects on preventing youth smoking are the establishment of smoke-free environments and cigarette tax increases. However, policies aimed at reducing youth access to tobacco do not show strong evidence of effectiveness. Increases in beer taxes and/or state minimum legal drinking age have been shown to significantly reduce youth motor vehicle fatalities. There is also evidence that making family planning services more available can increase contraceptive behavior, particularly among girls during middle and late adolescence.	The adoption of evidence-based policies and legislation could significantly contribute to the promotion of healthy behaviors among adolescents and the prevention of health-compromising lifestyles. Although ideally behavior change should be voluntary, regulatory measures are necessary when specific behaviors become a threat to the collective health and well-being of the community as a whole. This is the case with second-hand smoke exposure, excessive alcohol drinking and its related consequences (e.g., reckless driving, interpersonal violence), and availability of firearms. Policies are also essential to facilitate voluntary choices and to overcome potential barriers to behavior adoption (e.g., through availability of condoms and contraceptives, recreation facilities for increased physical activity, plentiful and affordable healthy foods). Many health promoters agree that policies, whether community-based or emanating from the national government, are key to instilling positive adolescent behavior change, reasoning that if the policies are well implemented, they can profoundly influence the way people live, by making healthier choices easier and unhealthy choices more difficult.

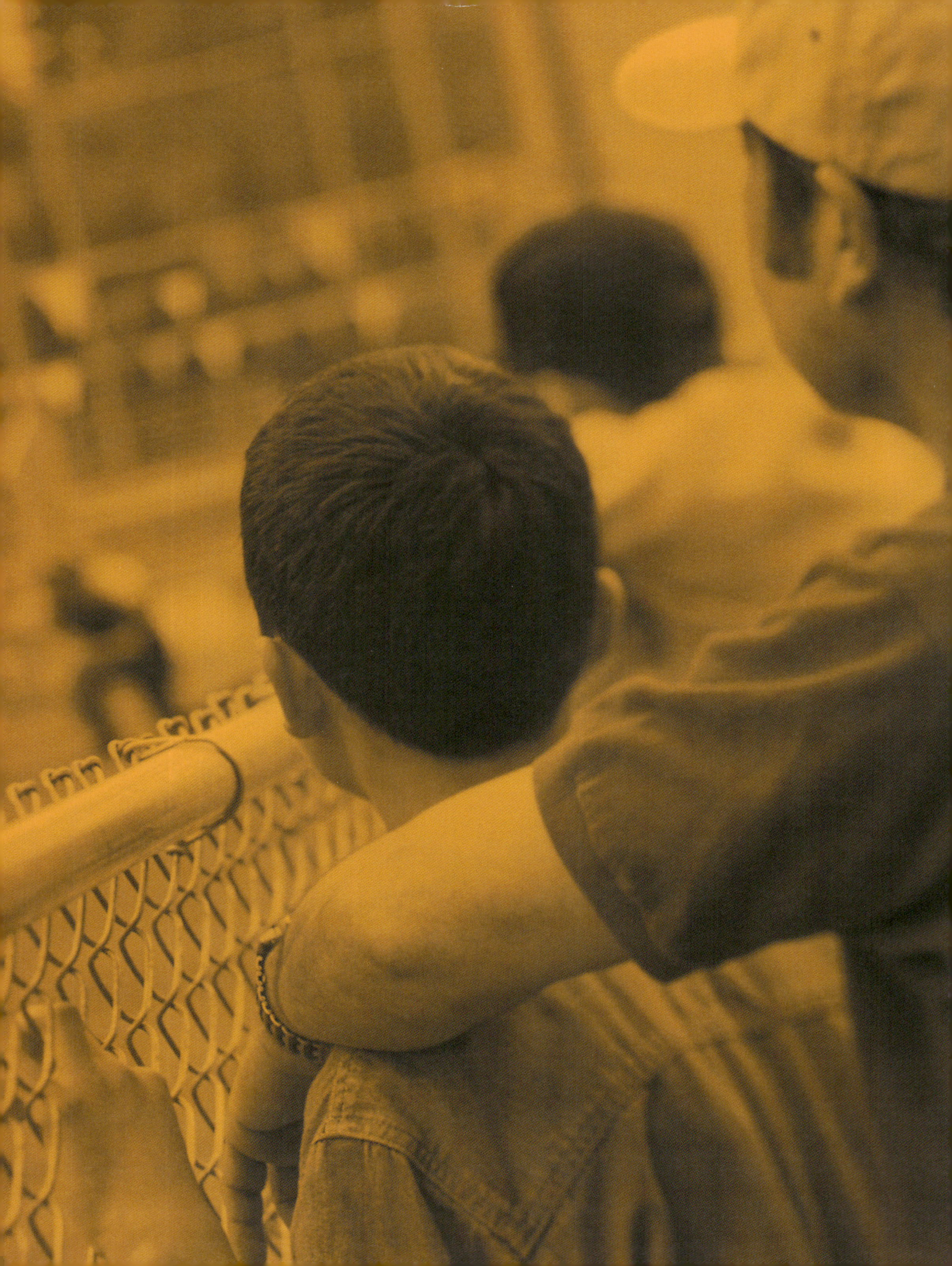

[Section Three]

Adolescent Developmental Changes and Goals: The Importance of Early Intervention

Introduction

While many of the classical behavioral change and health promotion theories and models presented in the first two sections of this book hold great potential in their applicability to adolescent health concerns, they represent only part of the puzzle in designing effective interventions. Section Three will present a series of other considerations that have received less attention, yet are critical ingredients that may determine success or failure in the achievement of the intervention's desired result. These missing pieces include consideration of the various adolescent developmental stages and their accompanying physical, cognitive, and socio-emotional changes; the pre- and early adolescent's changing needs and wants; the impact of early intervention; gender differences within a developmental context; and how the achievement of developmental goals contributes to the adolescent's ability to adopt protective, health-promoting behaviors.

Another piece of the puzzle often overlooked by intervention designers is the fact that behavior change theories have been traditionally developed by behavior learning theorists who tend to focus more on analyzing *cognitive* aspects of behaviors rather than the underlying *emotional* and *developmental* processes of behavior. Therefore, as noted in Chapters Six and Sixteen, learning theorists consider the basic processes of human behavior to be the same during adolescence as they are during other periods of life. Chapter Six points out the flaws of a "theories-only" approach to adolescent health interventions and discusses the need to link theoretical constructs to the particular *developmental* stage of the adolescent target group, a strategy whose importance has already been emphasized in health promotion literature (Juszczak and Sadler 1999, Dryfoos 1998). Yet for far too long, this crucial link has been ignored or underutilized—a key message of this book—and a phenomenon also observed by various other authors (Mummery, Spence, and Hudec 2000; Bush 1996; Sturges and Rogers 1996; Petosa and Jackson 1991).

To understand and be able to influence adolescent behavior, it is important to understand the world in which adolescents live and how that world affects their development, behavior, and social relationships. These contexts—family, peer groups, school, work, and leisure settings—are at the same time in a state of constant flux. In Chapter Four, the complexity of these multiple levels of influence is highlighted, as is the need to choose theories that blend individual and environmental approaches, in view of the interactions within and between these multiple settings and their continually evolving dynamics. In this sense, says Dr. Laurence Steinberg, "we need to understand how these changes are changing the nature of adolescence" (Steinberg 1999).

Aware of the challenges in developing effective interventions and programs to instill health-promoting behaviors in young people, the Pan American Health Organization presents the Youth: Choices and Change Model in Chapter Seven. The framework's components—a developmental and gender perspective, the identification of adolescent needs and wants as well as those of other actors, a problem-driven psychological approach to select appropriate theories, intervention at the individual level supported by inputs from other levels of influence, and the development of measurable variables enabling problem assessment and outcome evaluation—together form a roadmap allowing health promotion initiatives to not only target specific adolescent health behavior determinants, but also promote the strengthening of developmental capacities, focusing on the critical preadolescent and early adolescent periods and the development of skills and assets instead of preventing deficits or overcoming problems. The nature of the beginning of adolescence and why interventions during this period hold the greatest potential for positive and sustained behavior change will be the focus of Section Three.

[Chapter Twenty-six]

A New Approach to Classifying Adolescent Developmental Stages

The word *adolescence* is Latin in origin, derived from the verb *adolecere*, which means "to grow into adulthood" (Steinberg 1999). In all societies, adolescence is a time of evolution and maturation; of moving from the less developed cognitive skills and emotional experiences of childhood toward the—ideally—fully developed cognitive skills and more emotionally balanced experiences of adulthood. Adolescence is a period of transitions: biological, psychological, social, and economic. Although there is significant literature analyzing this period from different perspectives, there is little agreement on when adolescence begins and ends, and what the boundaries for this determination are (Steinberg 1999). A biologist might place the greatest emphasis on the attainment and completion of puberty; an attorney might look instead at important age breaks designated by law; an educator might focus on cognitive skills levels among students in different grades in school. Among adolescents themselves, acquiring such abilities as assuming responsibility for their own actions and making their own decisions are generally seen as more important considerations distinguishing adulthood from adolescence than more role-related transitions (e.g., using public transportation alone, finishing high school). Of the role-related transitions, being able to support oneself financially is viewed as the most important defining criterion of adulthood by adolescents themselves (Arnett 1994).

Although adolescence may span 10 years or more, most social scientists and practitioners recognize that, given the significant psychological and social growth that takes place during this decade, it makes more sense to view the adolescent years more as a series of phases than as one homogeneous stage (Steinberg 1999). In this sense, interests and tastes regarding music, television programs, movies, and magazines read, as well as the range of problems shared with friends, will be completely different for an 11-year-old than for a 13- or 15-year-old, as we will see in Chapters Twenty-eight and Twenty-nine of this book.

Different authors and organizations have proposed different ways of dividing this long period of adolescence. Furthermore, there is little agreement on this matter. Some sources refer to 11-year-old boys or girls as "preadolescents," while others call them "early adolescents," as shown in Table 26-1.

The authors and entities depicted in Table 26-1. are merely a small and somewhat random sample of those who have produced textbooks and other types of informational resources that are widely consulted by professionals working with adolescents. When seen together, these sources provide a clear illustration of the ongoing disagreement that exists regarding developmental classifications by age. Dan Acuff is the author of *What Kids Buy and Why*, an excellent resource for better understanding the marketing strategies that the corporate world utilizes to reach the adolescent consumer population. The Centers for Disease Control and Prevention (CDC) (U.S. Department of Health and Human Services 2004) has developed

Table 26-1. **Variances in Developmental Stage Classifications, Ages 8–14**

Sources \ Ages	8	9	10	11	12	13	14
Acuff (1997)	Preadolescence					Early Adolescence	
U.S. Youth Media Campaign (U.S. Department of Health and Human Services 2004)		Preadolescence					
National Youth Anti-Drug Media Campaign (Office of National Drug Control Policy 2002b)		Early Adolescence					
Steinberg (1999)				Early Adolescence			
Neinstein (2002)			Early Adolescence				
Juszczak and Sadler (1999)			Early Adolescence				

Source: Breinbauer and Maddaleno 2004

a Youth Media Campaign in the United States to encourage preadolescents ages 9–13 to engage in and maintain high levels of regular physical activity. Informational resources and updates on this campaign can be found at the CDC's Web site (http://www.cdc.gov/youthcampaign/research/resources.htm). Campaign developers refer to the preadolescent stage as "tweens," a term also used by Acuff. On the other hand, the U.S. National Youth Anti-Drug Media Campaign, in its publication on the scientific and situational bases for the Campaign's strategy (U.S. Office of National Drug Control Policy 2002b) refers to 9–11-year-olds as early adolescents.

Other sources in Table 26-1. include Laurence Steinberg, the Distinguished University Professor and Laura H. Carnell Professor of Psychology at Temple University, Philadelphia, Pennsylvania, with a Ph.D. in human development and family studies. Steinberg is the author of *Adolescence* (1999), a very comprehensive textbook on this age group. Lawrence Neinstein is Professor of Pediatrics and Medicine at the University of Southern California (USC), with a specialty in adolescent medicine. He is also Executive Director of the USC University Park Health Center and author of the excellent textbook *Adolescent Health Care: A Practical Guide* (Neinstein 2002). Linda Juszczak and Lois Sadler are the authors of "Adolescent Development: Setting the Stage for Influencing Health Behaviors," an outstanding review on this topic published in *Adolescent Medicine: State of the Art Reviews* (Juszczak and Sadler 1999). All of these individuals are widely recognized and published research authorities in the area of adolescent health and development.

As noted in this book's Foreword, the Pan American Health Organization (PAHO) and the World Health Organization have defined adolescence as the period between 10 and 19 years of age, youth as the period between 15 and 24 years of age, and the young population as the period between 10 and 24 years of age. Traditional approaches to dividing adolescent stages correspond in general to the way in which society groups young people in educational institutions (i.e., elementary, middle, high school, university, as well as individual school grades). As an example, the U.S. National Youth Anti-Drug Media Campaign also refers to its primary youth target audience as *middle school-aged adolescents* (11–13 years old) and to its secondary youth audiences as *late elementary school-aged children* (9–11 years old) and *high school-aged adolescents* (14–18 years old) (U.S. Office of National Drug of Control Policy 2002c). Nevertheless, this approach can differ enormously from culture to culture and country to country, and it does not adequately address the situation of adolescents in many parts of the world who do not attend school at all.

However, there is agreement on three features of adolescent development that occur universally. These are:

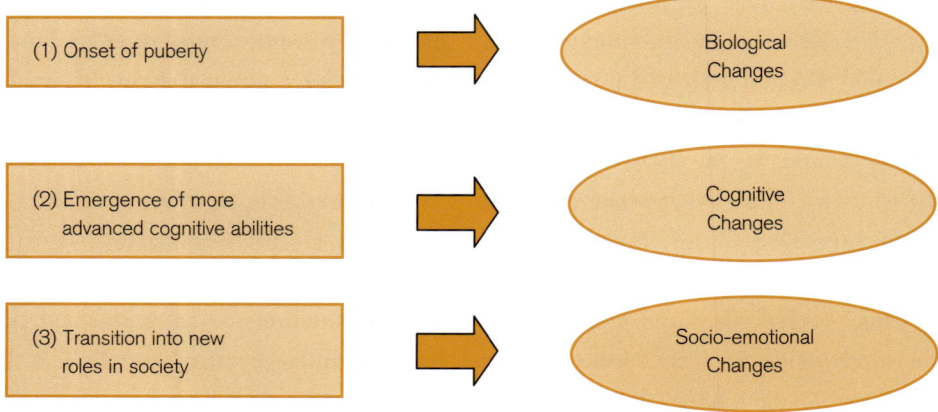

Figure 26-1. **Universal Features of Adolescent Development**

- the onset of puberty;
- the emergence of more advanced cognitive abilities; and
- the transition into new roles in society.

Without exception, all adolescents in every society go through these three stages (Hill 1983). These features have been further organized under the categories of the biological, cognitive, and socio-emotional changes which accompany each (Steinberg 1999).

These universal features do not occur at a specific given point in time, thus separating childhood from adolescence, but instead introduce themselves gradually over the continuum of the adolescence period. The accompanying biological, cognitive, and socio-emotional changes also increase in complexity as the adolescent moves from one developmental stage to the next.

Steinberg and Morris (2001) conducted a literature review for the publications on adolescent development released between 1988 and 2001. The main conclusion that emerged from this review, according to the authors, is the need for a comprehensive theory of both normative and atypical adolescent development that would integrate the current collection of "mini-theories" that explain only fragments of the larger puzzle.

Traditionally, adolescent development has been divided into three main categories—early, middle, and late adolescence—without a clear understanding of where they start and where they end. The most agreed-upon starting point has been puberty age, marked by the menarche milestone for girls and full genital development for boys. Adolescent development has also been described within the framework of different theories focusing on specific areas of development (e.g., psychodynamic theories on emotional development, the work of Harry Stack Sullivan on interpersonal development, Jean Piaget on cognitive development, Erik Erickson on psychosocial development, Lawrence Kohlberg on moral development, and Carol Gillberg on gender differences and female development). In addition, Urie Bronfenbrenner's *The Ecology of Human Development* (1979) has contributed to a better understanding of the impact of the environmental context on adolescent development and behavior.

Although each one of these theorists has left a major legacy, development is a complex phenomenon, and in the final analysis, all elements must be integrated into a theory of the whole person. Furthermore, significant findings have emerged in recent years from the impact of the environment, as well as from other studies on sensation-seeking theory, brain development, information-processing, and neuropsychological functioning. There is a particularly urgent need to integrate these fragmented findings into a comprehensive model of adolescent development. A theory of the whole person—one that can explain the needed changes and competencies at each developmental period to successfully negotiate the challenges of increasingly complex social, cultural, and economic environments—continues to elude researchers. There is a need, then, for more comprehensive and in-depth research, analysis, and descriptions of the different stages of adolescence, to enable us to better understand the different *needs and wants* and *developmental goals* of adolescents, as they progress through this long transition.

Table 26-2. presents a new approach developed by PAHO to classifying adolescent stages. This classification organizes progressive adolescent stages, starting with preadolescence and ending with young adulthood, according to the changes that traditionally occur between 10–24 years of age, into five domains: body, brain, sexual, emotional, and social development. This approach is a first attempt to integrate the most recent and still somewhat fragmented contributions of different theories in an evolutionary approach which PAHO and the authors of this book hope will stimulate the further refinement of theoretical constructs promoting the perspective of the whole person and the adoption of this lens to study adolescents as they navigate through the successive growth and developmental stages.

The age range for each of the adolescent development stages, as shown in Table 26-2., correlates to the average ages at which the developmental changes occur in these five domains, taking also in consideration frequently described gender differences for the earlier stages. However, there will always be exceptions to the age segmentation boundaries, with extremely precocious adolescents at one extreme and their late-maturing counterparts at the other. Particular differences will be found for sexual development and behaviors, the domain in which the environment holds significant impact. Abma and Sonenstein (2001), for example, have noted that environmental factors such as level of education, income, and access to health care account for many

Table 26-2. A New Approach to Classifying Adolescent Developmental Stages

Developmental Domains	Adolescent Stages (Average Ages)	Preadolescence 9–12 years (Girls) 10–13 years (Boys)	Early Adolescence 12–14 years (Girls) 13–15 years (Boys)	Middle Adolescence 14–16 years (Girls) 15–17 years (Boys)	Late Adolescence 16–18 years (Girls) 17–18 years (Boys)	Youth 18–21 years	Young Adulthood 21–24 years
Body Development		The growth spurt starts, and the body gradually acquires secondary sex characteristics. There is an increase in body fat and weight, as well as a redistribution of these to reflect secondary sexual characteristics. There is a gradual increase in sensation-seeking.	Girls acquire menstruation (mean age = 12.4 yrs.), and boys ejaculation (mean age = 13.4 yrs). There is a significant growth spurt and a marked increase in sensation-seeking, particularly among boys.	The body continues to grow and change. The need for sensation-seeking reaches its peak by the end of early adolescence and the beginning of middle adolescence.	The body is completing its period of growth and change, particularly among girls. Sensation-seeking begins to gradually decrease.	By the end of this period, full body maturation is reached among both girls and boys. Sensation-seeking continues to decrease.	Full body maturation reached among girls and boys. Sensation-seeking is decreased.
Brain Development		A gradual shift occurs from egocentric to socio-centric thought, with more concrete logical thinking. Conservation tasks[1] are in the process of being acquired. There is an increased craving for new information, but language is still concrete. There is still little development of prefrontal lobe and executive functions.	More abstract thinking (formal operations) and less concrete thinking are used. Most adolescents will acquire all conservation tasks during this stage. There is still little development of prefrontal lobe and executive functions, particularly among boys.	There is a major opening to abstract thinking and full meta-cognitive functions. There is also increased problem-solving, planning-ahead, and impulse-control abilities among girls.	Completion of prefrontal lobe development occurs during this stage, particularly among boys, who acquire increased problem-solving, planning-ahead, and impulse-control abilities.	Higher stages of cognitive and moral development are achieved in most youth, given that they possess adequate biological potential and social and emotional support.	Higher stages of cognitive and moral development are achieved in most young adults, given that they possess adequate biological potential and social and emotional support.
Sexual Development		Boys and girls explore more differentiated masculine and feminine roles compare to previous years. For girls, androgyny is a viable alternative to exclusive femininity, while for boys exclusive masculinity is still	Sexual arousal increases, and so does the need for masturbation. Other auto-erotic behaviors, such as sexual fantasies and wet dreams, occur. While gender identity is developed in the first years of life, its	More experience in dating and in engaging in some sexual experimentation is acquired. Socio-sexual behaviors evolve from less intimate to more intimate. This progressively involves necking and petting above	Socio-sexual behaviors continue to evolve toward intercourse.	Most youth have experienced sexual intercourse by this stage, regardless of race, gender, or socioeconomic status. Usually homosexuality is not internally assumed until this stage.	Most young adults have experienced sexual intercourse by this stage, regardless of race, gender, or socioeconomic status.

Sexual Development (continued)	the alternative that is socially most expected.	stability becomes increasingly challenged with the development of sexual orientation, preference, and exploration involving another person during this age period, including at times the emergence of confusing homosexual feelings.	the waist, genital touching through the clothing, direct genital contact, oral sex, and/or intercourse.[2]	
Emotional Development	A gradual increase in self-consciousness occurs, with fluctuations in self-image and increasing feelings of embarrassment. There is an emerging need for greater privacy, individuation, and more emotional autonomy from parents: to feel individuated within the relationship with parents (e.g., to feel that parents don't know some things about the adolescent), to depend more on oneself rather than on one's parents, and to gradually de-idealize parents. Fluctuations occur in verbal and nonverbal expression (facial gestures) of intense	A high level of self-consciousness and fluctuations in self-image are present. The level of stress increases, particularly among girls. The need for more emotional autonomy from parents continues, fueled by a stronger de-idealization of one's parents and increased defining of the adolescent's own opinions. At the same time, there is an increase in emotional dependency on one's friends. Intimacy, loyalty, and shared values and attitudes assume a greater weight in friendship. There is an increase in empathy	There is intense development of more differentiated self-conceptions, an increase in self-reliance, and the ability to reflect on feelings in relationship to an internalized sense of self. Feelings of homesickness previously experienced as anxiety and depression lessen. Greater emphasis is placed on security in friendship (e.g., concerns about loyalty and anxieties over rejection), particularly among girls. There is an increase in empathy and responsiveness toward close friends. The presence of a conventional morality still exists	There is once again a gradual increase in intimacy with parents, given that there was a positive relationship with them during previous years. Intimate friendships with opposite-sex peers become more important than in previous years, which were more dominated by intimate same-sex friendships. There is a gradual increase in value autonomy and in some cases the development of a post-conventional morality (i.e., in which society's rules are seen as being relative to support and serve human ends). Related changes	Emotional autonomy continues to increase, with the emerging capacity to see one's parents as individuals beyond their roles as parents. There is an increased stabilization in intimacy with one's parents, given that there was a positive relationship during previous years. There is an increase in feelings of loneliness, particularly among youth without strong best friends. Value autonomy and sometimes post-conventional morality are achieved. Interest and concerns with future plans intensify.	Higher stages of emotional and value autonomy, and in some cases post-conventional morality, are achieved in most young adults, given that they possess adequate biological and cognitive potential and social and emotional support. Concerns with having economic independence increase.

[1] Conservation tasks: Piaget has described a series of experiments to identify the point at which a child or preadolescent is no longer bound by the configuration perceived at a given moment. The classic example is for conservation of quantity, in which the child is asked to estimate which cylinder has more water, the tallest and thinnest or the shortest and widest (both having the same amount). The concept of weight conservation is acquired at ages 9–12 years (Lewis 1997).

[2] The described orderly progression of sexual activity varies among races, regional areas, and socioeconomic status (e.g., African-Americans move toward intercourse at an earlier age and without as many intervening steps as their other U.S. counterparts). Boys engage in these activities at a somewhat earlier age than girls. Differences will also be attributable to ethnic culture, religious beliefs, and other factors that vary around the world.

Table 26-2. A New Approach to Classifying Adolescent Developmental Stages—*(continued)*

Developmental Domains	Adolescent Stages (Average Ages)	Preadolescence 9–12 years (Girls) 10–13 years (Boys)	Early Adolescence 12–14 years (Girls) 13–15 years (Boys)	Middle Adolescence 14–16 years (Girls) 15–17 years (Boys)	Late Adolescence 16–18 years (Girls) 17–18 years (Boys)	Youth 18–21 years	Young Adulthood 21–24 years
Emotional Development *(continued)*		emotions (e.g., aggression, frustration, excitement, boredom). The ability emerges to explore multiple reasons for a feeling, to compare feelings, and to understand triadic interactions among feeling states. This is accompanied by the capacity to differentiate shades and gradations among feeling states (e.g., "I feel a little angry."). There is a gradual shift from pre-conventional morality (rewards and punishments) to conventional morality (society's rules).	and responsiveness toward close friends and an emerging ability to reflect on feelings in relationships with an internalized sense of self ("I shouldn't feel this angry."). A conventional morality is assumed.	among most middle adolescents.	include an increase in reasoning capability, hypothetical thinking, and emotional autonomy, as well as a heightened interest in making plans for one's future.		
Social Development		The need emerges for a same-sex best (or similar) friend with whom to have fun and share secrets. Academic and social demands and expectations increase. Time is still spent with parents, and parental supervision is still present, but these start to gradually decrease, accompanied by a gradual increase in conflicts between the preadolescent and parents. Susceptibility to peer pressure increases.	More time is spent with social subgroups (cliques) and/or alone. There is an emerging interest in opposite-sex ("different") friends. Less time is spent with parents, parental supervision decreases, and conflicts about independence increase. New social privileges are expected (e.g., watching more movies with adult plots rated for those 13 years and older). Susceptibility to peer pressure reaches its peak.	More time is spent with large mixed-sex groups (crowds) and/or alone. Less time is spent with parents, with less parental supervision. Academic and social demands and expectations increase. While perceptions of the strength of peer pressure continue to grow, susceptibility to peer pressure begins to gradually decrease.	There is a decrease in the perceived importance of peer group as well as decreased susceptibility to peer pressure. At the same time, interest in one-to-one intimate relationships grows. A genuine increase in behavioral autonomy occurs in relation to increased problem-solving, planning-ahead, and impulse-control abilities, together with a decline in conformity both to parents and peers.	This stage marks the emergence of some legal privileges and responsibilities. Economic independence, while not complete, continues to grow, as does behavioral autonomy.	The acquisition of full legal privileges and responsibilities is attained. Economic independence increases, even though some young adults still remain somewhat economically dependent upon their families, particularly in areas with proportionately high unemployment rates among the young population.

Source: Breinbauer and Maddaleno 2004

of the differences in sexual and contraceptive behaviors among white, black, and Hispanic youth in the United States.

For the reasons presented in the preceding paragraphs, at the current time, disagreement continues among developmental researchers about what would constitute a definitive classification, although most would agree that the development of an instrument capable of measuring specific body, brain, social, emotional, sexual, and other similar changes would signify tremendous progress toward being able to safely and accurately establish age delineations based on these indicators. This direction for future research will most likely yield important baselines upon which to construct effectively targeted, developmentally appropriate adolescent health promotion interventions. In the meantime, until an instrument of this type is developed, program designers will need to rely on the current age classifications, which, albeit imperfect and perhaps incomplete, nonetheless provide importance guidance in planning and implementing interventions tailored to the different adolescent developmental stages.

Adolescence is a stage of life when, with the exception of infancy, the body grows and changes more dramatically than at any other point in life. As adolescents become biologically capable of reproduction and sexual arousal, issues related to sexual orientation become one of their principal concerns. Throughout adolescence, reasoning capabilities rise to new levels of complexity, accompanied by a greater sophistication in language skills, the possibility of more advanced moral development, and improved abilities in overall organization, self-regulation, time management, and impulse control. With these developmental tools, adolescents interact with others, expose themselves to new experiences and lifestyle choices, build their identity, and find their role in society, during a period in which parental influence is decreasing and exposure to peer, media, and cultural influences is continually increasing.

The stage progression is not simply biologically determined, but also depends on the joint interactive effect of both environmental experience and endogenous factors, as shown in Figure 26-2. Furthermore, the speed with which an individual progresses through these stages and achieves certain developmental tasks depends upon individual biological differences, cognitive abilities, and educational, emotional, and life experiences, as well as the cultural and social contexts in which the progression occurs. The effect of social interactions on cognitive processes and development has been well delineated by L.S. Vygotsky (1978). He uses the term *zone of proximal development* to describe the difference between an adolescent's actual development and his or her level of potential development when given the opportunity to engage in problem-solving with the guidance of parents, other adults (e.g., teachers), or more expert peers (e.g., peer educators). The critical role of positive

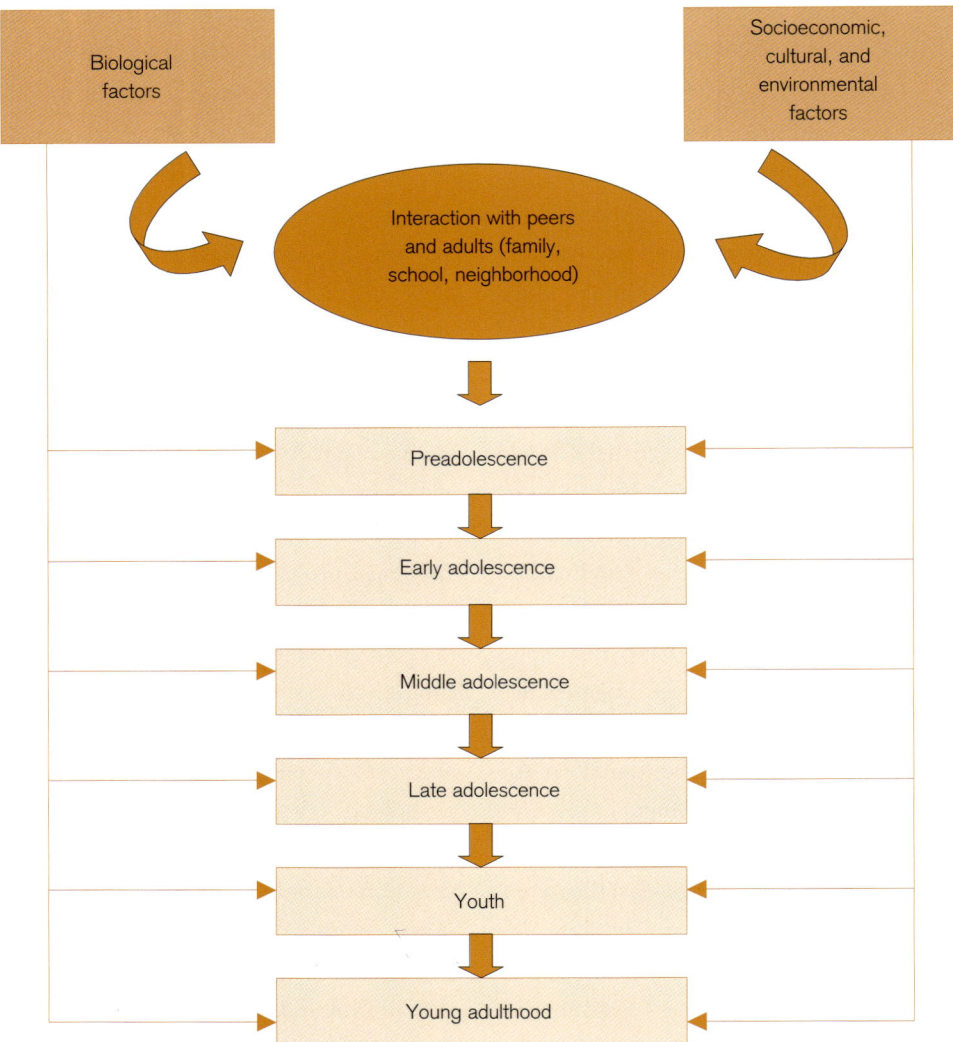

Figure 26-2. **Factors in Adolescent Stage Progression**

Source: adapted with permission from *The Functional Emotional Assessment Scale (FEAS): Clinical and Research Applications,* by S.I. Greenspan, G. DeGangi, and S. Wieder. Interdisciplinary Council on Development and Learning Disorders, Bethesda, Maryland, 2001.

affect and emotions in these types of social interactions was later introduced by Greenspan (1997a).

According to Bronfenbrenner (1979), "the psychological impact of the biological, cognitive, and social changes of adolescence is shaped by the environment in which the changes take place." Psychological development during adolescence is a product of the interplay between the very basic and universal changes (body, brain, social, emotional, and sexuality) and the contexts (families, peer groups, school and work environment, and leisure settings) in which these changes take place. The contexts of adolescence are, in turn, themselves shaped and defined by the larger society in which young people live.

Growing up under adversity (e.g., extreme poverty, domestic violence, parental mental illness, loss of one or both parents, catastrophic events, political violence, civil war) has been associated with an earlier transition into adult roles and behaviors. However, whether "earlier" signifies "better" is a matter of some debate. Growing up in poverty, for example, may profoundly impair youngsters' ability to transition easily from adolescence into adulthood. Poverty is associated with failure in school, unemployment, and early pregnancy, all of which contribute to transition difficulties (Steinberg 1999).

Throughout the various developmental stages, adolescents will not only need to adjust to and assimilate the universal changes depicted in Table 26-2.; at the same time they will need to master a series of *biological, cognitive,* and *socio-emotional goals*. As will be further shown in Chapters Twenty-eight and Twenty-nine of this book, the full attainment of these goals in each stage will support the development of new goals to be achieved during the next stage. Yet it is important to note that socio-emotional development may not always keep pace with physical and cognitive changes occurring at the same time. Also, while there may be a *biological predisposition* for the level of cognitive skills an adolescent may achieve, the optimal development of these abilities requires an interactive and stimulating social environment that includes parents, teachers, and other adult actors willing to actively engage the adolescent and challenge his/her thoughts and feelings in a positive manner. Support structures such as these provide a healthy backdrop against which adolescents whose chronological age and physical development are well synchronized may secure the necessary stimuli to achieve the corresponding levels of cognitive and socio-emotional development for their age group.

Following the concept of audience segmentation introduced by social marketing, increasingly used in the field of public health, PAHO and the authors of this book propose the differentiation of the transition between childhood and adulthood describing these smaller, more homogeneous subgroups to which the intervention programs will be designed and delivered. When designing an intervention it is not only important to know the 11-year-old girl or boy's interests, which can be obtained through questionnaires or focus groups; it is also necessary to be aware of the girl or boy's developmental challenges at that age (body, sexuality, cognitive, social, and emotional), so that the intervention may be tailored to the developmental level and experiences the adolescent is living at the moment of the intervention. This information is necessary, since, as is shown in Table 26-2., the cognitive skills, social interests, and biological capabilities of a 14-year-old will be significantly different than those of a 10-year-old adolescent.

For many of the reasons already suggested in this chapter, as well as those that will be further discussed in Chapters Twenty-eight and Twenty-nine, the preadolescence and early adolescence stages are a strategically critical entryway for interventions encouraging the adoption and maintenance of health-promoting lifestyles during adolescence, particularly those related to healthy and safe sex practices. Early intervention beginning during the preadolescence period allows for greater emphasis to be placed on protecting one's health and preventing the negative consequences of risky sexual behaviors. By waiting until adolescents grow older, health-compromising practices may already be well established and thus harder to change.

Despite this fact, the preadolescent and early adolescent age groups have been frequently overlooked by adolescent health programs, particularly in developing countries, where the tendency observed by this book's authors has been to focus principally on adolescents 15 years of age and older. This is particularly the case for programs which promote safer sex practices. Program developers and facilitators often feel uncomfortable and lack the skills to address topics of sexuality development with adolescents younger than 15 years old. Nevertheless, approximately one in every three to five adolescents worldwide has experienced intercourse by this age, and a higher percentage has been actively involved in sexual exploration. Furthermore, preadolescence and early adolescence are the stages at which young people are most susceptible to sexual coercion and abuse. Despite this situation, most of the information currently available on the global status of adolescent health and development focuses on the middle and late adolescence periods, and comparatively little is known about their earlier-stage counterparts (World Health Organization, UNAIDS 2003). Chapters Twenty-eight and Twenty-nine will review in further depth the needs and challenges of these first two stages of adolescent development.

[Chapter Twenty-seven]

Gender Differences and Adolescent Behaviors

While both girls and boys move through the various developmental stages and experience similar changes, there are significant gender-based differences that need to be considered when planning health-promoting interventions among adolescents. Whereas the term *sex* refers to the biological dimension of being male or female, *gender* refers to the sociocultural dimension of these differences. Few aspects of adolescents' development are more central to their identity and their social relationships than gender considerations. A *gender role* is a set of expectations that prescribes how females or males should think, act, and feel. Biology and sociocultural experiences together shape gender development.

In his book *Boys and Girls Learn Differently!*, Michael Gurian (2001) uses brain-based research to explain the origins of gender differences. He points out that, although our cultural environment shapes children and adolescents, this culture does not arise in a vacuum, but is instead the result of a history of neural responses to natural surroundings and processes. Biological differences are evident at a very early age. From birth on, the body movements of males are more vigorous and less refined than those of females, which are more precise and accurate and more confined to small muscle groups than those of their male counterparts. As males grow, their muscular structure becomes larger and more powerful, giving them greater physical strength (Acuff 1997). For their part, girls take in more sensory data than boys. On average, they hear better, smell better, and take in more tactile information through their fingertips and skin. After a few weeks of age, females will pay attention more to sound and tonal patterns than to visual patterns. Throughout life, they are better able to localize sounds and differentiate between their intensities. Females are faster in their processing of verbal information and demonstrate a more accurate understanding of social clues. Females have better clarity and quality of speech throughout childhood than males. By age 3, females are more responsive to new playmates and, in general, they show greater interest in playmates than in objects (Acuff 1997).

Researchers, such as Ruben Gur (Gur et al. 1995) at the University of Pennsylvania, have discovered functional differences using positron-emission tomography (PET) scans. In most cases, and in most aspects of the developmental chronology, girls' brains mature earlier than those of boys. Girls, for example, may acquire their complex verbal skills as much as a year earlier than boys. The myelination of the brain, which enables electrical impulses to travel down a nerve quickly and efficiently, is one of the last steps in the brain's growth into adulthood. Myelination continues in all brains into the early 20s, but in women the process completes itself earlier than in men. The size of the corpus callosum, which is the bundle of nerves that connects the brain's right and left hemispheres, is up to 20% larger in females than in males. Both prefrontal lobes, which are responsible for the development of executive functions and self-regulation capacity, and the occipital lobes, where sensory processing often occurs, mature earlier and with greater intensity in females than males (Gurian 2001).

Males tend to have more development in certain areas of the brain's right hemisphere, which provides them with better spatial abilities for activities such as measuring (e.g., mechanical design) and geographical orientation (e.g., map-reading). After a few weeks of age, boys will also be more readily attentive to visual patterns than will girls (Acuff 1997). The male advantage on many spatial performance tests emerges before age 10 and remains more or less constant during the adolescent years. Casey and colleagues (1995) propose that any observed differences between males and females in mathematical aptitude are entirely due to this small sexual difference in spatial ability.

A wide variety of empirical studies show that boys' play is much more physical than that of girls. Boys are more physically aggressive than girls, though girls show greater relational aggression. On the other hand, females often tend to be better than males at controlling impulsive behavior (Maccoby 1998).

Interestingly, the behaviors and interactions of both female and male adults toward boys and girls are different, beginning at the infancy stage. Male adults are more physical and aggressive with boy infants and children and more cautious and gentle with girls. Female adults are more likely to react to their sons and physically pacify them, whereas they spend more time talking to their daughters (Acuff 1997).

Despite the gender differences that have been found in brain development, Gurian (2001) proposes that this process is best understood as a spectrum of development rather than two poles, female and male. Many girls lean toward the female extreme, and many boys lean toward the male, but there are boys and girls who possess nearly equal qualities of both the male and female brain traits. According to Gurian, these boys and girls with the most "bi-gender" brains are, in a sense, the bridge between male and female cultures.

Despite possible sex differences in mental abilities, boys and girls learn gender roles through imitation and observational learning by listening to what other people say and watching what they do. Cultural beliefs and attitudes, as well as those found in the school environment, and expressed by peers, the media, family members, and particularly parents, are important influences on gender development.

Parents, by action and by example, influence their children and adolescents' gender development. Social learning theoretical constructs have been especially important in understanding social influences on gender, emphasizing that children and adolescents' gender development occurs through observation and imitation of gender behavior, and through rewards and punishments they experience for what are considered gender-appropriate and -inappropriate behaviors. By observing parents and other adults, as well as peers—at home, at school, in the neighborhood, and in the media—adolescents are exposed to a myriad of models that display masculine and feminine behavior (Santrock 1998). Consciously or unconsciously, parents often use compliments and reprimands to teach their daughter traditional versions of how to be feminine and their sons how to be masculine.

The messages about gender roles carried by the mass media also are important influences on adolescents' gender development. Early adolescence may be a period of heightened sensitivity to television messages about gender roles. Young adolescents increasingly view programs designed for adults that include messages about what is considered gender-appropriate behavior, especially in heterosexual relationships.

Nevertheless, certain traditional versions of masculinity and femininity by which children and adolescents are socialized can have harmful consequences for their health and development. Society sends strong social messages to girls to stay "innocent and virginal" and to control their sexual arousal at the same time that it encourages boys to seek sexual experience with girls and downplays the boys' need to regulate and control sexual arousal. Girls report often being pressured by boys to have sex as a proof of their love and commitment to the relationship. In the male adolescent culture, youths perceive themselves to be more masculine if they engage in premarital sex, drink alcohol, use drugs, and participate in delinquent activities (Santrock 1998). Pleck and O'Donnell (2001) studied the gender attitudes and health risk behaviors among urban African-American and Latino early adolescents. The results showed that after controlling socio-demographic and family variables, males' violence-related behaviors and substance use were associated with traditional beliefs about masculinity. Among these adolescents, females contribute to the traditional version of masculinity by positively associating being sexually active with traditional beliefs about masculinity.

Traditional beliefs about masculinity development were also explored through a qualitative research study supported by the Pan American Health Organization (Aguirre and Güell 2002) in which focus groups were conducted among 10–24-year-old young boys living in nine Latin American and Caribbean countries (Brazil, Colombia, Costa Rica, El Salvador, Guatemala, Honduras, Jamaica, Mexico, and Nicaragua). The study concludes that adolescent boys approach and undergo masculinity development by accepting a series of traditional mandates imposed by male culture organized into four domains:

(1) Body and character development:
Masculine males are expected to be stronger, physically and emotionally, than women and children, so that they will be respected by others. They are also expected to be able to tolerate hard work and be attractive to women. In the countries studied, masculinity was believed to be especially proven on the soccer field, where one's body and personal character are required to respond to the sport's competitive demands of resistance, mental and physical agility, aggression, and tolerance of aggression in order to win against the opponent.

(2) Family relationships:
Masculine males are expected to establish physical and emotional distance from their mothers or else risk the perception by others that they might be homosexuals. Soccer, in this context, symbolizes leaving the mother's world to enter into the father's world. Masculine males are expected to produce children. Those who do not do so are considered to be incomplete males. Masculine males are expected to provide financial support for their families; those who are not financially self-sufficient are considered to be worthless. Because of their ability to provide the family's income, masculine males are also expected to act as the family's principal authority figure.

(3) Intimate partner relationships:
Masculine males are expected to sexually possess, satisfy, and subordinate women. Women's infidelity is not tolerated, since this is viewed as a threat to one's masculinity, and as a possible justification for initiating acts of physical violence against intimate female partners. On the other hand, masculine males are considered to have a heightened sexual arousal level, and masculinity is gauged by the number of

women that men can sexually seduce and subordinate.

(4) Peer relationships:
Masculine males are expected to spend time away from the home, with their peers, beyond the reach of parental protection. Masculinity is developed when males explore, take risks, and accept challenges proposed by their peers. Masculine males prove their autonomy and capacity by handling uncertainties without parental protection.

Rodrigo Aguirre and Pedro Güell, the authors of this study, suggest that the most imminent risk felt by male adolescents when adopting new behaviors is the perceived threat to the development of their masculinity, which is considered to be of much greater importance than the more distant consequences of these new behaviors (e.g., practicing unprotected sex, alcohol and drug exploration, participation in violent gangs). Given this fact, the authors recommend that any intervention that seeks to reduce risk behaviors among adolescent males in Latin America and the Caribbean should take into account the needs related to consolidation of a masculinity identity and should propose alternative behaviors that satisfy these needs in healthier and more positive ways (e.g., excelling in sports, respecting sexual limits set by girls, striving for economic security by making plans for the future).

While male peer relationships and friendships often are based on companionship and joint activities, girls' peer relationships and friendships tend to be characterized by high levels of self-disclosure, intimacy, and emotional support. Several lines of research support the proposal that adolescent girls are at increased risk for stress in their relationships. Adolescent girls report more interpersonal strain and anxiety, including negative events and problems that involve family, peer, and intimate relationships than do boys, who report finding events of self-relevance (e.g., performing well in a sporting event) more stressful than do girls. Almeida and Kessler (1998) support the idea that gender differences in stress levels and types are real and not due to reporting bias. For example, adolescent girls have been found to perceive negative interpersonal events as more stressful than do boys. Adolescent girls are more likely than adolescent boys to be preoccupied with negative thoughts about their friends and to experience negative affect within peer and family contexts.

Kaplan, in his book *Adolescence* (2004), observes that women are often socialized to balance their needs against those of others and to focus more on others' needs than on their own, whereas males are often socialized to confront issues directly and to fulfill their needs by acting upon them. Women often have to be more empathetic and assume roles that require them to support others, which may increase their own stress. In this sense, women might feel they have less control than men over important areas of their lives (Nolen-

Hoeksema, Larson, and Grayson 1999). Women are also more likely to use rumination as a coping style, tending to focus on negative feelings, which prolong the distress (Nolen-Hoeksema 2000). The tendency of women to ruminate more than men is first observed during early adolescence and continues throughout adulthood (Nolen-Hoeksema and Girgus 1994). Levels of stress tend to increase from preadolescence into early adolescence, the stage at which gender differences become more obvious, indicating that this transition represents a period of particular vulnerability for girls (Rudolph 2002).

The types and patterns of aggression and abuse experienced during the adolescent years do appear to differ by gender. Adolescent girls experience higher rates of sexually-related and relational manipulation and abuse, whereas adolescent boys experience more overt forms, such as bullying and physical aggression. Interestingly, this correlates with the different patterns by which boys and girls, at a younger age, express their aggressive feelings, in which boys are more physically aggressive and girls show greater affective aggression. It is not clear if there are gender differences in adolescence for total exposure to victimization but there *are* gender differences during childhood: sexual abuse is more common in females, and physical abuse is more common in males. When subjects who have experienced both sexual and physical childhood abuse are compared by gender, females outnumber males by more than two to one (Hayward and Sanborn 2002).

Unfortunately, the identification of the particular needs and wants of boys and girls has been obfuscated by the unresolved discussion of whether gender differences are natural or imposed by society. While this debate continues, the most effective way to discover these differences will be through focus groups held with the actual adolescents themselves who are being targeted. This valuable input will enable program developers to discern not only gender differences, but within these, variances in the needs and wants by developmental stages, when planning, implementing, and monitoring health promotion interventions.

Girls and boys both share certain particular needs (e.g., love, acceptance, success) during pre- and early adolescence, which will be described in the next two chapters of this book. Both want to have fun and seek novelty and "grown-up" experiences. Nevertheless, boys and girls develop different interests and ways of having fun with their friends, with similarities and differences across cultures. The challenge for parents, teachers, and others who provide support to adolescents is to help them find out what they need, want, and enjoy, rather than allowing cultural and environmental forces to define who they should be and become according to traditional, and, at times, harmful versions of masculinity and femininity.

Adolescent girls and boys need to be listened to, given opportunities, encouraged to have new experiences, and yet be provided with value systems, guidance, and limits. What they need, want, and enjoy must be acknowledged and taken seriously. They need opportunities to attain their needs and most of their wants. They need values and guidance to recognize harmful temptations and in choosing "wants" that are safe and will lead to a healthy development. They need boundaries to discourage and/or curb harmful behaviors.

Girls and boys also need help in mastering gender-specific developmental goals during pre- and early adolescence that will protect them from the harmful effects of traditional and dominant versions of masculinity and femininity that, in turn, may affect the way they approach sexual activity and relationships. Furthermore, adults need to recognize that most adolescent lifestyle decisions (e.g., sexual practices; tobacco, alcohol, and drug use; physical activity and nutrition; anger expression) are influenced at least in part by the anxieties surrounding male-female interactions and gender-related expectations.

The *Young Men's Sexual and Reproductive Health: Toward a National Strategy, Framework, and Recommendations* was prepared by an interdisciplinary working group of experts and edited by Freya Sonenstein (2000) for the Urban Institute, a social and educational research organization. It emphasizes the importance of forming a new vision of men's sexual health in which "all males will grow and develop with a secure sense of their sexual identity, an understanding about the physical and emotional aspects of sexual intimacy, and attitudes that lead to responsible behavior." Achievement of these developmental goals, the report emphasizes, "will result in men postponing sexual intercourse until they are emotionally mature enough to manage the physical and psychological aspects of sexual intimacy. When they have sexual intercourse, it will occur with as little risk as possible to either themselves or their partner."

To achieve the described results, the above-mentioned framework proposes that all young men need access to a range of services that, in combination, fulfill five goals: they will promote sexual health and development; promote healthy intimate relationships; prevent and control STIs, including HIV; prevent unintended pregnancy; and promote responsible fatherhood. To attain each of these goals, the working group suggests that a comprehensive reproductive health strategy for young men should ensure access for them to the necessary information, foster skills development, promote self-concept, help men to identify and develop positive values and sufficient motivation to act on those values, and provide access to clinical care, as needed (Sonenstein 2000).

The Pan American Health Organization shares this new vision of male sexual and reproductive health. Yet, at the same time, PAHO considers that the developmental goals proposed by Sonenstein and colleagues need to be further refined into gender-specific goals for each of the different adolescent developmental stages. As will be shown in the next two chapters, this further refinement takes into account the differences in how boys and girls approach and adjust to the changes characteristic of each successive developmental stage.

[Chapter Twenty-eight]

Early Intervention during Adolescence: The Preadolescent Period

In the transition from childhood to adulthood, the stages of *preadolescence*[1] and *early adolescence*[2] are extremely relevant to our discussion of adopting and maintaining health-promoting lifestyles. As has been previously noted, the Pan American Health Organization considers these two groups to be the most overlooked by adolescent health programs, and it emphasizes the importance of early intervention beginning with preadolescence, instead of waiting until later, when health-compromising behaviors have already begun and may be more difficult to change. This chapter, focusing on preadolescence, and Chapter Twenty-nine, focusing on early adolescence, will present an analysis of the needs and wants of each age group, as well as of age-appropriate developmental goals, which can contribute to adolescents' ability to foster and sustain positive and protective health behaviors. By recognizing and understanding the universal biological, cognitive, and socio-emotional changes that characterize the two developmental stages, as well as lifestyle- and gender-specific development goals appropriate for each group, health promotion program developers can set the stage for a *respectful intervention* that responds to adolescent needs and wants and encourages them to become agents in their own positive behavioral change.

In their award-winning comic strip *Zits*, Jerry Scott and Jim Borgman chronicle the life of Jeremy Duncan, a 15-year-old aspiring rock musician, "riddled with angst, boredom, and

---

[1] Ages 9–12 (girls) and 10–13 (boys)
[2] Ages 12–14 (girls) and 13–15 (boys)

parents who don't understand anything." Jeremy must deal with parents trying to figure out "the mysterious science of parenting a teenager" and live up to the "dreadfully perfect example" of his "glowing college-student brother," all the while honing his "advanced hangin' out techniques" with his best friend Hector. In one adventure, Jeremy waxes particularly philosophic about the at-times incompatible wants and needs of youth and the difficulties in reconciling them when he says: "Fitting in. Being different. Growing up. Staying a kid. Breaking away. Settling in. Needing help. Wanting out. Adolescence bites. . . ."

Not surprisingly, the response to the comic series by its youthful audience has been overwhelming since its debut in 1997. Perhaps its appeal lies in the deft mixture of Jeremy's projection of comedy and irony, understatement and overkill, frustration and indifference, joy and suffering—all typical adolescent reactions to the oftentimes bewildering world that surrounds them. And Jeremy feels caught in the middle of it all.

The road to adulthood, from the perspective of those who are just preparing to make their way onto it, inspires both anticipation and apprehension. This period is the transitional phase from childhood into adolescence, which many have come to call preadolescence or "preteen," meaning, literally, "before becoming 13 years old." During preadolescence, physical, cognitive, sexual, and socio-emotional changes occur, with a permanent interaction between these new aspects, as we saw in Chapter Twenty-six. Physical transformations involve all the bodily changes associated with puberty. Cognitive changes include the use of more concrete, logical, reality-based thinking, with a shift from egocentric to socio-centric thought, which enables preteens to begin to place themselves in others' situations and understand better the feelings and viewpoints of other people. Socio-emotional changes are marked by a newly emerging need for an intimate one-to-one relationship with a companion of the same sex ("best friend"). As preadolescents' bodies start to change, so do their interests, the type of friendships and other relationships they establish, the ways in which they choose to have fun, and their strategies for analyzing new situations using emerging cognitive skills.

Preteens' physical changes begin with the first signs of a growth spurt and the redistribution of body fat, which transform the shape and look of the child's face and body. Parents become aware of the need to buy new clothes for their growing children, while the latter begins to show distinct preferences in what she/he wants to wear, choosing popular brands and styles usually worn by other friends. During the preteen years, boys and girls realize the effect clothing can have in making them more attractive and mature-looking. How preadolescents wish to express themselves through their clothing choices may be a frequent topic of negotiation and/or argu-

Table 28-1. **Universal Changes during the Preadolescent Stage**

Body Development	— Appearance of secondary sex characteristics
	— Increase in and redistribution of body fat and weight
	— Emerging signs of significant growth spurt
	— Heightened need for sensation-seeking
Brain Development	— Shift from egocentric to socio-centric thought
	— Capacity for more concrete, logical thinking, with conservation tasks[3] in the process of being acquired
	— Accelerated information-craving, although language is still concrete
	— Little development of frontal lobe and executive functions
Sexuality Development	— Exploration of more differentiated masculine and feminine roles by boys and girls compared to previous years
	— For girls, androgyny is a viable alternative to exclusive femininity while for boys exclusive masculinity remains most socially expected role
Emotional Development	— Gradual increase in self-consciousness and fluctuations of self-image with increasing feelings of embarrassment
	— Emerging need for greater privacy, individuation, and more emotional autonomy from parents: to feel individuated within the relationship with parents (e.g., to feel that parents don't know things about them), to depend more on themselves rather than on their parents, and to gradually de-idealize their parents
	— Fluctuations in verbal and nonverbal expression (facial gestures) of intense emotions (e.g., aggression, frustration, excitement, boredom)
	— Ability to explore multiple reasons for a feeling, compare feelings, and understand triadic interactions among feeling states
	— Ability to differentiate shades and gradations among feeling states (e.g., "I feel a little angry")
	— Gradual shift from pre-conventional (rewards and punishments) to conventional morality (society's rules)
Social Development	— Emerging need for a same-sex best friend
	— Emerging need to have fun and share secrets with best friend
	— Time spent with parents and parental supervision still present but begins gradually to decrease
	— Gradual increase in conflicts with parents
	— Increase in academic and social demands and expectations
	— Increase in susceptibility to peer pressure

ments with their parents. Girls become more interested in experimenting with makeup, nail polish, and hair styles, in some cases attempting to imitate older girls they know, television and music personalities, fashion magazine role models, and "popular" girls at school. Preadolescents, particularly girls, will begin to spend more time in the bathroom and their bedrooms studying their appearance in the mirror and picking out their wardrobe. Both males and females will be concerned about pimples and have mixed feelings about the emergence of body hair.

---
[3] See Table 26-2 footnote.

Preteens' faces also change due to the eruption of new permanent teeth (canine, first and second premolars). This is the period when dentists generally recommend braces, if necessary. Preadolescence is also characterized by the appearance of secondary sex characteristics (breast bud around the nipple in girls; larger testes with redder scrotum in boys). Boys and girls become aware of how their bodies are changing, and in many cases wish to compare these changes with those experienced by their friends. The re-proportioning of body fat might trigger significant concern in girls (and, to a lesser extent, boys) if they feel that their new body shape makes them look overweight.

During this time, girls will discuss with their friends when is the time to begin wearing a bra. They might also show apprehension about the beginning of menstruation, especially if they do not feel comfortable discussing this new experience with their mothers or if much of their information is gleaned from television, magazines, and/or other friends' experiences. Girls begin contemplating the idea of having a romantic relationship with boys and comparing the qualities and defects of their male peers among their same-sex friends, oftentimes developing a secret classification system for including or discarding candidates. As part of this, female friends will often confide in each other about who has a "crush" on whom. They also become more keenly aware of popular musical lyrics, often relating these to their own life experiences, whether the message refers to romantic ideas or the desire for empowerment and more freedom of expression.

Boys begin to use deodorants and will make fun of each other's underwear and other types of clothes. They tend to enjoy informal competitions among their friends regarding who is the "grossest," who has the capacity for louder flatulence and burps, and who possesses the most natural talent for incorporating obscenities of a sexual nature in their daily language. In general, during adolescence, the female's interest in the opposite sex is not reciprocated. Instead, boys prefer to trivialize and minimize the importance of girls in their environment by making fun of them and avoiding the formation of close contact and friendships with them.

As preadolescents' bodies change, they become aware that they feel, look, and move differently than before and experience feelings of clumsiness and poor motor planning as their bodies change and become bigger. Parents expect preadolescents to have greater autonomy with respect to aspects of daily living and self-care, such as personal hygiene and grooming, representing a transitional period in which preadolescents avoid these new responsibilities, particularly washing their hair and taking showers. These changes need to be absorbed by the preadolescent, so that he/she comes to feel that this new body is a part of him or her. The glamorous, polished, and self-assured male and female body images preadolescents see on television and in magazines tend to establish unrealistic and even false expectations.

In *Reviving Ophelia*, author Mary Pipher (1994) contends that the preoccupation with bodies at this age cannot be overstated. She contends that "generally girls have strong bodies when they enter puberty. But these bodies soften and spread out in ways that our culture calls fat. Girls feel an enormous pressure to be beautiful and are aware of constant evaluations of their appearance." Boys, on the other hand, feel pressured to have a strong body that projects their ideals of masculinity development, and the strength of their bodies has a direct impact on their self-image. It is therefore essential for parents to not only have a sufficient grasp of the biological facts of normal growth and development, but also to have a clear understanding and empathy for what these changes mean to their preadolescent.

Pubertal changes do not happen at the same age in boys and girls. A meta-analysis of U.S. growth statistics indicates that puberty now begins at an average age of 9 years in girls and 11 years in boys (Abbassi 1998). A difference among races has also been found. Pubertal changes begin by an average age of 10 in white girls, whereas puberty begins between 8–9 years of age in black girls (Herman-Giddens et al. 1997).

Although subtle body changes start earlier during preadolescence, it is in the middle of this period that growth spurts have the greatest impact. For girls, the average age at which the growth spurt becomes most apparent is 10. The average boy experiences significant growth at about age 12 (Pruitt 1999). They now have bigger bodies and more physical strength to carry out strenuous activities. Nevertheless, physical growth is not necessarily accompanied by cognitive and socio-emotional growth, as we saw in Chapter Twenty-six. Tall, physically well-developed preadolescents may have the emotions of children; more abstract thinkers may have the social skills of first graders. These differences in developmental levels within the same child confound adults. Very often, parents and teachers in their lives hold expectations for them based on physical appearance, forgetting the child's chronological age and current emotional functioning. More mature physical appearances make young adolescents more likely to associate with a chronologically older peer group, regardless of whether they possess similar levels of cognitive and socio-emotional development.

Because preteens enter and complete the biological changes associated with puberty at different times, their preparation for, and experiences with, the physical changes of adolescence are highly variable, as well. Early-maturing girls and late-maturing boys are at heightened risk for adjustment problems (Graber et al. 1997). Hormonal fluctuations occurring during puberty have been associated with mood and behavior changes. Hormones are instrumental in altering peripheral systems, such as the sensory system, and in changes related to the menstrual cycle that influence vision, smell, and general arousal. Hormonal changes also influence the central nervous system and neurotransmitter activity involved in the regulation of emotions and affective processing (Killgore, Oki, and Yurgelun-Todd 2001; Buchanan, Eccles, and Becker 1992). Nevertheless, there is evidence that social events and hormonal change together predict negative affect better than hormonal change alone (Brooks-Gunn and Warren 1989).

According to Brooks-Gunn and Paikoff (1993), the first developmental challenge concerning sexuality in adolescence is accepting one's changing body. The preadolescence years are a stressful time characterized by mood swings and a need for privacy, withdrawal, and confrontation. As they see themselves and their peers change, preteens start to worry about whether or not they are "normal" and whether they are developing into the person they would like to be. As children enter their preteen years, a necessary but difficult process of defining their own personality begins. They look to their peers as their measure of "normalcy." For the first time, preadolescents turn away from their parents and toward their peers to determine what behaviors and attitudes are acceptable and appropriate (U.S. National Youth Anti-Drug Media Campaign 1999).

During preadolescence, a new need for interpersonal intimacy with a playmate of the same sex emerges, as boys and girls move away from the broad need for a larger group of playmates which prevailed in previous years. There is also a need for the intimate sharing of thoughts, feelings, and ideas with just one playmate. This "best friend," who also becomes a confidant, is usually of the same sex and social status and approximately the same age. According to Sullivan and his Interpersonal Theory of Psychiatry (1953), the preadolescent experiences, often for the first time, feelings of genuine love and loyalty and opportunities for self-disclosure and intimacy, but in an atmosphere still relatively uncomplicated by the sexual arousal that will manifest itself with more intensity during early adolescence. As the preoccupation with the "best friend" relationship gains importance, preadolescents tend to distance themselves from the family. They begin to look at the family more objectively, and often more critically, and share these new perceptions with their best friend.

Preadolescents and their parents often find themselves on unfamiliar terrain, in which the issue of trust becomes emotionally charged. Preteens are still greatly dependent upon their parents' permission in a variety of aspects. However, this dependence is in conflict with their desire for greater freedom and autonomy. Their need for privacy makes them feel it is no longer acceptable for their parents to be aware of everything that is happening in their lives. Parents want to trust their child, but are reluctant to grant them the amount of freedom they request. Preadolescents, for their part, feel "entitled" to the level of trust they are requesting, and often feel that their parents' former trust in them is waning just at the time they most need it. These adjustments often result in parent-preteen interactions that are laden with conflict, power struggles, and ambivalence. These are the years in which an effective parenting style that incorporates the characteristics discussed in Chapter Eighteen can have a profound impact on whether adolescents adopt health-promoting or health-compromising lifestyles.

Preadolescents' lives are also more stressful because of external demands. Academic, social, and athletic competition becomes increasingly overwhelming. In many developing countries, dropping out of school has already begun among those in this age group, especially boys, with a strong association between those who drop out and subsequently enter the workforce. In Venezuela, 4% of boys fall into this category by the age of 12. Child labor at age 12 reaches almost 10% in Honduras (Filgueira, Filgueira, and Fuentes 2001). In rural areas, the situation is more severe. In Brazil, rural youth average 4.2 years of education (with the average dropout age being approximately 10.2 years) and 5.3 years in Honduras (with the average dropout age being approximately 11.3 years) (Comisión Económica para América Latina y el Caribe 1997). Unfortunately, child labor and dropping out of school are still a frequent reality for preadolescents living in several Latin American and Caribbean countries, although the principal international legal instrument that recommends minimum ages for labor, the International Labor Organization's Convention 138, states that the countries ratifying the convention should specify a minimum age for admission to employment or work, which "shall not be less than the age of completion of compulsory schooling and, in any case, shall not be less than 15 years" (International Labor Organization 1973).

Peer grouping becomes more defined towards the end of preadolescence (11–12 years old). By this age, preteens sense that they need to make the difficult choice of either attaching themselves to a specific group or being isolated and socially left out. This realization may result in a loss of confidence regarding social relationships and an intense desire to "fit in" at all costs. In preteen culture, the process of growing into adolescence is inextricably linked with taking part in risky behaviors, having secrets, and testing the limits and rules of authority. Peers see a preteen who is unable to take risks as one who is immature, unwilling, and/or incapable of growing up. These risks can take numerous forms, ranging from the more benign (e.g., mischievous pranks, playing jokes on others) to the more dangerous (e.g., physical/sports challenges, sexual adventurism, and/or cigarette, alcohol, or drug experimentation). In order to be perceived by themselves and others as "growing up," preadolescents often feel compelled to aggressively "push away" from supposedly childish concepts and activities. They may even feel the need to make these childish concepts "wrong" in order to establish themselves as "beyond them" (e.g., being told by parents what to wear, playing with toys, watching cartoons on television with younger siblings, joining in family sports, helping in family chores). It is also easier, at this stage of development, to rationalize breaking the rules. Along with greater concerns about right and wrong come more sophisticated reasoning powers that preteens employ to try to get around rules they previously might not have questioned (Acuff 1997).

During the preadolescent years, due to their sharpened thinking skills and opening to the outside world, boys and girls crave information. This new information, and the values they will develop based on it, will come not only from their parents, but also from friends, older siblings, other significant adults (e.g., teachers, guidance counselors, friends' parents, church leaders), and media messages (e.g., television, radio, magazines, books, Internet). Preadolescents are vulnerable to building their identity by focusing on pleasing others around them whom they admire instead of focusing on discovering their own inner strengths and weaknesses and likes and dislikes. At the same time, they are at risk of defining themselves through *not being* someone or something else instead of being who and what they are. For example, girls are expected *not to be* like boys, boys are expected *not to be* like girls, and both are expected *not to be* babyish and to instead become more mature. There is also a gray area regarding whether it is acceptable to notice and "like" members of one's own gender versus the opposite one. In any case, preteens are expected *not to be* too different from the rest, but different from their parents. This tendency to build identity based on *not being* versus *being* leaves them more vulnerable to peer pressure once they reach middle adolescence. Therefore, it is crucial that parents and teachers work with preadolescents and help them to define themselves by their own unique characteristics (e.g., sense of humor, consideration for others, shy, outgoing, smart, need to work harder in school) and interests (favorite foods, colors they like to wear, ideas about and plans for the future, sports and leisure-time activities that most appeal to them) instead of allowing this group to define itself solely through the influence of peer groups and the media. This support will help boys and girls create internal standards based on a more stable and secure sense of self and provide a basis to judge experiences and further reflect upon them independently.

Peer relationships for both boys and girls intensify with the increasing introduction of sexual interests and behaviors in the last two years of preadolescence. For girls, personal relationships become increasingly important, while boys tend to focus on sports and other types of competition (e.g., video games). Talking with and about each other's friends and schoolmates on the phone, online, and in person becomes a favorite activity. As boys measure their physical and intellectual characteristics by their performance in sports, video games, and best "gross" jokes, girls become focused on virtually every aspect of their appearance, using products such as makeup, skin and nail care items, and hair accessories for the first time to bolster their self-confidence. The telling of dirty jokes; perusal of magazines, books, movies, and Internet sites with explicit sexual content; and increased shyness around the opposite sex are all part of the eagerness for, and fear of, the physical and sexual changes about to occur. During preadolescence, girls and boys attempt to differentiate themselves from the opposite sex by choosing different interests (e.g., sports versus fashion magazines, action movies versus love stories) and by making fun of the other gender's behaviors and physical appearance. There is a competition for power and recognition between genders that might develop further into disrespectful sexual advances and even use of physical force during the next stages of adolescence.

Despite this new distress and turmoil, preteens reap the benefits of integrating themselves into a group and defining themselves as group members. They gain an enormous ability for complex thinking. To negotiate successfully the intricacies of multiple relationships within a group, preteens must learn to reason on a very sophisticated level. This ability to diagnose group dynamics helps preteens to develop cognitive and social skills that will be very valuable in their immediate school environment and beyond, since much of the adult world in which they will eventually perform will involve many of these same dynamics. By the end of the preadolescent stage, most boys and girls will have begun to embrace their own beliefs and to develop their own set of internal values, and they also start to think about the future. They can now hold on to two realities at once: their external peer group reality and their emerging inner reality of values and attitudes (Greenspan 1993).

Within this context, the most successful health promotion and prevention programs will be those that not only tailor their interventions to the biological, cognitive, sexual, and socio-emotional changes occurring during the preadolescent period, but also *motivate* this age group to use the pertinent information and services available to achieve the skills and assets they need to prepare for the even more complex changes lying immediately ahead. By grasping this idea early, adolescents over time come to intuitively understand the desirability of moving away from negative influences and situations and learn to confidently make choices of this type as a statement of personal empowerment and self-preservation.

The Needs of Preadolescents

Different authors (Brazelton and Greenspan 2000, Acuff 1997) have identified some fundamental requirements that children and adolescents need for a healthy development. In many ways they complement and enhance the broad considerations first presented in Chapter Five of this book. All of these are needs that parents, teachers, and the community at large should respond to so that society's younger members may grow, learn, and be healthy and productive future adults. Any health promotion and prevention intervention aimed at young people—and particularly those in the first stages of adolescence—should incorporate a targeted response to these needs in its design. A literature search by the authors of this book revealed several overarching needs that are particularly important to preadolescents. (The needs themselves are very similar for early adolescents, as we will see in the following chapter. Yet in each case, the way in which these needs may be met or responded to will take into account distinct developmental characteristics.)

- **Love, ongoing nurturing relationships, and acceptance:** Relationships are essential for regulating human behavior, moods, and feelings, as well as for intellectual stimulation and development. Any effort to promote the adoption of healthy lifestyles requires the presence of ongoing nurturing relationships with the actors involved in this task (e.g., parents, teachers, role models, peer facilitators). The preteen's need for acceptance is essentially the need to feel "OK" and approved of by the important people in his or her life, including parents, siblings, and peers. Preadolescents also need reassurance that they are still going to be loved and accepted by their parents and other significant others, even though this is the stage at which disagreements in opinions and about likes and dislikes usually first emerge. This need for continued acceptance as a human being is particularly strong during preadolescence due to an expanded cognitive awareness (e.g., ability to read nonverbal cues) and the social sensitivities that accompany that sharpened awareness. The majority of these anxieties may occur unconsciously and be imperceptible to others, including parents and teachers. During this period, communication with caring adults is essential to bring many of these formational conclusions about the child's identity to the surface so that they may be adequately defined and dealt with (Acuff 1997). Preadolescents may pretend to be more emotionally independent, but insecurity nonetheless surrounds them when confronted with changes and new decisions to make. They need to know that they can come back to their secure base (home, parents, and involved teachers) and feel protected, loved, and cared for by supportive adults. Even more, they crave positive reinforcements and the feeling of being admired by their parents and teachers, which is related to the need for success described below.

- **Developmentally appropriate experiences and success:** During this stage, preteens begin to concern themselves, consciously or unconsciously, with what conditions and requirements might be needed to survive on their own and succeed in the real world. To help them do this, they need to establish a *sense of industry*, by learning how to produce things and do a job well, thereby winning the recognition and approval of others, and gaining a feeling of success. The need for success drives them to search for answers to key questions: what are the rules and how can I deal with them? What is good, bad, right, and wrong? What roles are out there in society, and which of these do I want to emulate? Despite the conclusions they reach, preteens are still quite malleable and open to influence. They do not yet have the ego strength or sense of self to completely "think for themselves." Much of the learning that takes place during this period is through experience and emulation of role models in real life and in entertainment and sports (Acuff 1997). Parents and teachers play a crucial role in helping preadolescents acquire the ability to "think for themselves" and increase their ego strength and sense of self by providing developmentally appropriate experiences and challenges that will allow them to successfully master these challenges.

■ ***Opportunities, guidance, limits, values, and expectations:*** As preadolescents explore new behaviors and define their identities with new and changing bodies, they need opportunities, guidance, clear limits, and expectations. Parents will need to define in which areas of life preadolescents may make their own decisions, in which they still need guidance, and in which they need firm limits to protect them from harm. Adolescents need to be aware of their parents' values and expectations. They need opportunities to express their likes and dislikes and to be involved in choosing their own clothes, after-school activities, and ways to have fun. Preadolescents need guidance regarding what is socially appropriate, but should still be able to express their uniqueness within set social limits. They also need guidance on how to interact with other boys and girls; how to be appropriately empathetic, assertive, and distrustful; how to protect themselves from temptations and dangers; and how to spend and save money according to their economic circumstances. Preadolescents need to experience the consequences for trespassing minor limits. But most importantly, they need firm limits for behaviors that can cause them harm. Parents need to enforce these limits by anticipating situations that can expose their children to the option of trespassing those limits and helping them avoid these situations by redirecting their behavior, offering other alternatives to satisfy the need for exploring risky behaviors, and increasing communication with children about the risks involved.

■ ***Safe and supportive environments at home, school, and in the neighborhood:*** Preadolescents need to feel a sense of physical safety and security where they live, play, and work. They need to live in a safe and secure house with safe and secure relationships that contribute to their overall sense of well-being. Being a witness to or a victim of domestic or neighborhood violence has detrimental effects on their development and health and significantly decreases the possibilities that they will adopt health-promoting behaviors. Preadolescents also need to receive an adequate academic education, which will be optimized in a safe, caring, and protective school climate. Finally, preadolescents need to feel that the homes of their neighbors, the commercial establishments they go to, and the public spaces they visit (e.g., playgrounds, parks, beaches, churches) will not place them in danger or cause them harm.

- **Structures to provide healthy nutrition, physical activity, and proper sleep:** Preadolescents are growing at a rapid pace, since this is the period when the most significant growth spurt occurs. They need to adopt and maintain healthy nutrition and physical activity not only to prevent future obesity and heart disease, but also to fuel their body with the necessary nutrients to support their current development. Preadolescence, along with lactation, is the period when the largest amounts of calcium are required by the body. During preadolescence, boys and girls need between 1,200 and 1,500 mg of calcium per day. Weight-bearing exercise (i.e., any sport except for swimming or cycling) helps not only to build muscle, but also to build and strengthen bones. If preadolescents do not receive sufficient supervision and encouragement, their eating, physical activity, and sleeping habits will become unpredictable and erratic. Their life is now driven by the search for novelty, fun, and sensation-seeking, which takes priority over eating, sleeping, and exercise considerations. At the same time, their appetite, particularly for snack foods, increases considerably. Preadolescents enjoy watching late-night television and no longer go to bed early. They will also tend to sleep in until the late morning hours, not rising until long after all the other family members. Parents should allow some flexibility in these areas while at the same time providing structure. Preadolescents need adult help in organizing their schedules to include not only new age-appropriate experiences, but also adequate attention to the body's nutritional, exercise, and sleep requirements.

The series of preadolescent needs described in the preceding paragraphs should be taken into account in the design of all health promotion and prevention programs targeted to this group. Whenever possible, the parents of preadolescents should also be active participants in the health-promoting intervention. In determining how best to respond to preadolescent needs, the interpersonal level theories for behavior change presented in Chapters

Sixteen to Twenty, and particularly the Authoritative Parenting Model (Chapter Eighteen), can provide much practical insight into the necessary components to be included in the intervention.

The Wants of Preadolescents

Preadolescents want to have fun. Almost every parent of a preteen will have heard their son or daughter say on more than one occasion: "I am bored." Compared to previous ages, preadolescents now have more developed skills to explore and participate in new experiences, but still not enough autonomy to do this on their own. This stage is also characterized by an increase in high sensation-seeking behaviors, as we saw in Chapter Fourteen.

Preadolescents want to have fun alone and with their friends. In general, the higher sensation-seeking preadolescents with well-coordinated motor skills will want to engage in sports and outdoor activities. Less well-coordinated and sensation-seeking preadolescents will prefer indoor activities, such as computer and video games. Both groups will enjoy different types of media entertainment (e.g., television, music, magazines, movies, Internet) than in the past. The type of sports, outdoor activities, and peer group and media entertainment they choose will vary in different cultures and countries.

Any health promotion and prevention intervention that seeks successful results should provide preteens opportunities for novelty, fun, humor, and social interactions. Furthermore, this group is more likely to engage in activities that allow them to share their interests and likes and dislikes first, before dealing with topics imposed by an adult agenda (e.g., drug resistance skills). Lastly, but equally important, understanding media preferences at each adolescent stage will help program designers to better analyze existing media messages and develop and deliver age-appropriate health messages. The literature shows that there are several wants that seem to attract preadolescents across the board, although cultural variations may determine the actual way in which these wants are acted out:

- ■ *Novelty*: Preadolescents seek novelty, through new television shows, movies, video games, magazines, leisure activities, sports, music, and new friendships. They also explore new ways to "reinvent" themselves, to appear unique in the eyes of their peers. Most preadolescents also want to change the appearance of their rooms and make them more reflective of their new interests by adding personal touches (e.g., new paint color, posters, photos, bedspread and sheets, other mementos they highly prize).

- ■ *Social interaction*: Preadolescents enjoy get-togethers with their best friends. Sleepover birthday parties and spending the night at their best friend's house are very attractive panoramas for most preadolescents. At this age, preadolescents also begin using the telephone more frequently and independently to share experiences with their best friends.

- **"Grown-up" experiences:** Preadolescents want to differentiate themselves from younger children. They also want to explore new experiences previously "forbidden" to them. Most girls want to dress like older girls in school and popular television and musical personalities, use cosmetics and nail polish, and be able to spend long periods of time unsupervised with their best friends in their room. Most boys want to play more mature (T [teen]-rated) video games, stay up late watching television, and not have to share in competitive sports (e.g., football, soccer, basketball, baseball) with younger children. Both want "grown-up experiences," such as drinking coffee, earning their own money, buying things with personal earnings, having their own cell phone, and watching PG-13 movies.

- **Television shows and movies**: Preadolescents want to watch television and be the first in their peer group to see the latest popular movie. The types of television shows and movies that most appeal to this age group are essentially comedy and action-oriented. Girls will also be interested in romantic comedies, while boys will tend to like sport themes. Both sexes also enjoy light situation comedies and dramas, preferably family- or relationship-based. Preteens are eager to discover and learn the rules and roles of how to get along in society. They want to identify themselves with characters that are similar to themselves or have characteristics preteens aspire to emulate.

- **Humor in the media**: The ability to understand more abstract humor is fast developing at this age. Preadolescents begin to enjoy darker, edgier, "irreverent" forms of media humor (sarcasm, ridicule) such as gross jokes, the humiliation of other characters, and depictions of the outwitting of authority figures (e.g., parents, teachers, school principals, police, judges). For boys more than girls, humor with a dark side holds significant appeal. "Gross-out" humor is also entertaining at this age because it is considered a taboo. The irreverent actions of certain cartoon characters, or the latest "bad-boy/bad-girl" antics of a rebellious sports hero or musical star, appeal to the preadolescent's desire for independence and for the freedom to be similarly daring. In general, however, preteens are still not ready to enjoy more sophisticated forms of humor that deal with political issues, ethnicity, or sexuality (Acuff 1997).

- **Magazines and books:** There are a number of publications whose contents are oriented toward preteen interests and feature a variety of role models for them to emulate. Comic books and sports and video game magazines are usually targeted toward boys. Girls tend to prefer magazines dealing with the latest news and gossip about their favorite "teen idols" from the worlds of music, television, and film, as well as teen beauty magazines that provide skin care and makeup tips and show the latest clothing and hairstyle trends. Many girls at this age also enjoy how-to magazines or books dealing with pet care; principally dogs and cats, but also horses, a particular attraction for preteens.

- *Music*: Interest in pop music is increasing during this stage, usually occurring in girls earlier than in boys. Girls tend to prefer pop songs with danceable rhythms and simple melodies, whereas boys tend to prefer harder-edged and less mainstream types of music with action-based lyrics that are laced with black humor and at times even violent themes.

- *Video and computer games*: Boys are more avid game players than girls, the latter of whom account for only about 20% of electronic game play (Acuff 1997). These electronic types of entertainment provide the challenge, competition, complexity, stimulation, variety, and rewards boys and girls seek at this age.

- *Sports*: Preteens, especially boys, become passionate about sports. This activity offers them the opportunity to challenge their own abilities and gain skill over time; it enables them to compete with others and gauge their relative level of physical prowess; and it provides time to just have fun with their friends and schoolmates. As professional sports teams (particularly football, soccer, basketball, and baseball) become a major source of interest, boys want to acquire all types of sports paraphernalia for their personal use and to share with their closest friends. Girls' sports involvement increases during this period, but remains lower than that of boys. Sixty-one percent of boys reported playing at least one sport on an organized team, compared to only 38% of girls (U.S. National Youth Anti-Drug Media Campaign 1999, Sports Illustrated for Kids 1998).

Preadolescents also experience changes in their beliefs and attitudes regarding drug usage while moving into early adolescence. Because a dramatic upswing in drug awareness and experimentation has been found in the United States among this group (Partnership for a Drug-Free America 1999), it is the primary youth target for the National Youth Anti-Drug Media Campaign. From sixth grade (average age 12 years) to eighth grade (average age 14 years), a steady erosion of anti-drug feelings has been shown, with a clear shift to greater acceptance of illicit substances, particularly marijuana. While three-quarters of fifth graders (i.e., still preteens) feel that "taking drugs scares me," less than two-thirds of sixth graders and only one-third of eighth graders (early adolescents) feel that way. The great majority of seventh (80%) and eighth (82%) graders do not perceive any major risk in experimenting with marijuana. In sixth grade, about 20% have at least a few friends who use marijuana or inhalants. The percentage of preadolescents who have friends who use marijuana increases significantly, reaching 40% in seventh grade and 59% in eighth grade.

Based on these findings, the U.S. National Youth Anti-Drug Media Campaign has incorporated into the design of its messages the four Sensation-Seeking Targeting (SENTAR) principles described in Chapter Fourteen, as well as elements from the Social Cognitive Theory, the Health Belief Model, and the Theories of Reasoned Action and Planned Behavior. The messages are particularly geared toward high sensation-seekers, although they have also been proven to be successful with low sensation-seekers (Palmgreen et al. 2001, 1995).

The *wants* of preadolescents described in the previous paragraphs should be given as equally serious consideration as this group's *needs* when health promotion interventions are being developed for them. Given that a general upswing occurs in sensation-seeking during preadolescence, the authors of this book recommend that those working with this age group gain a full understanding of the principles discussed in Chapter Fourteen and recognize that while preadolescents *need* outlets for novelty and fun, they often confuse this with *wanting* to try experiences (e.g., smoking marijuana) that are potentially harmful and dangerous to them. By understanding that increased sensation-seeking among preadolescents is a normal reflection of their growth and development process, program designers may better learn how to provide youth with satisfying and safe health-promoting alternatives. When planning interventions, the most effective way to identify preadolescent wants is to develop questionnaires at the local level and encourage the target group members to express their own preferences regarding media entertainment, social activities, and types of food, physical activities, and sports they most enjoy.

The Health-Promoting Developmental Goals of Preadolescence

In developing health promotion and prevention programs for this age group, designers need to include not only the particular health goals of their interventions (e.g., increase physical activity among preadolescent girls, improve nutritional intake among preadolescent male athletes), but also a series of *developmental goals* that will contribute to the preadolescent's ability to adopt health-promoting behaviors. These goals may be divided into five categories: (1) biological changes and developmental goals; (2) cognitive changes and developmental goals; (3) socio-emotional changes and developmental goals; (4) lifestyle-specific developmental goals; and (5) gender-specific developmental goals.

The first three basic goals are related to the biological, cognitive, and socio-emotional changes universally experienced by preadolescents, as discussed in Chapter Twenty-six. Although separated to facilitate the reader's comprehension, these goals are in reality interrelated and constitute the foundation for achieving health-promoting behaviors. The fourth category addresses the specific developmental goals that preadolescents should master to help them adopt specific health-promoting lifestyle behaviors. These include safer sex practices, responsible and reasonable drinking, tobacco and drug resistance skills, nonviolent anger expression and conflict resolution, and healthy nutrition and adequate physical activity. The fifth category identifies gender-specific developmental goals that will help boys and girls adopt health-promoting lifestyles.

Preadolescents need to learn and adopt a series of beliefs, attitudes, and behaviors that will protect them from health-compromising behaviors as they grow older. Unfortunately, acquiring these beliefs, attitudes, and behaviors is not automatic; parents, teachers, and other adults should not assume that preadolescents will learn them on their own. Instead, they will need guidance from caring and supportive adults and through age-appropriate interventions and programs that appeal to preadolescent needs and wants and actively engage them in the mastery process. This mastery should include the following stage-specific goals:

Biological changes and developmental goals:

- to accept and enjoy themselves and their changing bodies (Brooks-Gunn et al. 1993)
- to develop the capacity to become aware of, regulate, and satisfy increasing high sensation-seeking needs by identifying activities that are fun, yet safe and healthy, to try
- to achieve a greater autonomy with respect to aspects of daily living and self-care, such as personal hygiene and grooming
- to be able to identify a supportive adult with whom to share their curiosity and questions about body changes

Cognitive changes and developmental goals:

- to master and apply basic concrete logical operations (logic of classes and of relations, principle of conservation, and reversibility of thought processes) to actual life situations (e.g., understanding that while it is normal for preteens to gain weight, they will also become taller and perhaps look thinner)
- to shift from egocentric thought to socio-centric thought, enabling them to place themselves in other people's situations and understand their points of view as well
- to develop the capacity to engage in self-reflective thinking, or *reciprocal perspective-taking*, by making inferences about other people's perspectives, thus reflecting on their own behavior and their own motivation from the other person's point of view (Selman 1977)
- to begin to develop the ability to accurately read nonverbal and verbal cues that will help them to decide whom to

trust and whom not to trust (e.g., among peers, older schoolmates, neighbors)
- to understand the consequences of actions they are frequently involved in at this age (e.g., body image consequences of eating impulsively or increasing physical activity; another person's feelings after being physically or verbally mistreated)
- to establish a *sense of industry*, by learning how to produce things and do the job well, thereby winning the recognition and approval of others and gaining a feeling of success (Erikson 1968)
- to develop more autonomy in organizing their daily schedule to responsibly fit in their home and school obligations (e.g., sports practices, homework, household chores) and leisure time (getting together with friends, enjoying hobbies)
- to be aware of how parents earn money and to improve impulse control skills to save and spend money responsibly

Socio-emotional changes and developmental goals:
- to develop the capacity to regulate and appropriately verbalize the mood changes and intense emotions (e.g., anger, frustration, fear, envy, disappointment) that accompany puberty
- to be able to identify at least one supportive adult with whom to share intense feelings (e.g., excitement, anger, sadness, apprehension, jealousy)
- to develop the capacity to engage in *reflective empathy*, or the ability to experience how another person feels and compare it to one's own feelings. This is the basis for emotionally understanding the feelings of others and reasoning about others' feelings in relationship to one's own personal experiences and an internalized sense of self (Greenspan and Shanker 2003, 2002).
- to take responsibility for one's own behavior by learning when and how to apologize and repair damage
- to be able to define oneself by one's qualities (e.g., nice, cool, smart, strong, considerate, humorous, athletic, good student) and own interests (type of foods preferred, favorite colors and styles of clothing, pastime activities enjoyed) rather than seeing oneself only through peer group perceptions (Greenspan 1993). This developmental goal facilitates the creation of internal standards based on a sense of self that is more stable and provides a basis upon which to judge experiences and further reflect upon them.
- to be assertive with parents by expressing likes and dislikes in appropriate ways
- to be able to identify enjoyable activities they would like to share with parents
- to develop social skills that allow them to interact and practice the give-and-take process for achieving agreement among their peers
- to develop the capacity to establish an intimate one-to-one relationship with a playmate of the same sex ("best friend") (Sullivan 1953)
- to start developing a strong value for respecting the trust given by a close friend by being loyal to him or her (e.g., not

- telling secrets to another person, caring for her/his safety and well-being)
- to be able to successfully negotiate the intricacies of multiple relationships within a group and be able to hold on to two realities at once: the peer group reality and their emerging inner reality of values and attitudes, including a strong internal sense of what is right and wrong, even if this disagrees with the peer group reality (Greenspan 1993)

Lifestyle-specific developmental goals:
Safer sex practices:

Preadolescents are exposed to sexual coercion and media messages that glorify casual and frequent sexual experiences. During this developmental stage, girls particularly begin to have romantic ideas and to show interest in the opposite sex. However, preadolescents in general feel embarrassed about discussing sexual issues with adults, and preteen girls, in particular, are embarrassed to talk about sex in front of boys. Oftentimes, parents as well feel uncomfortable talking about sexual relations with their children, feeling unsure about how much information to provide and about their own ability to completely and accurately answer questions about the biological and hormonal changes taking place in their children's bodies. In this light, the success of the preadolescent's learning process may perhaps be best ensured by school- and other community-based programs that supplement, support, and reinforce parental messages and aim for the mastery of the following developmental goals:

- to be able to read nonverbal and verbal cues that suggest inappropriate sexual intentions from others
- to be able to anticipate, react to, and protect themselves from unwanted sexual advances and coercion by seeking help from one or more supportive adults
- to be able to identify at least one supportive adult with whom to share questions about sexuality development and experiences
- to know their parents' values and expectations regarding appropriate behaviors when interacting with the opposite sex
- to develop the capacity to critically analyze messages about sex and sexuality as depicted on television and in music videos, films, magazines, and books (media literacy skills)
- to believe that girls and boys should possess equal rights and responsibilities
- to be empowered to explore sexuality and express affection through behaviors such as kissing and holding hands, yet holding a personal conviction about not moving into sexual relationships until one feels emotionally ready
- to demonstrate respect for girls and boys who have interests and manners of self-expression that are different from the ones traditionally expected of the respective genders (i.e., girls who are tomboys, boys who are effeminate)

Responsible and reasonable alcohol experimentation:

Because their growth and development process is far from complete, preadolescents should not drink alcohol. Nevertheless, this is a frequent reality in many countries of the Americas at all socioeconomic levels and, indeed, around the world. Given that the use of alcohol is widespread and enjoys general cultural acceptance in many societies, promoting alcohol abstinence among adolescents might not be a realistic goal to set. Yet parents, other adults, and health promotion and prevention programs can and should work together to help equip preadolescents for how best to approach and handle themselves in situations where alcohol is available. Not only is this age group the most vulnerable to peer pressures; it is also the most critical point at which interventions should begin preparing adolescents to master resistance skills, so that as they mature they will more easily and readily adopt safe and responsible drinking habits. The developmental goals to be achieved during preadolescence include:

- if choosing to experiment with alcohol, to be willing to do so only on certain social occasions (e.g., New Year's Eve, family celebrations) and under adult supervision
- to know their parents' values and expectations regarding appropriate behaviors when experimenting with alcohol
- to develop the capacity to identify and adopt safer and healthier alternatives to drinking alcohol when hanging out with friends
- to develop the capacity to critically analyze messages about alcohol drinking as depicted on television, in music videos and movies, and in print and electronic advertising (media literacy skills)
- to develop the capacity to critically analyze role model behaviors that include excessive and irresponsible alcohol consumption (including media role models and relatives)
- to develop the capacity to recognize and critically analyze social pressures to initiate drinking as a rite of passage, as well as the skills to resist them
- to understand the varying alcohol contents of beer, wine, and mixed drinks; how varying amounts of alcohol affect the body and brain; and the community's social and legal limits associated with what is considered "reasonable and responsible" drinking

Nonviolent anger expression and conflict resolution:
In modern life, forms of random and gang violence have invaded nearly every community to some extent, while remaining a serious public health problem in their most traditional enclave: large poor and urban areas. Not only are children today more exposed to violence in their daily lives, but they are also increasingly exposed to expressions of explicit violence in media programming tailored to the youth market.

Home, school, and community activities should encourage preadolescents to master violence prevention skills and understand the benefit to their own safety and well-being, as well as that of others, of learning how to work through situations that provoke anger utilizing peaceful dialogue and negotiation techniques. These promotion and prevention activities should aim to help preadolescents achieve the following developmental goals:

- to be able to identify feelings of anger, frustration, jealousy, envy, and other negative feelings and what causes them, as well as to adopt nonviolent strategies to express these feelings in socially acceptable ways (e.g., discussing them with parents, teachers, peers, other trusted individuals in the community)
- to develop the capacity to critically analyze messages about violence as depicted on television, and in movies, musical videos, books, and magazines (media literacy skills)
- to develop the capacity to critically analyze role model behaviors that use violence as a strategy to express anger or solve conflicts (including media role models, peers, and relatives)
- to develop the capacity to critically analyze and apply learned skills to resist social pressures to use violence as an expression of manhood (boys) or strength and toughness (girls)
- to be able to identify at least one supportive adult with whom one feels comfortable sharing anger and other intense feelings of distress
- to know their parents' values and expectations regarding appropriate behaviors for anger expression and conflict resolution

Healthy nutrition:

Weight gain increases and peaks during the adolescent growth spurt. Pubertal weight gain accounts for about 50% of an individual's ideal adult body weight (Neinstein 2002). Preadolescents, especially girls, need to accept that weight gain during this period is a normal and necessary part of the growth and development process. On the other hand, boys and girls also need to learn how to maintain a healthy optimal weight through increasing physical activity levels and acquiring a sufficient degree of self-control over impulsive eating behaviors.

In order to help preadolescents adopt and maintain healthy eating habits as they mature, the following developmental goals should be promoted:

- to be able to identify foods and food combinations they enjoy eating that are nutritionally balanced and accessible, and provide the necessary calories to maintain a healthy body weight
- to be able to identify nutritional snacks available at home and school that will satisfy their appetite and serve as healthier alternatives for foods high in sugars, carbohydrates, and/or fats
- to be able to identify one or more supportive adults who can guide them in the choice of satisfying and healthy meals and snacks
- to know their parents' values and expectations regarding appropriate behaviors for satisfying their appetite and maintaining a healthy weight

- to be able to regulate and control daily consumption of sugars, carbohydrates, and fats
- to understand the growth curve, be aware of the ideal weight for their age and height, and understand how food choices contribute to achieving and maintaining this ideal weight
- to be aware of the interrelationship between healthy nutrition and positive body image
- to develop the capacity to critically analyze messages about impulsive eating, eating disorders, and fast food consumption as depicted on television, and in movies, music, magazines, and promotional advertising (media literacy skills)

Adequate levels of physical activity:
The easy access to and appeal of fast food, television viewing, and computer and video games, as well as sedentary classroom and/or work-related activities, provide distractions from and even obstacles to the need for preadolescents to achieve and maintain healthy levels of physical activity in their daily lives. As girls and boys progress through the adolescent years, they experience a steady decline in the levels of physical activity, coinciding with an increase in academic and/or job demands and a growing focus on other types of personal interests. Due to the significant weight gain that naturally occurs during puberty, it is essential that parents and the community at large provide appealing incentives for preadolescents to achieve and maintain sufficient levels of physical energy exertion to counteract and balance this increase in body weight.

Girls are particularly affected by the inevitability of weight gain due to concerns related to body image and because teen culture (classmates, fashion magazines, media role models) frowns upon young bodies that are not thin. The natural tendency of preadolescent girls, influenced by traditional messages from society, (e.g., parental chiding and other expressions of concern, school nutrition curriculum) has been to focus on increasing self-control over caloric intake and digestion, instead of increasing physical activity levels, which is more commonly associated with boys. There is an urgent need for educational curricula, health promotion and prevention interventions, the media, and even parenting techniques to shift from this classical approach that places preadolescent girls at risk for eating disorders to more evidence-based strategies which promote healthy weight management through an emphasis on enhanced physical activity versus rigid eating behaviors.

In order to encourage preadolescents to discover enjoyable activities involving physical exercise and sports participation, health promotion and prevention efforts should help this age group to achieve the following developmental goals:

- to be able to organize, with their parents' support, their after-school time

and determine the optimal amount of physical activity that should occur during this period of the day
- to become aware of their natural abilities and skill regarding particular sports or other related activities involving physical exercise
- to be able to identify sports or activities they enjoy that are accessible to them and provide adequate physical exercise to maintain a healthy weight
- to be aware of the interrelationship between physical activity and positive body image and of the individual activity level necessary to achieve and maintain a healthy body weight
- to understand the growth curve, be aware of the ideal weight for their age and height, and understand how different types of physical activity enable the body to burn excess calories
- to develop the capacity to critically analyze activities (e.g., watching television, doing homework, studying or playing on the computer) and technologies (e.g., elevators, escalators, motorized transportation) that promote sedentary behaviors and determine how to alternate or combine these with activities that promote physical energy exertion
- to identify physical activity as a healthy strategy for reducing levels of stress and anxiety (Norris, Carrol, and Cochrane 1992)

Tobacco/drug resistance skills:
At the same time that preadolescents are targeted by the tobacco industry, they are also increasingly exposed to illegal drug offers, especially marijuana. In order to help preadolescents adopt strong resistant skills against tobacco and drug use, families and communities should work together to help this age group master the following development goals:

- to understand the short- and long-term health consequences of tobacco and drug use and develop the resistance skills to refuse them. If preadolescents can provide meaningful reasons, related to their actual lives, to refuse involvement with these products, they develop *personal convictions*, which last longer than attitudes. Therefore, a change in peer attitudes may cause a preadolescent's negative attitude toward tobacco and drugs to change, whereas a personal conviction will be more resistant to peers' changes in attitudes.
- to be able to identify at least one supportive adult with whom to share questions and concerns about tobacco and drug use, as well as experiences of having been offered these products
- to know their parents' values and expectations regarding appropriate behaviors when dealing with tobacco and/or drug offers
- to develop the capacity to critically analyze tobacco industry promotional messages in the mass media, as well as depictions of tobacco and drug use on television and in films, music videos, books, and magazines (media literacy skills)
- to be empowered to exercise their right to enjoy smoke-free environments where they live, learn, work, and play

Gender-specific developmental goals:

In addition to the four groups of developmental goals described on the previous pages, preadolescent girls and boys need guidance in mastering gender-specific developmental goals which will raise their awareness regarding traditional and pervasive stereotypes of masculinity and femininity and help protect them from their harmful effects. Preadolescence is a period of development when boys and girls still tend to spend the majority of their time with same-sex friends. Opposite-sex interactions are often loaded with competition and various degrees of anxiety caused by shyness, awkwardness, uncertainty, and inadequate communication. These difficulties may be translated into practical joke-playing and making fun of the other sex, which often rely on the perpetuation of unfair, uninformed, and/or inaccurate beliefs about masculinity and femininity and which in turn may interfere with the development of healthy male-female relationships at this and future stages. By the end of this period, girls and boys should have mastered the following developmental goals:

Girls:

- to develop the ability to quickly identify nonverbal behaviors and social contexts that might expose them to sexual coercion. This requires strengthening girls' visual and spatial skills, which are generally weaker than those of boys, as seen in Chapter Twenty-seven.
- to develop the ability to be assertive without using harmful interpersonal aggression
- to identify at least one supportive female adult with whom to critically analyze socially expected gender roles and behaviors
- to develop the ability to analyze traditional versions of femininity and reflect upon how they feel about them, within the context of their own personal needs and wants
- to develop media literacy skills that allow them to critically analyze media messages concerning body image and feminine appearance and reflect upon them, based on their sense of self and their individual needs and wants
- to develop a high approach coping style to deal with daily challenges and stresses, and avoidance coping abilities when confronted with uncontrollable and/or overwhelming stressors. (For more information on these styles, see Chapter Twenty of this book.)
- to identify and practice sports or other forms of physical exercise they enjoy as a way to improve their body image and assertiveness and reduce stress

Boys:

- to develop the ability to listen to girls' needs and wants. This requires strengthening boys' listening skills, which are generally weaker than those of girls and are the basis for developing empathy.
- to develop the ability to speak and be assertive with girls without the use of verbal, emotional, or physical violence
- to develop the ability to regulate and control impulsive behaviors by recog-

nizing the underlying emotions and developing a plan for how to express or channel those emotions through dialogue and safe behaviors (e.g., conversation and negotiation) instead of impulsive physical actions (e.g., hitting, slapping)

- to develop the ability to identify high sensation-seeking needs and fun, but healthy and safe, behaviors that satisfy those needs (e.g., different types of sports and hobbies)
- to identify at least one supportive male adult with whom to critically analyze socially expected gender roles and behaviors
- to develop the ability to analyze traditional versions of masculinity and reflect upon how they feel about them, within the context of their own personal needs and wants and their emerging internal standards for caring and protecting (this latter being a product of the cognitive and socio-emotional changes occurring during preadolescence)
- to identify traditional masculine obligations and expectations that can lead to risky behaviors, as well as viable alternatives that can lead to a healthier masculinity development (Aguirre and Güell 2002)
- to incorporate alternative expectations, viewpoints, paths, and behaviors in the construction of masculinity that are acceptable for young boys and are not perceived as unmanly by their peers (Aguirre and Güell 2002)
- to develop media literacy skills to critically analyze media messages concerning physical aggression and masculinity and reflect upon them within the framework of their own lives and sense of self

This chapter has presented a series of universal changes related to body, brain, social, emotional, and sexuality changes that occur during the preadolescent years, followed by the needs and wants specific to this stage of adolescence. It concludes with a discussion of the five categories of health-promoting developmental goals this group should master before moving into early adolescence, taking into account universal biological, cognitive, and socio-emotional changes occurring upon entering into adolescence, as well as lifestyle behaviors and gender-specific tasks.

The Pan American Health Organization considers preadolescence to be the most critical juncture at which health promotion and prevention endeavors should begin activities promoting the importance of healthy lifestyles and environments. If these efforts are postponed until later on, their focus will most likely be less on prevention and more on how to control health-compromising behaviors that have already become well-entrenched and will therefore present greater challenges.

While the initial goal of these health promotion and prevention initiatives may be to increase access to health information and preadolescents' knowledge about health risks, program designers need to be aware of the gap existing between knowledge and behavior change and develop innovative, creative, and appealing strategies that motivate this age group to master the developmental goals presented in this chapter. This mastery, in turn, will help preadolescents successfully navigate the increasingly challenging years of change ahead through a sense of empowerment and the personal conviction that they have the capacity to make conscious choices about their lives, including the desirability of moving away from harmful and negative influences and situations as a means of achieving their own self-set goals and life plan.

Box 28-1. **Summary of Preadolescence Basic Developmental Goals**

- **Biological changes**
  - to accept and enjoy themselves and their changing bodies
  - to achieve greater autonomy in self-care aspects (e.g., hygiene, grooming)
  - to become aware of and learn to regulate increased sensation-seeking needs
  - to identify healthy new activities that will satisfy these sensation-seeking needs
  - to identify a supportive adult with whom to share curiosity and questions about body changes during this period

- **Cognitive changes**
  - to master and apply basic logical operations to real-life situations
  - to shift from egocentric to socio-centric thought
  - to engage in self-reflective thinking and reciprocal perspective-taking
  - to develop the ability to read nonverbal and verbal cues to decide whom to trust and whom not to trust
  - to understand the consequences of actions typical of this age
  - to establish a sense of industry
  - to increase autonomy in responsibly organizing their daily schedule
  - to be aware of how parents earn their money
  - to improve impulse control skills to responsibly save and spend money

- **Socio-emotional changes**
  - to become aware of, regulate, and verbalize mood changes and intense feelings
  - to identify a supportive adult with whom to share intense feelings
  - to engage in reflective empathy
  - to take responsibility for one's own behavior
  - to be able to define self by one's own qualities and interests
  - to be assertive with parents, expressing likes and dislikes in appropriate ways
  - to identify enjoyable activities they would like to share with parents
  - to develop social skills to interact and practice the give-and-take process for achieving agreement among peers
  - to develop the capacity for a one-on-one relationship with a same-sex friend
  - to develop a strong value for respecting the trust given by a close friend by being loyal to him or her
  - to successfully negotiate multiple relationships within a group
  - to have a strong internal sense of what's right and wrong

Box 28-2. Summary of Preadolescence Lifestyle Developmental Goals

- **Safer sex practices**
  - to be able to read nonverbal and verbal cues that suggest inappropriate sexual intentions from others
  - to be able to anticipate, react to, and protect themselves from unwanted sexual advances and coercion
  - to identify a supportive adult with whom to share questions about sexuality development and experiences
  - to know parents' values and expectations regarding appropriate behaviors when interacting with the opposite sex
  - to develop media literacy skills for messages and advertising with sexual content
  - to believe that girls and boys should possess equal rights and responsibilities
  - to be empowered to explore sexuality and express affection through behaviors such as kissing and holding hands
  - to have a personal conviction against early sexual relationships
  - to demonstrate respect and acceptance for those whose interests and manners of self-expression are different from the ones traditionally expected of their gender

- **Responsible and reasonable alcohol experimentation**
  - if choosing to experiment with alcohol, to be willing to do so only on certain social occasions and under adult supervision
  - to know parents' values and expectations regarding appropriate behaviors for alcohol experimentation
  - to be able to identify and adopt alternative options to hanging out with friends and drinking alcohol
  - to develop media literacy skills for alcohol messages and advertising
  - to critically analyze role model behaviors that involve excessive and irresponsible drinking
  - to critically analyze and resist social pressures to begin drinking as a rite of passage
  - to understand the varying alcohol contents of different beverages and the social and legal limits of "reasonable and responsible" drinking

- **Tobacco and drug resistance skills**
  - to understand the consequences of tobacco and drug use
  - to develop skills to refuse tobacco and drugs from peers
  - to have a personal conviction against tobacco and drug use
  - to identify a supportive adult with whom to share questions and concerns about tobacco and drug use and experiences of having been offered them
  - to know parents' values and expectations regarding tobacco and drug use
  - to develop media literacy skills for tobacco and drug messages
  - to be empowered to exercise the right to enjoy smoke-free environments where adolescents live, learn, work, and play

- **Nonviolent anger expression and conflict resolution**
  - to identify feelings of anger and other negative feelings and to adopt nonviolent strategies to express these feelings in socially acceptable ways
  - to develop media literacy skills for messages and advertisements depicting violence
  - to critically analyze role model behaviors involving violence
  - to critically analyze and resist social pressures to use violence as an expression of manhood (boys) or strength and toughness (girls)
  - to identify a supportive adult with whom to share intense negative feelings
  - to know parents' values and expectations regarding appropriate behaviors for anger expression and conflict resolution

> **Box 28-2. Summary of Preadolescence Lifestyle Developmental Goals**–*(continued)*
>
> - **Healthy nutrition**
>   - to identify foods that are healthy, enjoyable, and easily available that will help them to maintain a healthy body weight
>   - to identify nutritional snacks available at home and school that will satisfy appetite and serve as healthier alternatives to foods high in sugars, carbohydrates, and/or fats
>   - to identify a supportive adult who can guide them in the choice of satisfying and healthy meals and snacks
>   - to know parents' values and expectations regarding appropriate behaviors for satisfying their appetite and maintaining a healthy weight
>   - to be able to regulate and control daily consumption of sugars, carbohydrates, and fats
>   - to understand the growth curve, be aware of the ideal weight for their age and height, and understand how food choices contribute to achieving and maintaining this ideal weight
>   - to be aware of the interrelationship between healthy nutrition and positive body image
>   - to develop media literacy skills for messages and advertising involving impulsive eating, eating disorders, and fast food consumption
>
> - **Adequate levels of physical activity**
>   - to be aware of their natural abilities and skill regarding particular sports or other related activities involving physical exercise
>   - to identify sports or other physical activities they enjoy that are accessible to them and provide sufficient exercise to maintain a healthy weight
>   - to organize, with parents' support, after-school time and determine the optimal amount of physical activity that should occur during this period of the day
>   - to be aware of the interrelationship between adequate levels of physical activity and positive body image
>   - to understand how different types of physical activity enable the body to burn excess calories
>   - to critically analyze activities and technologies promoting sedentary behaviors and determine how to alternate or combine these with more physical activities
>   - to identify physical activity as a strategy to decrease stress or anxiety

Box 28-3. **Summary of Preadolescence Gender-Specific Developmental Goals**

- **Girls**
  - to be able to quickly identify nonverbal behaviors and social contexts that might expose them to sexual coercion
  - to develop the ability to be assertive in expressing needs and wants, without using harmful interpersonal aggression
  - to develop a high approach coping style to deal with daily challenges and stresses, and avoidance strategies for uncontrollable and/or overwhelming stresses
  - to identify at least one supportive female adult with whom to critically analyze socially expected gender roles and behaviors
  - to be able to analyze traditional versions of femininity and reflect upon how they feel about them, within the context of their own needs and wants
  - to develop media literacy skills for messages about body image and feminine appearance
  - to identify and practice sports and other forms of physical exercise they enjoy as a way to improve body image and emotional assertiveness and reduce stress

- **Boys**
  - to develop the ability to listen to girls' needs and wants
  - to develop the ability to dialogue and be assertive with girls without the use of verbal, emotional, or physical violence
  - to identify at least one supportive male adult with whom to critically analyze socially expected gender roles and behaviors
  - to develop the ability to control impulsive behaviors involving sensation-seeking, anger expression, conflict resolution, and food cravings
  - to be able to analyze traditional versions of masculinity and reflect upon them
  - to identify traditional masculine obligations and expectations that can lead to risky behaviors, as well as viable alternatives that can lead to a healthier masculinity development (Aguirre and Güell 2002)
  - to incorporate alternative expectations, viewpoints, paths, and behaviors in the construction of masculinity that are acceptable for young boys and are not perceived as unmanly by their peers (Aguirre and Güell 2002)
  - to develop media literacy skills for messages revolving around physical and sexual aggression and masculinity

[Chapter Twenty-nine]

Early Intervention during Adolescence: The Early Adolescent Period

Early adolescence begins around the time of the "eruption of genital sexuality," roughly coinciding with menarche for girls and the occurrence of first ejaculation in boys. Early adolescence is a period of new biological, cognitive, sexual, and socio-emotional changes. Early adolescents will be challenged to learn how to deal with a variety of new experiences related to menstruation, ejaculation, nocturnal emissions ("wet dreams"), and with regulation of feelings of sexual arousal. It is the stage at which understanding and accepting that sexual activity is voluntary, and learning how to reflect this in one's behavior, become crucial. Early adolescents will be developing the potential for more abstract types of thinking and will begin to look beyond what they have been told up to this point by their parents and other adults and start to think for themselves. Early adolescents also begin to explore the world with more independence and less parental supervision and to spend more time with their friends in small same-sex subgroups, or *cliques*, as discussed in Chapter Seventeen. As their bodies continue to change, so will their interests, the type of relationships and friendships they establish, the ways they choose to have fun, and their strategies for analyzing new situations using emerging cognitive skills.

The average age of menarche varies from race to race. Less than 10% of U.S. girls start to menstruate before 11 years, yet 90% are menstruating by 13.75 years of age, with a median age of 12.43 years (Chumlea et al. 2003, Neinstein 2002). African-American girls have their menarche at an average age of 12.1–12.3 years (Freedman et al. 2002; Wu, Mendola, and Buck 2002; Herman-Giddens et al. 1997). The average age for white girls in the United States is between 12.6–12.88 years (Freedman et al. 2002, Herman-Giddens et al. 1997), while Mexican-American girls have their menarche at an average age of 12.2 years (Chumlea et al. 2003; Wu, Mendola, and Buck 2002). The median age at menarche found among Italian girls was 11.9 (range = 11.4 to 12.4 years) (Bona, Castellino, and Petri 2002). The median age at menarche for Brazilian girls ranges between 11 and 12.6 years in different studies (Borges and Pires Junior 2000, Tavares et al. 2000). Borges and colleagues described in their Brazilian study

Table 29-1. **Universal Changes during the Early Adolescent Stage**

Body Development	— Beginning of menstruation (median age = 12.4 years) — Beginning of ejaculation (median age = 13.4 years) — Increase in sexual arousal, masturbation — Experiencing of most significant growth spurt — Marked increase in desire for sensation-seeking experiences, particularly among boys
Brain Development	— Capacity for more abstract thinking (formal operations), accompanied by more abstract language — Use of less concrete thinking, with conservation tasks expected to be acquired by most early adolescents — Still little development of executive functions, particularly among boys
Sexuality Development	— Increased feelings of sexual arousal and need for masturbation — Occurrence of other types of autoerotic behaviors (e.g., sexual fantasies and wet dreams) — Stability of gender identity becomes increasingly challenged by development of sexual orientation, preference, and sexual exploration involving another person, including sometimes the emergence of confusing homosexual feelings
Emotional Development	— High self-consciousness and fluctuations in self-image — Increased levels of stress, particularly among girls — Continued need for more emotional autonomy from parents, stronger de-idealization of parents, and increased defining of one's own opinions — Increase in emotional dependency upon friends, with intimacy, loyalty, and shared values and attitudes holding great weight — Increase in empathy and responsiveness toward close friends — Emergent ability to reflect on feelings in relationship to an internalized sense of self ("I shouldn't feel this angry") — Assumption of conventional morality
Social Development	— More time spent with social subgroups (cliques) and/or alone — Emerging interest in opposite sex ("different") friend — Less time spent with parents, decrease in parental supervision, and increase in conflicts about independence — Enjoyment of new social privileges (e.g., watching more adult-plot movies for 13 years and older) — Peaking of susceptibility to peer pressure

that 12% of girls have their menarche at 10 years of age, 40% at 11 years of age, and 30.6% at 12 years of age, while the majority (85%) have had their menarche by the time they reach age 13.

The median age of first ejaculation has been less studied. Neinstein (2002) describes this event as occurring at a median age of 13.4 years (range = 11.7 to 15.3) in boys in the United States. Guizar-Vázquez and colleagues found similar results for Mexican boys, where first ejaculation also occurs at approximately 13.4 ± 1.01 years (Guizar-Vázquez et al. 1992).

Studies of girls' attitudes and beliefs about menstruation revealed that 40% were both pleased and scared about what was happening to their bodies and 20% had negative feelings. The girls more likely to have negative feelings are those who experience unpleasant physical symptoms during their period, those who begin menstruating relatively early, those who were not sufficiently prepared for the event, or those who received information about the process from a person who expressed negative feelings. During their adolescent years, three out of four teens develop acne. Girls often notice an aggravation of their acne condition prior to their menstrual period each month, another source of negative feelings (American Academy of Child and Adolescent Psychiatry 1999).

During early adolescence, there is also a universal progression into a new dimension of thinking, in which teens begin employing more *formal operations* (i.e., more abstract reasoning) and less concrete operations in their daily routine. They now turn to manipulating ideas internally, seeking hypotheses, experimenting, and utilizing both deductive and inductive reasoning. As they achieve increasing autonomy, they want to begin dating and to explore more in depth their sexuality and "forbidden" behaviors (e.g., experimentation with tobacco, alcohol, and/or drugs).

Early adolescents who did not develop a strong *personal conviction* (see Chapter Twenty-eight section on developmental goals) against drug use during preadolescence experience a clear shift toward greater acceptance, starting with tobacco use. In Chile, the minimum average age for first-time smoking is 12.9 years for tobacco and 14.4 years for marijuana (Pan American Health Organization 2002c). In one study in Argentina, 35% of adolescents ages 12 to 15 reported having used alcohol and tobacco within the past 30 days (Pan American Health Organization 2002b). In the United States, 80% of 14-year-olds reported not seeing any great risk in trying marijuana (Partnership for a Drug-Free America 1999).

The beginning of this adolescent stage also marks the advent of increased independence. Parental supervision and direct monitoring decrease. Early adolescents often go unsupervised to the movies, shop on their own more frequently, and make their own decisions about item and brand purchases much more independently than ever before. During this time, teens also move rapidly toward adult tastes and choices. Brand consciousness and discernment increase as a direct result of growing peer influence.

Early adolescents are social creatures who tend to gravitate toward friends and social-group activities far more than in previous years. They seek out support from and affiliation with a social subgroup or clique (e.g., school athletes, student leaders, those who rebel against authority, those who are unstylish and socially inept). They will gravitate toward the type of group that best satisfies their own needs for acceptance, self-esteem, and assertion. Their choice will be based on matching their own emerging sense of self, and their abilities and interests, with those of other individuals they perceive to share similar characteristics.

Although identity is being constructed constantly throughout the course of life, early adolescence is a key period of identity formation in terms of teens' future sexual and intimate relationships and their role in society. The importance of the peer group in helping the early adolescent to answer key identity questions (i.e., "Who am I?" "How does my background define me?" and "What do I want to become in life?") cannot be underestimated. The answers to these questions depend on social feedback from peers who provide the adolescent with their perception and evaluation of him or her. In this sense, identity is based on *psychosocial reciprocity*.

In this process of establishing his/her own separate identity, distinct from established family and social values, there are three sets of *competencies* that are key to a healthy adolescent development. Although these are always evolving competencies, early adolescence is the period when practicing these competencies becomes crucial for future relationships and behaviors (Greenspan 2002, Steinberg 1999).

The first of these sets of competencies is the capacity to *develop autonomy and at the same time accept dependency*. Early adolescents need to establish a healthy sense of independence from their parents and increasingly come to depend upon their peers for approval and sense of identity. At the same time, in many cases, they still depend upon their parents for comfort even if they consciously resist acknowledging this fact. Accepting the need for autonomy and dependency, then, is a process fueled with ambivalent feelings of learning when to ask for autonomy and when to accept dependency.

Secondly, early adolescents are confronted with learning the dual capacity for *controlling aggression* on the one hand, and *practicing empathy* on the other hand. They need to learn how to regulate their intense feelings of anger and yet be assertive in expressing their emotions. They also need to practice empathy, a competency that allows them to better understand and show concern for other people's strong emotions.

Thirdly, early adolescents will develop competencies to gradually explore *sexual-*

ity, together with the capacity for developing respectful *intimacy*, with other boys and girls. This is the stage when young people start to form close and caring relationships with other people, express sexual feelings, and enjoy physical contact with others.

These competencies are extremely relevant in our discussion of adopting and maintaining health-promoting lifestyles during adolescence, especially as regards the development of healthy safe sex practices. Following is an expansion of these important abilities and how they relate to behavior change.

- **Autonomy and dependency:** From the viewpoint of the adolescent, establishing a sense of autonomy is a very important part of becoming an adult. From the perspective of human development, becoming an autonomous person is one of the fundamental developmental tasks to be mastered during the adolescent years. The struggle of adolescents to establish themselves as independent, self-governing individuals—in their own eyes and in the eyes of others—is a long and occasionally difficult process, not only for young people themselves, but also for those around them, particularly parents, teachers, and other figures of authority. Furthermore, this growth of autonomy during adolescence is often misunderstood. Autonomy is often confused with rebellion, and becoming an independent person is often equated with breaking away from the family (Steinberg 1999).

The emergence of expressions of autonomy by early adolescents often causes great anxiety in parents as well, since it forces them to deal with their own feelings of dependency towards their children. During this period, parents begin feeling a vague sense of rejection from their early adolescents, who show increasingly less interest in family activities, a greater tendency to make plans for the weekend or vacations that do not involve their parents, and a decided preference for hanging out with friends instead. Parents find themselves missing that interaction with their children, and many come to the realization that they will have to discover new ways of engaging their adolescents' attention and interest. Early adolescence indeed marks the beginning of a long process of parent-child separation that reaches its peak when late adolescents or youth leave home, thus creating the "empty nest syndrome" for the parents being left behind. Ideally, however, early adolescence should be a period of "mutual letting-go," in which both child and parent maintain close emotional connections that may be easily accessed as needed.

Adolescents in today's world probably spend much more time away from the direct supervision of adults, either by themselves or with their peers, than ever in the past. Therefore, learning how to govern one's own behavior in a responsible fashion is a crucial task for contemporary youth, many of whom feel pressured—by parents, by friends, and by the media—to grow up quickly and to act like adults at an earlier age than ever before.

Psychologists generally differentiate three types of autonomy in adolescence: *emotional autonomy*, which refers to emotional independence in relationships with others, especially parents; *behavioral autonomy*, which refers to the development of independent decision-making abilities; and *value autonomy*, which concerns the development of independent beliefs.

Emotional autonomy develops best under circumstances that encourage both individuation and emotional closeness. Adolescents whose parents use a great deal of enabling techniques and relatively few constraining techniques are more likely to develop in healthy ways. They are more confident in themselves and score higher on measures of ego development and psychosocial competence. This finding coincides with other research indicating that healthy identity development is more likely to occur within families in which adolescents are simultaneously encouraged to be connected to their parents and to express their own individuality. In authoritarian households, where rules are rigidly enforced but seldom explained to the child, adjusting to adolescence is more difficult for the family as a whole. Authoritarian parents have a greater tendency to view the child's increasing emotional independence as a sign of rebelliousness or a lack of respect, and they may resist their adolescent's growing need for independence, rather than accepting it openly. When closeness is absent as well, the problems are compounded. In families in which excessive parental control is accompanied by extreme coldness and excessive discipline, the adolescent may rebel explicitly against parental standards, in an attempt to assert his or her independence in a visible and unequivocal fashion. Fuhrman and Holmbech (1995) have suggested that adolescents from particularly hostile or stressful family environments may do best when they actively detach themselves from their parents.

One of the most tangible ways in which the development during adolescence of *behavioral autonomy* is evident is in the growth of decision-making abilities. As individuals mature, they become better able to seek out and weigh the advice of individuals with different degrees of expertise and to use this information in making independent decisions. The prefrontal lobe, as discussed in Chapters Nine, Twelve, and Thirteen of this book, controls executive cognitive functioning, such as increased problem-solving capacity, ability to plan for the future, and impulse control. Studies of the development of executive functions in children and adolescents illustrate the probable differential timing for the maturation of these functions. Levin et al. (1991) found significant increases in a number of executive function measures as a function of age. Differences in sensitivity to feedback, problem-solving, concept formation, and impulse control between 7-to-8-year-old and 9-to-12-year-old age groups of developmentally normal children were found. Further significant developmental advances were noted in memory strategies, memory efficiency, planning of time, problem-solving, and hypothesis-seeking between 9-to-12-year-old and 13-to-15-year-old age groups. The final development of the prefrontal lobe occurs during late adolescence, reflected by progressive cellular maturational events, such as increased myelination and synaptic pruning, determining the ultimate density of mature frontal lobe gray matter (Sowell et al. 2001).

Consequently, even though by early adolescence the development of executive functions is underway, this group will still continue to need effective supervision and guidance in learning how to organize itself in issues related to time, space, problem-solving, and decision-making, since final prefrontal lobe maturation will not occur until several years later.

At the same time, genuine increases in behavioral autonomy occur only in middle and late adolescence (between ages 15 and 18), when conformity both to parents and to peers declines even though peer pressure continues to increase (Steinberg 1999). During early adolescence, peer pressure is particularly high in a variety of issues related to day-to-day activities. This susceptibility achieves its peak around 14 years of age and then falls during middle and late adolescence. *Perceptions* of the strength of peer pressure increase throughout the early adolescence period, while *susceptibility* to parental pressure decreases. Adolescents whose parents are extremely authoritarian or extremely permissive are the most easily influenced by their friends, especially in antisocial situations.

Erickson (1982) described a particular strength of early adolescents, *fidelity*, the search for something and somebody to be true to. Fidelity can only emerge through the interplay of social experiences in the individual's development and incarnates the capacity to sustain freely given loyalties even when confronted with inevitable contradictions between one's own and other people's value systems. In this sense, fidelity can become a dimension of adolescent ego strength. It defines what we are faithful to, what we identify with, and what in turn we are identified by. It implies having strong personal convictions about different behaviors (e.g., drug use, early sexual experimentation, physical aggression). Fidelity is essential for the development of autonomous behavior (Muss 1996).

Early adolescents whose sense of self has enabled them to develop internal standards and strong personal convictions will nonetheless find themselves challenged to assess their standards and convictions as the world around them begins to open even further (Greenspan and Shanker 2003). They will judge new experiences and further reflect on them. They will use abilities of multiple-cause thinking, which is the ability to give multiple reasons for a behavior or feeling and set up multiple hypotheses for it. Early adolescents will have the ability to identify multiple angles to problem-solving. Gray-area thinking ability will also help early adolescents to realize that there exist different degrees of emotions within the realm of anger, love, excitement, and disappointment, and to describe their own feelings in terms of these degrees. They will begin to reflect on momentary feelings or experiences and, at the same time, compare these to a more long-term view of themselves and their experiences, values, and goals or ideals. Early adolescents will need to develop effective coping skills to deal with the anxiety that can accompany these new experiences, in order to counteract feelings of intimidation, insecurity, and rigidity in their response to the events.

According to Lawrence Kohlberg's development of moral reasoning theory (Kohlberg 1976), adolescence is a time of potentially internalizing right and wrong on the basis of one's own basic moral principles and not only in terms of society's rules and consequences. This shift traditionally does not tend to occur until late in adolescents who have not previously developed internal standards and strong personal convictions, suggesting that unfortunately, the development of *value autonomy* occurs later than the development of either emotional or behavioral autonomy.

- ***Aggression and empathy:*** Aggressive behavior is generally learned at home from an early age but is often enhanced by the sociocultural environment. Teens whose parents used corporal punishment may be more likely to resolve conflicts with aggression, too. Many movies and television programs feature violence in casual and even humorous situations, inferring that violence is normal behavior—an idea that is particularly dangerous for children already predisposed to aggression. The American Psychological Association has estimated that the average child or teenager in the United States views 10,000 murders, rapes, and aggravated assaults per year on television alone, or approximately 200,000 by the time the person reaches adulthood (Huston et al. 1992). New technology capabilities enable cable television to reach the farthest edges of the earth, bringing this content to new viewing audiences and cultures. Physical aggressiveness is also praised and rewarded in many sports, at all levels, beginning on the practice fields of schools and extending all the way up to professional sports. Violence is also an unfortunate reality in many neighborhoods where poverty is a factor. Children who grow up with these messages from family, coaches, the media, and the streets may have greater difficulties controlling their aggressive or violent impulses than those who are less exposed to these factors (American Academy of Child and Adolescent Psychiatry 1999).

Anger, aggression, rivalry, and competition are not necessarily unhealthy emotions. As long as they are balanced with feelings of warmth and empathy, anger and rivalry can have a positive effect, by energizing children and providing the motivation to perform better than was thought possible. They even help to define the sense of self, differentiating children from their parents, siblings, and friends (Greenspan 1993). A growing number of health promotion and violence prevention programs have been devised for use in the schoolroom that teach children and adolescents nonviolent conflict resolution skills. These strategies, despite their positive intentions, may not be effective in the long term, however, if they are taught only in hypothetical or role-playing situations with the automatic assumption that the techniques learned will be practiced outside the context of real emotions. These programs, when not successful, are also a classic example of how information provision and knowledge-gaining may not be enough to assure actual behavioral change. Early adolescents need to learn to identify their real-life feelings of anger and frustration, create an emotional idea of them, and then express these feelings in play or through words in non-hurtful ways, balanced with feelings of warmth and empathy.

- **Intimacy and sexuality:** A half century ago, H.S. Sullivan (Muss 1996) proposed that a need emerges in the normal pattern of social development that requires a shift in the object of intimacy during this period. For the preadolescent, that object or "best friend" is someone quite like oneself. During early adolescence, the need for a "best friend" changes, leading teens to choose someone who, in very significant ways, is quite different from oneself. This need spurs girls to show increased interest in boys and boys to turn to girls with new curiosity. However, the move toward opposite-sex intimacy initially involves a great deal of insecurity, fumbling, and unrealistic wishful thinking. It is complicated not only by adolescent anxieties about rejection by the opposite sex, but also by preconceived and stereotypical views of the opposite sex acquired during earlier periods of development. Gilligan, as well as other colleagues (Gilligan et al. 1992, Gilligan 1982), states that the intimate friendship between girls in early adolescence is a better preparation for love and heterosexuality than too-early and often shallow involvement with boys, in which there is less communication and emotional sharing.

The capacity for intimacy, which initially develops out of same-sex friendships, eventually is brought into cross-sex relationships. Today, adolescent girls begin dating around 12 or 13, and most boys between ages 13 and 14. The transitional period—between same-sex nonsexual relationships and opposite-sex sexual ones—oftentimes is a trying time for adolescents. This period usually begins with the peer group's gradual shift from same-sex cliques to mixed-sex crowds and then evolves into one-on-one boy-girl relationships during later adolescent periods. The interpersonal strains and anxieties inherent in the transition show up in the high levels of teasing, joking around, and overt discomfort young adolescents so often display in situations that veer toward being romantic or sexual (Steinberg 1999). For Sullivan (Muss 1996), early adolescence ends when interest and *actual intimacy* shift from a person of one's own sex to one of the opposite sex.

During the next stage (middle adolescence), girls may be more adept than boys at displaying certain types of intimacy, such as self-disclosure and interpersonal understanding. Studies describing the neurobiological correlates of emotional processing have found that during adolescence, males and females demonstrate different strategies in the processing of facial affect (Killgore, Oki, and Yurgelun-Todd 2001). Girls' cross-sex relationships may provide a context for further *expression* of intimacy, while for boys they may provide a context for the further *development* of intimacy.

Brooks-Gunn and Paikoff (1993) describe four developmental challenges of adolescent sexuality: (1) accepting one's changing body; (2) accepting one's feelings of sexual arousal; (3) understanding that sexual activity is voluntary; and (4) practicing safe sex with pleasure. Accepting one's changing body is a challenge that starts during preadolescence and continues through early adolescence, when the next two challenges, accepting one's feelings of sexual arousal and understanding that sexual activity is voluntary, become crucial. By the age of 15 (middle adolescence) many teens are beginning to engage in some form of sexual experimentation, which may include petting, oral-genital contacts, mutual masturbation, and even intercourse (American Academy of Child and Adolescent Psychiatry 1999).

Unfortunately, the reality in many societies today threatens the ability of early adolescents to address sexuality-related developmental needs at their own pace because of the prevalence of sexual coercion. Defined as physical or verbal pressure to engage in sexual activity, sexual coercion is a serious problem in many areas throughout the world. There is growing public awareness that a large proportion of teenagers are sexually harassed and that a significant minority are forced to have sex against their will (Lee et al. 1996). Estimates that include all forms of nonvoluntary sex suggest that about 25% of all females and close to 10% of all males have been victimized sexually before reaching adulthood. Adolescents as victims of dating violence reach similar rates in the United States (Foshee et al. 1998).

Cáceres, Vanoss, and Sid Hudes (2000) determined the prevalence and correlates of sexual coercion in adolescents and young adults in Lima, Peru. Over 40% of young women reported that their first heterosexual encounter occurred under pressure, and lifetime experiences of coercion were even higher. In multiple logistic regression analyses, men and women who reported having been coerced at heterosexual initiation also reported more sexually transmitted diseases in their lifetime and a lower age at first sex than those not reporting coercion. Age at first heterosexual encounter was not associated with sexual coercion for men, but for women, 62% of those who reported sexual initiation before age 15 reported coercion, compared with 28% of those reporting sexual initiation after age 22. In this survey, 11% of the males reported coercion at heterosexual initiation, and this group reported lower social economical status than those not coerced. For an adolescent girl, "a coercive initiation may disempower her, leaving her without the skills to resist pressure from partners or negotiate condom use. In many parts of the world, once a woman has had her first sexual experience, her reputation may make it difficult for her to refuse future sexual advances from the same or other partners. The term 'easy,' which refers to some men's sexual partners (but not women's), suggests this shift in reputation" (Cáceres, Vanoss, and Sid Hudes 2000).

Adolescents who have been sexually abused show higher-than-average rates of poor self-esteem, academic difficulties, anxiety, fear, and depression, and are more likely to engage in risky behavior (Biglan et. al 1995) and to become pregnant as teenagers. Kenney, Reinholtz, and Angelini (1997) examined the effect of adolescent sexual abuse on teenage pregnancy rates in the United States. In a sample of 1,900 women, twice as many women who were coerced into sex or raped also experienced a teenage pregnancy, compared with their non-abused peers.

Unfortunately, sexual coercion and abuse are not the only causes that threaten the ability of early adolescents to address the developmental needs of sexuality at their own pace. Early adolescents want more independence, autonomy, and money. Those living in extreme poverty desperately need to earn money, whether to support their families or because they live on the streets and/or are orphaned. For this reason, the exchange of money, favors, or gifts (clothing, food, electronic items) for sexual encounters is common in many countries. In recent years, the Internet has become a leading source for the advertisement of exchanges of this sort, with early adolescents—both boys and girls—being a principal target of adults seeking to initiate sexual activity, either through invitation and mutual consent or coercion and aggression.

Social pressure that encourages boys to engage in sexual activity early to prove their masculinity is also a frequent reality in many parts of the world. In Latin America, for example, the average age of first sexual intercourse is approximately 14–15 for boys (Camacho-Hubner 2000). The mixed messages regarding sexual activity that society imparts to early adolescents may be symbolized in the marked differences that are found between how the sexes feel after their first experience of sexual intercourse. A study, which involved more than 1,000 U.S. teens, found that boys were more likely to describe their first sexual partner in casual terms, and the majority said they were glad they had had sexual intercourse. Among the girls surveyed, 75% said their partner was their boyfriend, 61% said they had conflicted feelings after the experience, and 11% said they were sorry it happened (American Academy of Child and Adolescent Psychiatry 1999). The media, through newspapers, magazines, musical videos, and movies, also profit from the natural interest of human beings in sexuality by projecting a variety of messages that both implicitly and explicitly encourage the adoption of health-compromising behaviors (Strasburger and Wilson 2002).

The Needs of Early Adolescents

Just as in the case of preadolescents, early adolescents have a series of needs to which parents, teachers, and the community at large should respond in order to better ensure the healthy transitioning of young people from preadolescence into early adolescence and on into the next stage of middle adolescence. Any health promotion and prevention intervention aimed at early adolescents should incorporate a targeted response to the needs specific to this age group in its design. Research shows the following needs are of particular importance:

- ***Love in an ongoing nurturing relationship:*** A warm relationship between early adolescents and parents is crucial for behavior and mood regulation during these years. A stable emotional climate in the family and a significant amount of leisure time spent together will improve the chances that adolescents will positively interact with their parents and consider their input regarding the adoption of healthy lifestyles. Nevertheless, since early adolescents need to differentiate themselves from their parents, in many cases they will practice some form of rebellion in order to secure their new identity. Parents will need to discover new ways to interact and communicate positively with early adolescents, respecting their growing need for more "grown-up" activities. The *need for parental love* remains constant through early adolescence, although it may appear to "go underground" due to pressing peer acceptance and identity issues. That is, at this age, the teen will still need and want love from his/her parents, but may see as socially undesirable the display or acceptance of that love in public. Still, teens need to know that they are loved. Greenspan (2002) notes that "one of the key challenges for parents at this time is to sneak in the dependency (or the need for love) without embarrassing the teenager. The key is to provide the dependency on the child's terms. It is critical that dependency gets slipped in with respect." Receiving this love as a constant from their parents and family provides a solid emotional base and helps teens feel good about themselves and who they are.

- ***Self-esteem and acceptance:*** Adolescents most dramatically feel the *need for acceptance* during this period. They need this acceptance from peers, parents, and teachers, and—most importantly—from themselves. It is this strong drive toward acceptance from their peers, as well as the drive to establish their own identity separate from their parents, that often propels the adolescent toward "desirable" or "undesirable" subgroups. Early adolescents who are encouraged by their families to both be connected to their parents and to express their own individuality will have a greater ability to successfully negotiate the intricacies of multiple relationships within a group without losing their individuality.

- ***Developmentally appropriate experiences and success:*** While in many cases their need for acceptance may predominate, early adolescents also experience the *need to succeed*, although not as deeply or urgently as when they enter the late adolescent stage. Contemporary theories tend to stress the interaction between motives, beliefs, attributions, and goals as influencing adolescents' achievement orientation. Adolescents who believe that ability is malleable (rather than fixed), who are motivated by intrinsic (rather than extrinsic) rewards, who are confident about their abilities, and who attribute their successes and failures to effort (rather than to ability or luck) achieve more in school than their peers without these qualities. Early adolescents need developmentally appropriate experiences and challenges that allow them to put in place all their learned skills to successfully solve new problems and make appropriate decisions.

- ***Sexuality:*** There is an increased sexual awareness, arousal, and interest during early adolescence that demands to be dealt with during the coming years. Peer, parental, and religious beliefs, attitudes, and behaviors are some of the factors that will play a role in how the early adolescent will explore sexuality issues. Most schools today provide some form of sex education, but parents should not assume that all the questions their children have will be answered in the classroom. Furthermore, as seen in Chapter Twenty-three, teachers generally are not well prepared to provide effective sex education and often fail to fully implement sexual education curricula (Buston et al. 2002, Hallfors and Godette 2002). Students are also shy and embarrassed about addressing these topics with teachers, and their comfort level does not increase over time (Evans et al. 2002). Parental willingness and preparedness to discuss sexuality with early adolescents are therefore crucial. This discussion should include not only the risks of HIV/AIDS and other STIs and pregnancy prevention, but also the emotional aspects of physically intimate behavior, how to deal with natural sexual arousal, the advantages and limits of masturbation, the importance of respecting that sexual activity is voluntary, how to react and respond in situations of sexual coercion, and parents' personal feelings and values regarding early sex and casual sex.

- **Identity:** Adolescents' search for an identity involves the establishment of a meaningful self-concept in which past, present, and future are brought together to form a unified whole. During adolescence, young people will need to develop a commitment to a system of values—moral and religious beliefs, career and relationship goals, a general philosophy of life—and accept and understand their sexuality. Early adolescence falls in the middle of this process, where accepting one's own sexuality takes priority, while at the same time the individual is constructing the beliefs and values that will support his or her behaviors and goals in life. Conforming to the expectations of peers helps adolescents discover how certain roles fit them, but peer group conformity can also create a new kind of dependency, whereby the individual accepts the beliefs and values of others too easily without addressing the identity issue of how well these fit in with his or her own long-term goals. Eventually, adolescents must free themselves from their dependency on peers, which has just replaced their dependency on parents, in order to find their own selves. Healthy identity development is more likely to occur when parents encourage early adolescents to express their own individuality and strengthen their *fidelity* to themselves while maintaining closeness and connectedness within the family. Closeness and connectedness are vital for giving adolescents the emotional space and freedom to experiment, while at the same time, parents need to define the limits of acceptable behaviors and teach young people about accountability for their actions and decisions.

- **Opportunities, guidance, limits, values, and expectations:** In order for early adolescents to learn how to make responsible decisions, they need opportunities to make new decisions on their own with parental guidance, knowledge of their parents' values, clear expectations, and firm limitations. They still need guidance on how to interact with the opposite sex; how to be alternately empathetic, assertive, and/or suspicious as needed; how to protect themselves from temptations and dangers; and how to spend and save money according to their reality and that of their family. They need firm limits regarding behaviors that are potentially harmful or infringe upon the rights of parents, siblings, peers, and others. In order for limit-setting to be effective, parents need to maintain closeness, connectedness, and the capacity to have fun together. Having this basic emotional connection, parents need to make the rules clear, teach responsibility, demonstrate a willingness to negotiate when appropriate, avoid negative criticism of their children, and maintain self-control.

- **Safe and supportive environments at home, school, and in the neighborhood:** Early adolescents also need to have a sense of connectedness with their community and its leaders, to have the necessary supporting environments (e.g., home, school, church), public spaces (e.g., playgrounds, parks, other places they frequent alone and with friends), and freedom to safely explore the outside world with social regulations that protect them from potentially harmful behaviors. Safe and supportive neighborhoods will provide secure social networks that will contribute to their opportunities for adopting and maintaining health-promoting behaviors.

- **Structures to provide healthy nutrition, physical activity, and proper sleep:** Early adolescents' lives continue to be driven by novelty and having fun while hanging out with friends, which take priority over eating and sleeping. Interacting with their peers might not necessarily include activities that involve physical exercise. This is especially true in the case of girls, whose involvement in sports tends to be less than that of their male counterparts. Early adolescents find their lives full of social activity, spend more time away from home and unsupervised, and come home later than during their preadolescent years. Since they go to bed later, they will tend to sleep in during the morning. Parents will need to allow some flexibility in leisure time and sleeping patterns, while at the same time providing sufficient structure to help ensure that early adolescents balance the need for age-appropriate social experiences with adequate attention to nutritional, exercise, and sleep requirements.

The series of early adolescent needs described in the preceding paragraphs should be taken into account in the design of all health promotion and prevention programs targeted to this group. Whenever possible, parents should also be actively involved in these interventions. In determining how best to respond to the needs of early adolescents, the interpersonal level theories for behavior change presented in Chapters Sixteen to Twenty, and particularly the Authoritative Parenting Model (Chapter Eighteen), can provide practical insight into the necessary components to be included in the intervention.

The Wants of Early Adolescence

Early adolescents want to have fun, be accepted and loved by others, and enjoy success in their endeavors. They want to move away from childhood activities and interests of the past, and oftentimes will make this change clear to everyone around them by choosing new interests and behaviors. Those interests will involve larger challenges than in previous stages of their life as they explore novel and seemingly fun things to do with their friends. They might try their first cigarette or first beer, sneak into the girls' or boys' showers at school, or play a prank with the group on a neighbor, teacher, or other authority figure. Early adolescents will demand more autonomy from their parents to make decisions regarding the clothes they wear, the food they eat, the sports they play, the television programs they watch, and the leisure-time activities they participate in with their friends. The type of sports, outdoor activities, and peer group and media entertainment they choose will vary in different cultures and countries. Keeping in mind that cultural differences still remain, despite an increasingly globalized media industry, the main interests that attract early adolescents' attention and motivation at this age include:

- **Novelty**: Early adolescents are eager to use their growing independence to explore new experiences on their own and with their friends. New options that attract their attention will be those that help them to distance themselves from childhood activities; involve larger cognitive, motor, and/or social challenges; provide high sensations; and which can be done with their friends. They are also still exploring new ways to be seen as unique by their peers and thereby increase their acceptance in the group.

- **Social interaction**: Early adolescents like to hang out with their friends at fast-food restaurants, at the shopping mall, at the movies, or at get-togethers at peers' homes to watch rented videos or play video games. They spend less time with best friends and same-sex cliques, steadily moving on to bigger groups comprised of both sexes. Early adolescents increase the use of the telephone to stay in touch with their friends, relying on this form of communication even more than during the preadolescent years.

- **"Grown-up" experiences**: Early adolescents want to differentiate themselves from preadolescents. They are passing the barrier of the early teen years and feel socially entitled to do many more "grown-up" things than before. They also want to explore new experiences previously "forbidden" to them, including out-of-limit behaviors. They want to go to places alone, use public transportation on their own, and manage money independently. Early adolescence is also the stage at which many teens living in poor families in some Latin America and Caribbean countries assume new responsibilities towards their families, contributing with income obtained from formal types of employment, even though some of the poorest work for minimal pay in the informal sector in unhygienic and/or hazardous environments.

- **Television shows and movies**: Early adolescents are moving rapidly toward adult television programs. Especially attractive to the early adolescent are situation comedies that provide humor, as well as comedies and dramas that deal with adolescent and young adult issues. They now prefer television shows and movies that have adolescent and young adult stars and in which the characters and situations are more complex overall. Early adolescents are more capable of going beyond polarized, black-and-white thinking and are able to identify and appreciate the gray areas in between the two extremes. They are learning to process visual and auditory stimuli faster (Hale 1990) and more efficiently and are demanding greater levels of information to keep their attention. These newly acquired capabilities, combined with the fact that today's population of early adolescents has grown up exposed to highly compressed visual and auditory images and stimuli displays in the media—products of advances over the past decade in electronic digitalization technologies—have conditioned this age group to expect high-paced stimulation from all its information and entertainment sources (Acuff 1997).

- ***Humor in the media***: Early adolescents will increase their capacity to understand and appreciate more subtle forms of humor such as sarcasm, innuendo, and irony. They will lose interest in media programming that is too simple and does not deliver sufficiently complex characters, content, and humor. Boys in particular tend to prefer humor that is edgy and/or dark-sided, leans toward sexual and other taboos, and contains violent themes.

- ***Reading***: Early adolescents prefer reading magazines and newspapers to books. They are rapidly acquiring more adult tastes and choices in reading material and tend to prefer adult-marketed items. Early adolescents read fewer books than preadolescents but when they do read, their tastes gravitate more toward reality-based publications (e.g., newspapers, sports and entertainment magazines). Newspaper readership increases substantially during the early adolescent years.

- ***Music:*** Music preferences reflect, perhaps more than any other medium, the splintering of the early adolescent culture into different subgroups, each with distinct tastes. Early adolescents connect to messages in their favorite music, not just to the song's rhythm or melody.

- ***Video and computer games***: Males continue to enjoy electronic games during early adolescence, but the amount of time spent at individual play decreases. They tend to prefer multiplayer games, or at least two-player games (i.e., car racing), in which they may compete against each other. There is also a shift in the types of games preferred, with a growing preference for sports-related, reality-based games and challenging role-playing games. The electronic industry has also profited from early adolescent males' interest in sex, by incorporating subtle sexual innuendos in some of their products. Teen-rated (T) games tend to include more violence and stronger language.

- **Sports:** Boys, more than girls, continue to participate in organized sports (e.g., football, soccer, basketball, baseball). Independent or alternative sports that are chosen by early adolescents include rollerblading and skateboarding.

The Health-Promoting Developmental Goals of Early Adolescence

The ability of early adolescents to master the developmental goals presented in this section is directly related to the degree of success this group achieved as preadolescents in mastering the corresponding set of development goals for that stage, as described in Chapter Twenty-eight. As in the case of preadolescents, the goals for early adolescents are divided into five categories: (1) biological changes and developmental goals; (2) cognitive changes and developmental goals; (3) socio-emotional changes and developmental goals; (4) lifestyle-specific developmental goals; and (5) gender-specific developmental goals.

After identifying the target group of the intervention, health promotion developers should first determine to what extent its early adolescent members have not yet mastered the developmental goals of preadolescence and establish this objective as the program's initial priority. The program should then segue into mastery of the early adolescent goals, incorporating age-appropriate interventions that appeal to early adolescent needs and wants and actively engage the target group in mastering the following goals:

Biological changes and developmental goals:

- to accept positively and learn to manage new bodily changes (e.g., menstruation, ejaculation, voice changes)
- to learn how to regulate new eating and sleeping patterns in healthy ways
- to master healthy coping mechanisms for dealing with the increased anxiety levels characteristic of the early adolescence years
- to have learned how to satisfy increasing sensation-seeking needs in healthy and safe ways
- to continue to be able to identify at least one supportive adult with whom they feel comfortable sharing curiosity and questions about menstruation, ejaculation, wet dreams, and other new physical capabilities

Cognitive changes and developmental goals:

- to develop a preparatory stage of partial formal operations capacity (i.e., Piaget, stage III A), whereby the early adolescent is able to make correct conclusions and handle certain formal operations, even if not yet able to provide systematic and rigorous proof for his/her assertions
- to be able to adopt a *third-person* or *mutual perspective* (i.e., the capacity to abstractly step outside an interpersonal interaction and simultaneously and

- mutually coordinate and consider the perspectives of self and others) (Selman 1977)
- to have developed the ability to accurately read nonverbal and verbal cues that will help them to determine whom to trust and whom not to trust (e.g., among peers, older schoolmates, neighbors)
- to be able to give reasons for trusting or not trusting a particular person
- to recognize frequent temptations at this age and be able to understand the consequences of new actions in which they might be involved (e.g., flirting, having early sex, becoming pregnant, having unprotected sex, becoming infected with HIV/STIs)
- to develop increasing autonomy in organizing their daily schedule to responsibly fit in and balance their home, school, and work obligations (e.g., homework and special projects, household chores, sports practices, extracurricular activities, part-time job) and leisure time (hanging out with friends, enjoying hobbies)

Socio-emotional changes and developmental goals:

- to gradually shift interest from a person of one's own sex and same interests to one of the opposite sex and/or who is different from oneself (Sullivan 1953)
- to be able to identify and create a mental image of angry feelings and then express these angry feelings in play or through words in non-hurtful ways, balanced with feelings of warmth and empathy (Greenspan 1993)
- to continue to be able to identify at least one supportive adult with whom one may share intense feelings (e.g., excitement, anger, sadness, apprehension, jealousy)
- to be able to identify enjoyable activities, in keeping with new interests they have acquired during this stage, that they would like to share with their parents
- to establish a sense of personal identity in which the early adolescent is increasingly able to assess strengths and weaknesses and determine best how to deal with them (Erikson 1968)
- to achieve a greater *behavioral autonomy* (independent decision-making abilities), shown by going out with friends without parental supervision and by making safe and healthy choices in their absence
- to develop an "ego ideal" on which to model and evaluate oneself and be able to picture oneself in the future. The "ego ideal" permits early adolescents to envision themselves over time instead of simply living in the present—in which they react to daily events, respond to the needs of the moment (e.g., pleasure, affiliation, acceptance), and feel increasingly vulnerable to peer pressure (Greenspan 1993).

Lifestyle-specific developmental goals:

Safer sex practices:

- to learn to regulate and control feelings of sexual arousal (Brooks-Gunn and Paikoff 1993) by respecting and not forcing others into unwanted sexual experiences

- to be able to distinguish between feelings of sexual attraction, love, and intimacy
- to continue to be able to identify at least one supportive adult with whom one may share curiosity and questions regarding sexuality development, feelings of arousal, and experiences
- to know their parents' values and expectations regarding appropriate behaviors for sexuality exploration
- to be empowered to further explore sexuality and express affection through behaviors such as kissing and holding hands, yet holding a personal conviction about not moving into intercourse until one feels emotionally ready
- to have developed loyalty and caring for the other person's safety and well-being as strong values in close relationships
- to be able to identify personal goals that would be negatively affected by becoming an adolescent mother or father or by contracting STIs or HIV
- to believe girls and boys should possess equal sexual rights and responsibilities and be able to demonstrate this belief in their interactions with others
- to be able to set limits for a boyfriend or girlfriend in sexuality exploration and negotiate alternative behaviors to intercourse for channeling sexual arousal
- to develop the capacity to recognize and critically analyze social pressures to have sexual intercourse as a rite of passage, as well as the skills to resist these pressures
- to demonstrate respect and acceptance for boys and girls who do not possess characteristics associated with traditional gender roles (e.g., girls caring about makeup and appearance, boys being tough and strong), to avoid making fun of the appearance and behaviors of these individuals, and to consider including them in one's social group, despite the fact that they are "different"

Responsible and reasonable alcohol experimentation:
- to have the capacity to identify and walk away from unsupervised social gatherings or parties that involve alcohol in any form (e.g., beer, wine, mixed drinks)
- to be willing to experiment with alcohol-tasting only on certain social occasions (e.g., New Year's Eve, family celebrations) and under adult supervision
- to have developed the capacity to identify and adopt safer and healthier alternatives to drinking alcohol when hanging out with friends
- to be able to identify highly valued personal behaviors and opportunities (e.g., sports participation, driving privileges, employment, personal image) that might be negatively affected by drinking alcohol

Nonviolent anger expression and conflict resolution:
- to be able to identify the causes for feelings of anger, frustration, jealousy, and envy—particularly in new and more intimate types of relationships—and to

adopt nonviolent strategies to express these feelings in socially acceptable ways (e.g., sharing them with the other person involved, a parent, friend, other trusted individual)
- to have developed the capacity to identify and critically analyze heightened levels of PG-13-rated violence as depicted on television, and in movies, musical videos, books, and magazines (media literacy skills)
- to have developed the capacity to critically analyze and apply learned skills to resist social pressures to use violence as an expression of force, particularly when exploring new relationships with friends of the opposite sex
- to be able to identify a supportive friend with whom to share intense negative feelings (e.g., anger, jealousy, envy)
- to continue to identify at least one supportive adult with whom one feels comfortable sharing feelings of anger and other negative emotions
- to know their parents' values and expectations regarding appropriate behaviors for anger expression and conflict resolution, especially when interacting with the opposite sex

Healthy nutrition:
- to be able to identify tasty, yet healthy, foods and food combinations which are easy to obtain and/or prepare and that can be part of the food available when hanging out or meeting as a group at different friends' houses
- to be able to identify tasty and healthy snacks which are affordable and can be kept handy to eat and share with friends in moments of intense hunger
- to be able to identify at least one supportive adult to whom one may turn for help in selecting tasty, healthy foods and snacks for social gatherings with friends
- to be able to regulate and control, when alone or in a social group situation, the amount of sweets, carbohydrates, and fats eaten daily, without having adult supervision

Adequate levels of physical activity:
- to be able to identify sports or other physical activities that are attractive to oneself and one's friends that are also affordable and easy to do as a group after school or during weekends
- to be able to organize, with parental support, their after-school time to fit in opportunities for physical activity among other school-, work-, and home-related responsibilities

Tobacco/drug resistance skills:
- to be able to identify and walk away from unsupervised social gatherings or parties that involve tobacco and drug use in any form (e.g., marijuana, cocaine, speed, Ecstasy, other popular substances)
- to continue to be able to identify one or more supportive adults with whom to share personal experiences of drugs and tobacco being offered in social settings (e.g., parties, dances, dates)
- to have the capacity to identify and adopt healthier and safer alternatives to tobacco and drug use when hanging out with friends

- to be able to identify highly valued personal behaviors and opportunities (e.g., sports participation, driving privileges, employment, personal image) that might be negatively affected by the use of tobacco and drugs
- to be empowered to exercise their right to smoke-free environments where they live, learn, work, and play

Gender-specific developmental goals:

Girls and boys need help in mastering gender-specific developmental goals during early adolescence, which will help protect them from the social pressures of blindly accepting traditional and pervasive stereotypes of femininity and masculinity. This is a period when girls and boys are increasingly spending more time together. Sexual arousal, awareness, and exploration rise significantly in a period when adolescents are also most vulnerable to peer pressure. The developmental goals described below evolve naturally from the preadolescent gender-specific developmental goals described in the corresponding section of Chapter Twenty-eight. It is recommended that program designers determine the level of mastery by early adolescents of the preadolescence goals, and, if necessary, include these in their programs targeting early adolescents. By the end of this period, boys and girls should have mastered the following developmental tasks:

Girls:
- to strengthen their ability to identify not only their present needs and wants but also their future, long-term goals, so that they may envision themselves over time instead of simply responding to the needs and wants of the moment (e.g., pleasure, affiliation, acceptance)
- to practice the previously developed ability to be assertive in expressing their needs and wants
- to practice their developing capacity for dealing with anxiety through a high approach coping style for daily challenges and stresses, and avoidance coping abilities when confronted with uncontrollable or overwhelming stressors. (For more information on these styles, see Chapter Twenty of this book.)
- to continue to identify at least one supportive female adult with whom they may critically analyze socially expected gender roles and behaviors and discuss issues related to safe sex practices
- to have developed a heightened awareness regarding the inherent dangers of accepting traditional versions of femininity, which implicitly or explicitly encourage women to remain silent victims of verbal, emotional, and/or physical violence; sexual ignorance; and passivity; and, in some areas of the world, extend to the trafficking of young females for purposes of pornography, prostitution, sexual tourism, and other related criminal activities between and within countries

Boys:
- to understand and respect that sexual activity is voluntary
- to strengthen their ability to self-regulate and control sexual arousal

- to practice the ability, developed during preadolescence, to listen to girls' needs and wants
- to strengthen self-disclosure and interpersonal understanding abilities
- to continue to identify at least one supportive male adult with whom they may critically analyze socially expected gender roles and behaviors and discuss issues related to safe sex practices
- to have developed a heightened awareness regarding the inherent dangers of accepting traditional versions of masculinity, which implicitly or explicitly encourage early intercourse; sexual coercion; tobacco, alcohol, and drug experimentation; and displays of aggressive physical behavior, including violence, as a confirmation of manhood
- to practice their developing ability for impulse control and regulation of behaviors involving sensation-seeking, sexual and alcohol exploration, anger expression, conflict resolution, anxiety-coping, food cravings, and offers to try tobacco and drugs

---

Box 29-1. Summary of Early Adolescence Basic Developmental Goals

- **Biological changes**
    - to accept positively and learn to manage new physical capabilities (e.g., menstruation, ejaculation, voice changes)
    - to learn to regulate new eating and sleeping patterns in healthy ways
    - to master healthy coping mechanisms for dealing with increased anxiety characteristic of early adolescence
    - to learn how to satisfy increasing sensation-seeking needs in healthy and safe ways
    - to continue to be able to identify one or more supportive adults with whom to share questions about new bodily changes

- **Cognitive changes**
    - to develop a preparatory stage of partial formal operations capacity
    - to develop an "observing ego" and "mutual perspective" ability
    - to have developed the ability to accurately read verbal and nonverbal cues to help them determine whom to trust and whom not to trust
    - to be able to provide reasons for trusting or not trusting a particular person
    - to recognize frequent temptations and be able to understand consequences of new actions in which they might be involved (e.g., having early sex, becoming pregnant, having unprotected sex, becoming infected with HIV/STIs)
    - to be able to organize daily schedules in responsible ways and balance home, school, and work obligations

- **Socio-emotional changes**
    - to undergo shift in interest from person of same sex and interest to one of opposite sex and/or who is different from oneself
    - to be able to identify angry feelings and express them in non-hurtful ways, balanced with feelings of warmth and empathy
    - to continue to be able to identify one or more supportive adults with whom to share intense feelings
    - to be able to identify enjoyable and interesting activities to share with parents
    - to establish a sense of personal identity and be able to assess and accept one's own strengths and weaknesses
    - to achieve greater behavioral autonomy by making healthy choices when going out unsupervised with friends
    - to develop an "ego ideal" and be able to picture themselves over time and into the future

Box 29-2. Summary of Early Adolescence Lifestyle Developmental Goals

- **Safer sex practices**
  - to learn to regulate and control feelings of sexual arousal by respecting and not forcing others into unwanted sexual situations
  - to be able to distinguish between sexual attraction, love, and intimacy
  - to continue to be able to identify one or more supportive adults with whom to share questions about sexual arousal and exploration
  - to knows parents' values and expectations regarding appropriate behaviors for sexuality exploration
  - to be empowered to explore sexuality and express affection through behaviors such as kissing and holding hands, yet holding a personal conviction about not moving into intercourse until one feels emotionally ready
  - to have developed loyalty and caring for the other person's safety and well-being as strong values in close relationships
  - to be able to identify personal goals that would be negatively affected by becoming a mother or father or by contracting STIs or HIV
  - to believe girls and boys should possess equal sexual rights and responsibilities
  - to be able to set limits in sexuality exploration and negotiate alternative behaviors to intercourse for channeling sexual arousal
  - to have the capacity to recognize and critically analyze social pressures to have early sex as a rite of passage, as well as the skills to resist them
  - to demonstrate respect and acceptance for boys and girls who do not possess characteristics associated with traditional gender roles

- **Responsible and reasonable alcohol experimentation**
  - to have the capacity to identify and walk away from unsupervised social gatherings or parties that involve alcohol
  - to experiment with alcohol tasting only under adult supervision
  - to have the capacity to identify and adopt safer and healthier alternatives to drinking alcohol when hanging out with friends
  - to be able to identify highly valued personal behaviors and opportunities that might be negatively affected by alcohol consumption

- **Tobacco and drug resistance skills**
  - to be able to identify and walk away from unsupervised social gatherings or parties that involve tobacco and drug use
  - to continue to be able to identify one or more supportive adults with whom to share personal experiences of drugs and tobacco being offered in social settings
  - to be able to identify and adopt healthier and safer alternatives to tobacco and drug use when hanging out with friends
  - to be able to identify highly valued personal behaviors and opportunities that might be negatively affected by tobacco and/or drug use
  - to be empowered to exercise the right to smoke-free environments where adolescents live, learn, work, and play

- **Nonviolent anger expression and conflict resolution**
  - to be able to identify causes for feelings of anger, frustration, jealousy, and envy and adopt nonviolent strategies to express these feelings in socially acceptable ways
  - to have developed the capacity to identify and critically analyze PG-13-rated violence as depicted on television, and in movies, musical videos, books, and magazines (media literacy skills)
  - to have developed the capacity to critically analyze and apply learned skills to resist social pressures to use violence as an expression of manhood
  - to be able to identify a supportive friend with whom to share intense negative feelings

> **Box 29-2. Summary of Early Adolescence Lifestyle Developmental Goals**—*(continued)*
>
> - to continue to be able to identify one or more supportive adults with whom to share intense negative feelings
> - to knows parents' values and expectations regarding appropriate behaviors for anger expression and conflict resolution
>
> ■ **Healthy nutrition**
> - to be able to identify tasty, healthy foods and food combinations that are easily available when hanging out with friends
> - to be able to identify tasty, healthy snacks that are affordable and can be kept handy to eat and share with friends in moments of intense hunger
> - to be able to identify one or more supportive adults to whom to turn for help in selecting tasty, healthy foods and snacks for social gatherings with friends
> - to be able to regulate and control, when alone or in social group situations, and without adult supervision, the daily consumption of sugars, carbohydrates, and fats
>
> ■ **Physical activity**
> - to be able to identify sports and other physical activities that are fun, attractive, affordable, and easy to do with friends as a group after school or on weekends
> - to be able to organize, with parental support, their after-school time to fit in opportunities for physical activity among other school-, work-, and home-related responsibilities

Box 29-3. **Summary of Early Adolescence Gender-Specific Developmental Goals**

- **Girls**
  - to strengthen their ability to identify not only present needs and wants, but future, long-term goals
  - to practice their previously developed ability to be assertive in expressing their needs and wants
  - to practice their developing ability for dealing with anxiety through a high approach coping style for daily challenges and stresses, and avoidance coping abilities when confronted with uncontrollable or overwhelming stressors
  - to continue to identify at least one supportive female adult with whom to critically analyze socially expected gender roles and behaviors and discuss issues related to safe sex practices
  - to have developed a heightened awareness regarding the inherent dangers of accepting traditional versions of femininity, which implicitly or explicitly encourage women to remain the silent victims of verbal, emotional, and physical violence; sexual ignorance; and passivity

- **Boys**
  - to understand and respect that sexual activity is voluntary
  - to strengthen their ability to regulate and control sexual arousal
  - to practice the previously developed ability to listen to girls' needs and wants
  - to strengthen self-disclosure and interpersonal understanding abilities
  - to identify at least one supportive male adult with whom to critically analyze socially expected gender roles and behaviors and discuss issues related to safe sex practices
  - to have developed a heightened awareness regarding the inherent dangers of accepting traditional versions of masculinity, which implicitly or explicitly encourage early intercourse; sexual coercion; tobacco, alcohol, and drug experimentation; and aggressive physical behavior, including violence, as a confirmation of manhood
  - to practice their developing ability for impulse control and regulation on behaviors involving sensation-seeking, sexual and alcohol exploration, anger expression, conflict resolution, anxiety-coping, food cravings, and tobacco and drug offers

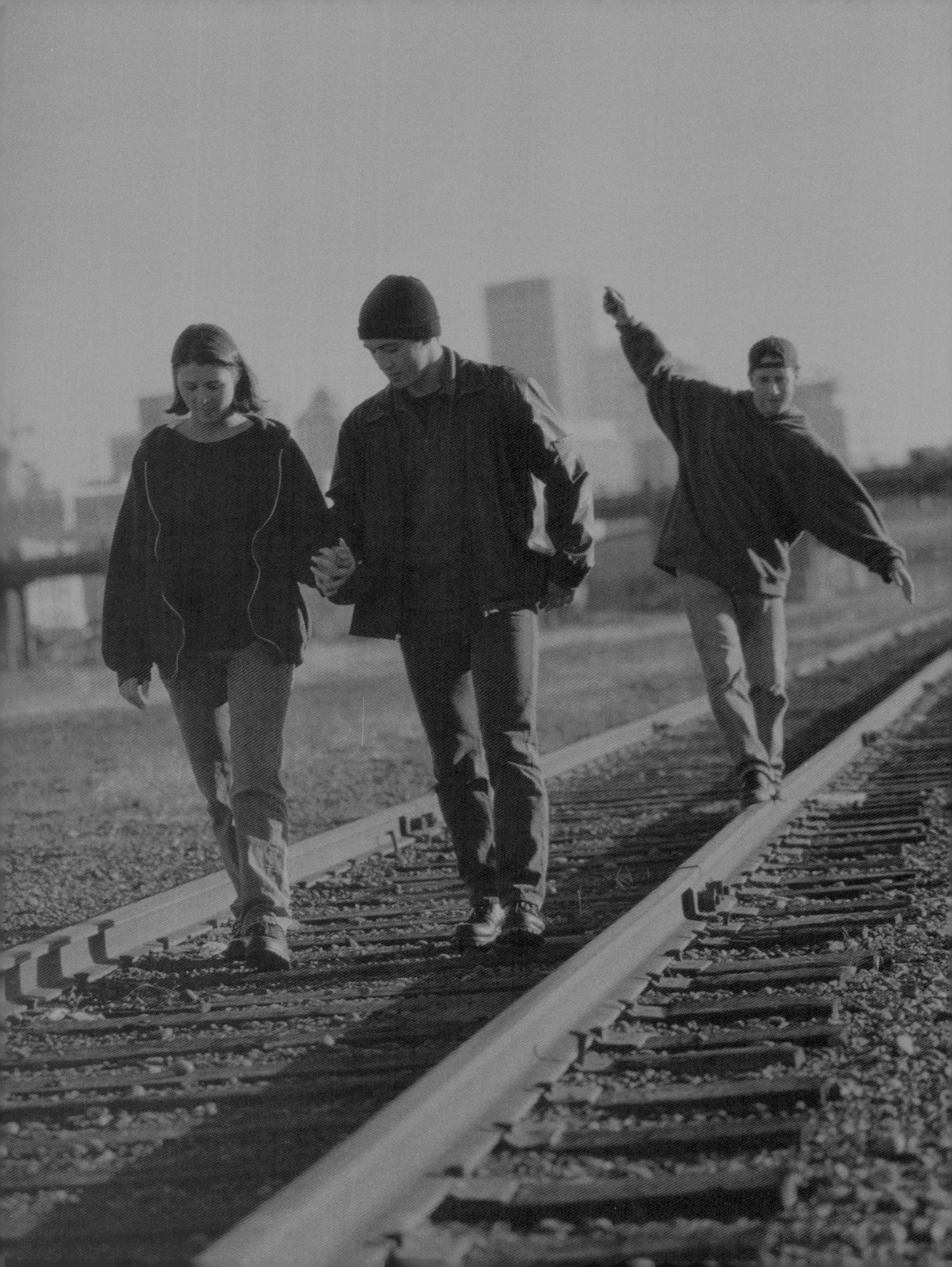

[Section Four]

Conclusions and Recommendations

Introduction

The Pan American Health Organization has developed the contents of this book to facilitate the design of more effective adolescent health programs and policies at all levels of society. By providing evidence-based examples of what works and what appears to have worked less well (or not at all), *Youth: Choices and Change* aims to provide cost-effective tools to those who are called upon to guide adolescent health policy and program development in order to ensure that finite economic resources yield the highest possible return on the investment made.

The theories and models presented in Section Two of this book have been utilized for several decades by social science researchers to study behavior change. However, their specific application to adolescent behaviors has received less attention than that accorded to other older age groups (e.g., the adult population). At the same time, as gleaned from the reference list accompanying this book, the findings of these theories-based applications to adolescents have, until now, been reported only in a rather disparate and fragmented fashion in journal articles, textbooks, and other forms of scientific literature. In this sense, *Youth: Choices and Change* represents a significant milestone: it presents a compilation of the current knowledge base on adolescent behavior change theories and practice and a systemized approach to the effective use of this comprehensive body of lessons learned and best practices. By incorporating this information in the choice of theoretical concepts and the construction of theoretical frameworks, developers of health promotion and prevention interventions will be able to achieve greater programmatic success strengthened by a more meaningful evaluation process.

As this book has shown, behavior change and health promotion theories and models need additionally to be applied within the appropriate context of adolescent development. Section Three presents a detailed discussion of the progression of adolescent developmental stages and their accompanying physical, cognitive, and socio-emotional changes, focusing in particular on the changing needs and wants characterizing the preadolescent and early adolescent years, gender differences as seen from a developmental perspective, and how the achievement of developmental goals contributes to the adolescent's ability to adopt protective, health-promoting behaviors. Much of the information regarding critical developmental distinctions between the preadolescent and early adolescent stages has been observed and shared informally by clinicians through years of working with these age groups, yet this book marks the first attempt to capture and compare these distinctions in a published source. This type of analysis allows those who work with adolescents to correctly identify and appropriately address differences in behavioral and socio-emotional capabilities between 12-year-olds, 14-year-olds, 16-year-olds, and 18-year-olds, for example, and be able to confidently and conscientiously design programs and interventions that effectively respond to the needs and wants of each specific target group.

One of this book's central lessons is that the foundation for successfully instilling life-long healthy behaviors among adolescents is early intervention, beginning in the preadolescence period, before health-compromising behaviors have become deeply rooted. A continuous approach, targeting key areas (e.g., physical activity and nutrition, sexual and reproductive health, and prevention of violence and of tobacco, alcohol, and drug use), should ideally begin during the early childhood years, mediated by the influence of positive role models whose presence remains palpable during the middle childhood period and particularly vigilant throughout adolescence and youth. This type of approach allows young people to practice skills learned during each successive development phase with greater feelings of self-efficacy and supportiveness, while at the same time increasing behavioral independence to positively confront peer, social, and media pressures.

Pipher (1994) has characterized adolescence as a critical period of marked internal development and massive cultural indoctrination. It is for this reason that PAHO so strongly urges early intervention, in contrast to the more prevalent current practice of focusing health promotion interventions on the 15- to 19-year-old age group. By following the suggested steps in this book, adolescent health program developers can provide a continuum of comprehensive support for young people through the provision of interventions at the individual, interpersonal, community, and policy levels and guidance in the mastery of developmental goals appropriate for each age group. Once young people learn how to protect and nurture their bodies and minds, and are sufficiently motivated to make conscious and independent decisions for healthy lifestyles and behaviors, they can confidently proceed toward their self-set goals for the future.

Chapter Thirty explores the current socioeconomic challenges and advantages facing youth in Latin America and the Caribbean, the principal focus of PAHO's technical cooperation efforts. This book's final chapter also presents a review of international commitments undertaken by the member countries of the United Nations designed to strengthen the health and development of young people in the Region of the Americas. It concludes with a series of recommendations for improving health and development opportunities for this group over the next decade.

[Chapter Thirty]

The Next Decade: Perspectives for Improving Adolescent Health and Development

The health of adolescents (10–19 years old) and youth (15–24 years old) is a key element for the social, economic, and political progress of all the countries and territories in the Americas. The future of the Region depends in great part on the participation of a healthy, educated, and economically productive population. Far too often, however, a consideration of adolescent needs and rights is absent from public policies and from the health sector agenda, except when adolescents behave in troubling ways. One contributing factor is that, compared to very young children and the elderly, adolescents suffer from few life-threatening conditions. Furthermore, most of the unhealthy habits learned during adolescence do not produce morbidity or mortality during the period of adolescence itself (Pan American Health Organization 1998).

Nonetheless, costs to governments and individuals are substantial when youth fail to observe healthy lifestyles prior to reaching adulthood. Cost analysis from the United States found that the country spends roughly $20 billion annually in payments for income maintenance, health care, and nutrition to support families created as a result of adolescent pregnancies (Schutt-Aine and Maddaleno 2003, Burt 1998). The World Bank (2002) estimates that a 1% reduction in juvenile crime would increase income from tourism by 4% in Jamaica and 2.3% in Barbados. Furthermore, it is estimated that the indirect costs of deaths from AIDS contracted during adolescence constitute 0.01% of the gross domestic product of Antigua and Barbuda and of Suriname, and 0.17% in the Bahamas alone in the year 2000 (Organización Panamericana de la Salud 2003b).

Thus, adolescence is a crucial stage in the life cycle and has a decisive impact on the health of present and future populations. The process of growth and development is cumulative as well as intergenerational: the successes or losses in each stage of life affect the future health of people and have an impact on the health of the next generation. It is during this stage of adolescence that human capital is developed; new understandings are acquired as well as new abilities and essential competencies to function in society. Adolescents progressively develop a coherent self-identity by internalizing values and attitudes and establishing commitments with the community. Adolescence is also a time when adolescents and those who support them should be attentive to the development of sexuality and the accompanying reproductive capacities. It is important, therefore, that adolescents learn how to identify and adopt health-promoting behaviors and consciously choose to avoid health-compromising behaviors, since the majority of harmful health habits are acquired during this stage of life (Organización Panamericana de la Salud 2003b).

Various countries in the Region of the Americas are faced with an opportunity for economic growth, known as the "demographic gift," thanks to the composition of their populations (Schutt-Aine and Maddaleno 2003, Bloom 2001). A cohort of young people ages 15 to 24 is entering the labor force in these countries without the pressure of a large cohort of children to follow it, nor an older population to maintain fiscally. However, in order to take advantage of this opportunity, young people will need to be healthy, acquire a good education, and have access to employment, as was the experience of Asian countries during the 1990s. With adequate support and appropriate investments by governments, this economically active young population will be able to become the motor for economic growth and an agent for positive social change in the Region (Schutt-Aine and Maddaleno 2003, Bloom et al. 1999, Jacinto et al. 1998). Developing effective interventions and programs to spur positive growth and development among the 15- to 24-year-old segment of the population, now and over the coming years, will therefore be crucial.

Given the importance of investing in adolescent and youth health and development in the Region, the member countries of the United Nations have signed a series of international agreements that have prioritized this topic to facilitate the allocation of resources and the elaboration of plans and programs for improving health and development opportunities for young people around the world. These include the following targets:

- United Nations General Assembly Special Session on HIV/AIDS (June 2001)
    - by the year 2005, reduce the prevalence of HIV infection in young men and women aged 15 to 24 by 25%
- United Nations General Assembly Special Session on Children (May 2002)

- by the year 2010, develop and implement national policies and programs for adolescent health
■ United Nations Millennium Summit/ U.N. Millennium Declaration/U.N. Millennium Development Goals (September 2000)
  - by the year 2015, reduce maternal mortality rate by 75%
  - by the year 2015, halt and begin to reverse the spread of HIV/AIDS

In addition to committing themselves to reducing the prevalence of HIV infections in young people by 25%, the countries have agreed to ensure that at least 90% of young men and women between the ages of 15 and 24 have access to the necessary information, education—including peer education and youth-specific HIV education—and services to develop the life skills required to reduce their vulnerability to HIV infection; this process is be carried out in full partnership with youth, parents, families, educators, and health care providers (Joint United Nations Programme on HIV/AIDS/World Health Organization/Pan American Health Organization 2001).

The Millennium Development Goals (MDGs), which focus on society's poorest segments and whose overarching goal is an extreme reduction of poverty, were adopted by 189 U.N. member nations and consist of an indivisible package of measurable goals and targets to be achieved by 2015. Four of the eight MDGs include indicators and targets for the 15-to-24-year-old age group, calling for universal education and a literate population, the promotion of gender equality and empowerment of women, and improving HIV/AIDS prevention strategies and socioeconomic opportunities for youth at the beginning of their economically productive years.

MDG-1, the reduction of maternal mortality by 75%, is particularly relevant to the global situation of young people, since the maternal mortality rate increases as the age of the pregnant woman decreases. Similarly, MDG-6, regarding the halt of the HIV/AIDS epidemic, will be achieved only through the development of more effective prevention strategies, since 50% of all new HIV infections occur between the ages of 15 and 24 (Joint United Nations Programme on HIV/AIDS 1998). Each year, an estimated 2 million young people continue to become infected with HIV, with women comprising two-thirds of this number. Young people form a large percentage of groups particularly vulnerable to infection, such as intravenous drug users and sexual workers. Likewise, young people represent a significant proportion of the parents of the estimated 2,000 children who become infected every day with HIV through vertical transmission. Finally, a large percentage of AIDS orphans are adolescents themselves (World Health Organization 2004a).

In addition to health, the MDGs include numerous references to the right of all children to have access to education and the need for regular school attendance. These, in turn, provide the basic foundation for opportunities later on for suitable employment and the ability of young people to economically support themselves and the families they create. Although the educational status of young people in Latin America and the Caribbean has improved significantly over the last decades, there continue to be geographical and socioeconomic inequalities. It is estimated that 50% of 20-year-olds living in urban areas and 75% of those living in rural areas drop out of school before completing their secondary education (Pan American Health Organization 2002b). The educational level of women has a great deal of influence on the number of children they have. Women with 10 or more years of education are four times less likely to initiate sexual activity before the age of 20 than women with fewer years of education (Schutt-Aine and Maddaleno 2003). Adolescent males ages 15 to 24 represent between 44% and 71% of the economically active population. However, economic conditions for young people are not optimal. It is estimated that 10 million children under the age of 14 work illegally, without social security benefits, receiving very low salaries, and frequently working under dangerous conditions. The official rate of unemployment for young people in Latin America is 16% and varies from approximately 35% in Colombia to 6% in Mexico. The most vulnerable groups are those young people who neither study nor work (World Bank 2002). It is estimated that between 12% and 40% of the poor families in Latin America and the Caribbean have adolescent children who do not study or work (Pan American Health Organization 2002b). In several countries, up to 25% of young people grow up in homes headed by single mothers and frequently characterized as poor.

PAHO is working on a number of fronts in support of MDG-2, the achievement of universal education, and MDG-3, regarding gender equality and the empowerment of women, in the belief that education is particularly important for young girls: it will help them to learn how to make better decisions regarding their health, their body, and the number and spacing of the children they have later on. At the same time, it will better protect them against partner abuse, improve opportunities for employment and remuneration equal with that of men, and increase their participation in decision-making roles at the community, national, and international levels.

"The health and development of adolescents and youth, and their active inclusion in daily life, are key elements for the social, economic, and political progress of the countries of the Americas," noted PAHO Director Dr. Mirta Roses at the XII Conference of First Ladies, Spouses, and Representatives of Heads of State and Government of the Americas, held in Santo Domingo, the Dominican Republic, in October 2003. At this meeting, whose focus was "Youth and Poverty," Roses also stated that special attention should be accorded to youth in special and/or precarious situations, such as the handicapped, the homeless, those who are wards of the State, and those who participate in gang violence and/or are involved in prostitution. "We must strengthen self-esteem and identity through harmonious and positive peer relations," she said, as she emphasized the importance of "building networks; creating spaces that facilitate and encourage creativity, originality, multicultural and multi-religious contributions, and a culture of tolerance; valuing diversity; and reducing stigmas and marginalization" (Organización Panamericana de la Salud 2003b).

Partnerships for Progress: Sharing What Works

Within the spirit of MDG-8, which calls for the creation of a global partnership for development, one of PAHO's objectives in publishing this book is to share best practices and lessons learned and to stimulate cross-country dialogues on how the public health sector, including community health promoters and practitioners, can design effective, well-targeted interventions, services, and programs to support the positive development of young people. As we have seen throughout this book, however, the health sector cannot work in isolation; actions must occur in much broader partnerships with the educational, economic, and political segments of society, as well. At the same time, as PAHO's Director noted at the Santo Domingo summit, the most effective interventions for improving health, education, and socioeconomic opportunities are those that "recognize the need to ensure full youth participation in defining policies, programs, and activities that affect and involve them" (Organización Panamericana de la Salud 2003b).

An excellent example of how this combination of strategies can bear positive fruit is happening in Canada, where Aboriginal peoples are one of the fastest growing segments of the population and more than half of this group is under the age of 24 (Pan American Health Organization 2002c). Although health and development indicators for Aboriginal people still reveal considerable gaps and inadequacies, as compared to the Canadian population as a whole, recognition is growing among leaders and decision-makers at all levels that creating socioeconomic opportunities for youth—particularly those who come from disadvantaged circumstances—contributes to the reduction of poverty and the creation of sustainable development, the essence of MDG-1 and MDG-8.

"Our youth are a large and dynamic population," First Nations National Chief Phil Fontaine told an Assembly of First Nations citizens in 2003. "They will be driving the economic and political life of this country in the coming years. We must harness that energy and provide education, employment, and hope. This makes for stronger First Nations and a stronger country for everyone" (Canada NewsWire 2003).

In recognition of the sizeable First Nations population under 24 years of age, in 2002 the Assembly established a National Youth

Council. When the Canadian Government's Standing Senate Committee on Aboriginal Peoples recently prepared a report on the health and educational status of First Nations youth living in urban centers, National Youth Council representatives from across the country provided input. Ginger Gosnell, Council representative from the province of British Columbia, told the 2003 Assembly: "Experience shows that the key factor for success in any initiative aimed at First Nations youth is that we be involved from the very beginning in the design, development, and delivery of these initiatives." Gosnell further indicated that the Council's coordinated and proactive response resulted in concrete improvements in the document when she observed that "the Senate report clearly benefited from the recommendations of First Nations youth, and we have to remain involved to make sure the follow-through is successful as well" (Canada NewsWire 2003).

The Canadian experience just described encompasses many of the values of the community organization models presented in Chapter Twenty-two of this book. By involving the target group in the development of interventions affecting their future and spurring the participation of First Nations youth across the country, the process of true community participation and positive change begins. The young members of this coalition gain empowerment, a critical consciousness of the root causes of their problems, collective self-efficacy, and the ability to select issues for political attention of most importance to them; in this case, health and education. The future of this group, to the degree that its individual members continue to believe in and practice the principles they are lobbying for today, holds great potential. They are coming to master the life skills that will transform them into agents for their own positive change.

Recommended Actions to Improve the Health of the Adolescent and Youth Population over the Next Decade

Adolescent health programs in Latin America and the Caribbean, as in many other parts of the world, have traditionally been geared toward specific negative behaviors and feature a problem-oriented approach that focuses on single issues, such as early maternity, drug abuse, or juvenile crime, in isolation. Such approaches focus on the individual and do not take into account other possibly related unhealthy behaviors or the broad social context within which the problem first arose. Nor are other actors in the adolescent's social environment (e.g., parents, siblings, other relatives, teachers, peers) normally called upon to provide input into the design or to participate in the intervention's execution. Furthermore, the interventions are usually curative in nature, and specific to the problem at hand, with relatively limited emphasis on positive health promotion and prevention principles. Such interventions are generally not coordinated (e.g., between health services, schools, and the family), causing costly duplication of efforts, even though numerous studies—a variety of them cited in this book—have shown that many adolescent behavioral problems have common origins and are interrelated. Finally, the needs, concerns, and rights of the adolescents themselves are often overlooked, as are gender- and culture-related considerations and the changing developmental needs of young people at different ages.

On the basis of these facts, PAHO proposes a new conceptual framework, in which approaches are based on prevention and health promotion, instead of the reduction of problems and their impact. This new health paradigm would focus on positive human development at the individual, family, and community levels, and encourage full participation by young people in the social, political, and economic life of their communities. Community health services can play a pivotal role in this empowerment process: by actively responding to the needs of adolescents and youth and forming effective linkages with other appropriate public and private local institutions, they can provide valuable support for the adoption of healthy behaviors and lifestyles, thereby preparing young people to become healthy, educated, and economically productive adults.

In summary, the new health paradigm should focus on the following components, with a view toward improving the health and development of young people over the next decade:

- disease prevention and health promotion principles
- early and integrated interventions
- strengthening of the individual-family-community series of relationships
- promotion of the political and social participation of young people in addressing their health and development needs

The following actions are crucial for creating a new paradigm of health and development for young people in the Americas and worldwide:

(1) **Improve the environment where young people live** through the formulation of broad-based, comprehensive policies addressing the determinants of good health and positive well-being for this group. At the national and community level, political leaders and decision-makers should preserve, support, strengthen, and empower families and communities by designing policies and laws that improve economic status, strengthen community services and resources, decrease exposure to violence and other unhealthy behaviors and conditions, foster positive social standards, and, above all, demonstrate a sustained commitment to health promotion. The mass media should be incorporated as a full partner in the promotion of positive, so-

cially responsible health promotion messages targeted to the adolescent and youth consumer markets.

(2) **Collect data, disaggregated by age and gender,** on the health situation of adolescents as a basis for policy formation and program development, both locally and nationally.

(3) **Improve access to health services.** Countries that are reforming their health sector should ensure the equitable access of all adolescents to a basic package of comprehensive health services that includes a component of health promotion and disease prevention. Furthermore, these services should ensure the legal right to confidentiality and to private care, based on individualized needs, that includes the target group's participation in the design and delivery of these services.

(4) **Improve access to education and strengthen the role of schools in adolescent health promotion.** Given that adolescents spend a majority of their time in the classroom and in school-related activities, the educational system can play a central role in helping to shape the attitudes of young people toward life and the future they envision for themselves. As we saw in Chapter Nineteen of this book, schools, along with parents and the family, can provide a key social environment where adolescents receive support and empowerment and learn boundaries and expectations and how to use their time constructively (external assets), at the same time that they develop a commitment to learning, positive values, social competencies, and a positive identity (internal assets). As earlier stated, it is the right of all children to have access to education, and there is a need for regular school attendance. Schools and the educational system can play a meaningful role in fostering the development of positive behaviors among children and adolescents by providing them with opportunities to learn what adults and society in general expect from them as they grow up and to practice adult roles in a positive learning environment. In this sense, schools provide a vital gateway not only to the adoption of strengths-based, protective behaviors but also to the achievement of the necessary academic, vocational, social, and emotional skills to become economically productive adults in an increasingly competitive world.

(5) **Design effective, evidence-based, developmentally and culturally appropriate interventions for adolescents of different ages and genders.** As has been noted and discussed throughout this book, adolescent health interventions and programs will be more effective if they are tailored to the different developmental stages (beginning with early intervention during preadolescence and early adolescence), instead of being targeted to

the entire adolescent age spectrum as a homogeneous group. Developmentally differentiated interventions and programs further require a gender perspective which takes into account the distinct wants and needs of girls and boys and the different rates at which each progress from one developmental stage to the next. Program designers also must be aware that adolescent needs and wants will vary in different geographical contexts and cultures, and that interventions succeed to the degree that they are locally based and responsive to their actual (versus theoretical) target group. Finally, effective interventions and programs will facilitate the learning and mastery of a series of developmental goals and growth competencies, described in Chapters Twenty-eight and Twenty-nine, that in turn strengthen the adolescent's ability to adopt protective, health-promoting behaviors.

(6) **Create intersectoral partnerships** at the grass roots, regional, and national levels, ensuring an appropriate and equitable distribution of roles and functions, for a well-coordinated, integrated response to adolescent health and development issues. The community organization models described in Chapter Twenty-two may be adapted for use at all levels of society and enable alliance members to collectively identify needs, problems, and goals; mobilize resources; and develop and implement strategies for reaching their mutually agreed-upon objectives. All of these stages should include the input and participation of adolescents and youth, in interaction with all alliances, coalitions, and networks whose members represent interests with a direct influence on the lives of young people, such as health, education, legislative, juridical, judicial, religious, community safety, the mass media, and others.

(7) **Develop an evidence base on the effects of globalization and new information technologies on youth and adolescent health** and incorporate effective responses to this issue in behavioral change interventions and programs. Today's generation of young people are the very first to experience the full impact of the numerous communication tools made possible by the Internet and globalized mass media capabilities. At the same time that these advances have made the world appear smaller and within reach of everyone, they have also created a "digital divide" between the world's wealthiest and poorest countries, resulting in new inequities for those individuals whose socioeconomic status prevents them from enjoying the benefits of these technologies.

Also, as noted in this book, youth are the primary market targeted by producers of emerging electronic and digital entertainment products, whether computer games, musical videos, or "reality television." The products' appeal to this age market results from their effectiveness in providing a satisfying response to youths' need for sensation-seeking and their ability to keep apace even as market tastes and expectations change. Oftentimes, however, the resulting messages promote and glamorize risk-taking behaviors, either implicitly or explicitly, thereby luring youth to move beyond boundaries that are safe and healthy.

Clearly, more research is needed to determine the ultimate extent to which the new global communication technologies influence youth's ability to make healthy choices and how the negative effects on adolescent health of these trends may be counteracted and even reversed with front-line, timely responses by health promotion advocates and public health policymakers. The building of an evidence base on how the information and entertainment needs of the youth market may be satisfied in healthier, more socially responsible ways will enable caring communities to secure better and more protective opportunities for self-empowerment of their young people and motivate them to confidently and consciously make personal choices that strengthen their physical, emotional, and socioeconomic well-being today and throughout adulthood.

Afterword

Throughout history, the world's greatest thinkers have mused on the mystique and powers of youth. "We have two lives," U.S. author Bernard Malamud once said. "The one we learn with, and the life we live after that." Clearly, adolescence is a period of learning, of trying out new experiences in life for size, fit, comfort, appeal.

"The fortune of our lives . . . depends on employing well the short period of our youth," Thomas Jefferson wrote in a 1787 letter to his daughter, suggesting that the adolescent years provide a brief window of opportunity for self-examination and the development of sufficient self-determination to carry us through to the eventual completion of our goals and dreams.

Ralph Waldo Emerson waxed philosophic when he wrote in 1870: "The youth suffers not only from ungratified desires, but from powers untried. . . . He is tormented with the want of correspondence between things and thoughts." Emerson's contemporary, British poet Mary Elizabeth Coleridge, wrote, on a lighter note: "We were young, we were merry, we were very, very wise; and the door stood open to our feast." The juxtaposition of these two very different views highlights the alternating feelings of turmoil and triumph every adolescent experiences. The depth of each emotion will remain etched in memory forever. That they stand at opposite poles as markers of human self-confidence testifies to the gamut and complexity of human emotions that characterize this time in life.

"To become aware in time when young of the advantages of age; to maintain the advantages of youth in old age: both are pure fortune," German poet and dramatist Johann Wolfgang Von Goethe wrote some two centuries ago. His message attests to the "usefulness" of that challenging period lying midway between childhood and adulthood. He and his other colleagues above, in essence, are saying that adolescence is a period to savor and enjoy, and at the same time till and cultivate sufficiently to provide fruit for life.

It is our job—as parents, teachers, faith leaders, health promoters, clinicians, policymakers, and politicians—to help and encourage youth to strike this critical balance during life's most self-defining juncture.

References

Abbassi V. Growth and normal puberty. *Pediatrics* 1998;102:507–511.

Abma JC, Sonenstein FL. Sexual activity and contraceptive practices among teenagers in the United States, 1988 and 1995. National Center for Health Statistics. *Vital Health Stat* 2001;23(21):1–79. http:/ www.cdc.gov/nchs/data/series/sr_23/sr23_021.pdf

Acuff D. *What Kids Buy and Why: The Psychology of Marketing to Kids.* New York: The Free Press; 1997.

Adih WK, Alexander CS. Determinants of condom use to prevent HIV infection among youth in Ghana. *Adolesc Health* 1999;24(1):63–72.

Aguirre R, Güell, P. *Hacerse hombres: la construcción de la masculinidad en los adolescentes y sus riesgos.* Washington, DC: OPS/WK Kellogg Foundation/FNUAP; 2002.

Ajzen I, Fishbein M. *Understanding Attitudes and Predicting Social Behavior.* Englewood Cliffs, New Jersey: Prentice Hall; 1980.

Ajzen I, Madden TJ. Prediction of goal-directed behavior: attitudes, intentions, and perceived behavioral control. *J Exp Soc Psychol* 1986;22:453–474.

Albrecht S, Payne L, Stone CA, Reynolds MD. A preliminary study of the use of peer support in smoking cessation programs for pregnant adolescents. *J Am Acad Nurse Pract* 1998;10(3):119–125.

Alexander C, Piazza M, Mekos D, Valente T. Peers, schools, and adolescent cigarette smoking. *J Adolesc Health* 2001;29:22–30.

Almeida DM, Kessler RC. Everyday stressors and gender differences in daily distress. *J Pers Soc Psychol* 1998;75(3):670–680.

Altman DG, Levine DW, Coeytaux R, Slade J, Raffe R. Tobacco promotion and susceptibility to tobacco use among adolescents aged 12 through 17 years in a nationally representative sample. *Am J Public Health* 1996;86(11):1590–1593.

American Academy of Child and Adolescent Psychiatry. *Your Adolescent.* Washington, DC: AACP; 1999.

American Legacy Foundation. Literature Review for American Legacy Foundation's Statewide Youth Movement against Tobacco Use. Draft report; September, 2000. www.americanlegacy.org.

American Psychiatric Association. *Diagnostic and Statistical Manual of Mental Disorders*. 4th ed. Washington, DC: APA; 1994.

Andreasen AR. *Marketing Social Change: Changing Behavior to Promote Health, Social Development, and the Environment*. San Francisco: Jossey-Bass; 1995.

Andrew G, Patel V, Ramakrishna J. Sex, studies or strife? What to integrate in adolescent health services. *Reprod Health Matters* 2003;11(21):120–129.

Andrucci GL, Archer RP, Pancoast DL, Gordon RA. The relationship of MMPI and sensation-seeking scales to adolescent drug use. *J Pers Assess* 1989;53:253–266.

Arnett J. Are college students adults? Their conceptions of the transition to adulthood. *J Adult Dev* 1994;(1):213–224.

Atalah E, Arteaga R, Rebolledo A, Delfín S, Ramos R. Prevalencia de obesidad en escolares de la región de Aysen. *Arch Argent Pediatr* 2001;99(1):29–33.

Averett SL, Rees DI, Argys LM. The impact of government policies and neighborhood characteristics on teenage sexual activity and contraceptive use. *Am J Public Health* 2002;92(11):1773–1778.

Ayres TS, Sandler IN, Twohey JL. Conceptualization and measurement of coping in children and adolescents. *Adv Clin Child Psych* 1998;20:243–301.

Azmier J. *Gambling in Canada: Triumph, Tragedy, or Tradeoff. Canadian Gambling Behavior and Attitudes*. Calgary, Alberta: Canada West Foundation; 2000.

Baker JG, Rosenthal SL, Leonhardt D, Kollar LM, Succop PA, Burklow KA, Biro FM. Relationship between perceived parental monitoring and young adolescent girls' sexual and substance use behaviors. *J Pediatr Adolesc Gynecol* 1999;12(1):17–22.

Bandura A. Self-efficacy: toward a unifying theory of behavioral change. *Psychol Rev* 1977;84(2):191–215.

Bandura A. *Social Foundations of Thought and Action: A Social Cognitive Theory*. Englewood Cliffs, New Jersey: Prentice Hall; 1986.

Bandura A. *Self-Efficacy. The Exercise of Control*. New York: WH Freeman; 1997.

Bandura A. Social cognitive theory: an agentic perspective. *Annu Rev Psychol* 2001;52:1–26.

Bandura A, Walters RH. *Social Learning and Personality Development*. New York: Holt, Rinehart & Winston; 1963.

Baranowski T, Davis M, Resnicow K, Baranowski J, Doyle C, Lin LS, Smith M, Wang DT. Gimme 5 fruit, juice, and vegetables for fun and health: outcome evaluation. *Health Educ Behav* 2000;27(1):96–111.

Barker C. *The Health Care Policy Process*. Newbury Park, California: Sage Publications; 1996.

Barkley RA. *ADHD and the Nature of Self-control*. New York: The Guilford Press; 1997.

Barrera M. Social support research in community psychology. In Rappaport J, Seidman E (eds.). *Handbook of Community Psychology*. New York: Kluwer Academic/Plenum; 2000.

Bartholomew LK, Parcel GS, Kok G, Gottlieb NH (eds.). *Intervention Mapping: Designing Theory-and Evidence based Health Promotion Programs.* Mountain View, California: Mayfield Publishing Company; 2001.

Basen-Engquist K, O'Hara-Tompkins N, Lovato CY, Lewis MJ, Parcel GS, Gingiss PH. The effects of two types of teacher training on implementation of a tobacco prevention curriculum. *J Sch Health* 1994;64(8):334–339.

Baumrind D. Child care practices anteceding three patterns of preschool behavior. *Genet Psychol Monogr* 1967;75(1):43–88.

Baumrind D. Current patterns of parental authority. *Devl Psychol Monogr* 1971;4(1):1–103.

Baumrind D. Parental disciplinary patterns and social competence in children. *Youth Soc* 1978;9(3):239–276.

Bejarano J, Carvajal H, San Lee L. *Consumo de drogas en Costa Rica. Resultados de la Encuesta Nacional de 1995.* San José: Instituto sobre Alcoholismo y Farmacodependencia; 1996.

Berk LE. Children's private speech: an overview of theory and the status of research. In Diaz RM, Berk LE (eds.). *Private Speech: From Social Interaction to Self-regulation.* Mahwah, New Jersey: Erlbaum; 1992.

Berk LE. Why children talk to themselves. *Sci Am* 1994;271(5):78–83.

Berkman LF, Glass T. Social integration, social networks, social support, and health. In Berkman LF, Kawachi I (eds.). *Social Epidemiology.* New York: Oxford University Press; 2000.

Bernstein Lachter R, Komro KA, Veblen-Mortenson S, Perry CL, Williams CL. High school students' efforts to reduce alcohol use in their communities: Project Northland's Youth Development Component. *J Health Educ* 1999;30(6):330–335.

Bettencourt T, Hodgins A, Huba GJ, Pickett G. Bay area young positives: a model of a youth-based approach to HIV/AIDS services. *J Adolesc Health* 1998;23(2 Suppl.):28–36.

Biglan A, Noell J, Ochs L, Smolkowski K, Metzler C. Does sexual coercion play a role in the high-risk sexual behavior of adolescent and young adult women? *J Behav Med* 1995;18(6):549–568.

Bilodeau A, Forget G, Tetreault J. Contraceptive self-efficacy in male and female adolescents: validation of the French version of the Levinson Scale. *Can J Public Health* 1994;85(2):115–120.

Bloom D. *Closing the Loop: Latin America, Globalization and Human Development.* United Nations Conference on Trade and Development/United Nations Development Programme; 2002.

Bloom D, Canning D, Evans DK, Graham BS, Lynch P, Murphy EE. Population Change and Human Development in Latin America. Background paper prepared for the Inter-American Development Bank in connection with *Economic and Social Progress in Latin America, 1999–2000 Report.* Washington, DC: IAD; 1999.

Blum RW, McNeely CA, Rinehart PM. *Improving the Odds: The Untapped Power of Schools to Improve the Health of Teens.* Minneapolis: University of Minnesota; 2001.

Bona G, Castellino N, Petri A. Secular trend della puberta. [Secular trend of puberty]. *Minerva Pediatr* 2002;54(6):553–557.

Borawski EA, Ievers-Landis CE, Lovegreen LD, Trapl ES. Parental monitoring, negotiated unsupervised time, and parental trust: the role of perceived parenting practices in adolescent health risk behaviors. *J Adolesc Health* 2003;33(2):60–70.

Borges GA, Pires Junior R. Idade da menarca em adolescents de Londrina-PR. [Menarche age in adolescents of Londrina-PR]. *Rev Bras Ativ Fis Saude* 2000;5(3):5–11.

Bosompra K. Determinants of condom use intentions of university students in Ghana: an application of the theory of reasoned action. *Soc Sci Med* 2001;52(7):1057–1069.

Boyer MR, Yanoff J. Working across difference to promote male involvement: one community's response. *SIECUS Rep* 1995;23(6):20–23.

Braithwaite RL, Bianchi C, Taylor SE. Ethnographic approach to community organization and health empowerment. *Health Educ Q* 1994;21(3):407–416.

Brazelton TB, Greenspan SI. *The Irreducible Needs of Children. What Every Child Must Have to Grow, Learn and Flourish*. Cambridge, Massachusetts: Perseus Publishing; 2000.

Breidablik HJ, Meland, E. Ung pa hybel-sosial kontroll og helserelatert atferd. [Adolescents living on their own—Social control and health-related behavior]. *Tidsskr Nor Laegeforen* 2001;121(3):287–291.

Brock GC, Beazley RP. Using the health belief model to explain parents' participation in adolescents' at-home sexuality education activities. *J Sch Health* 1995;65(4):124–128.

Brody G, Stoneman Z, Flor D. Parental religiosity, family processes and youth competence in rural, two-parent African-American families. *Dev Psychol* 1996;32:696–706.

Bronfenbrenner U. *The Ecology of Human Development*. Cambridge, Massachusetts: Harvard University Press; 1979.

Bronowski J. Human and animal languages. In *A Sense of the Future*. Cambridge, Massachusetts: MIT Press; 1977.

Brooks-Gunn J, Duncan G, Klebanov P, Sealand N. Do neighborhoods influence child and adolescent development? *Am J Sociol* 1993;99(2):353–395.

Brooks-Gunn J, Paikoff R. Sex is a gamble, kissing is a game: adolescent sexuality and health promotion. In Millstein S, Petersen A, Nightingale E (eds.). *Promoting the Health of Adolescents: New Directions for the Twenty-first Century*. New York: Oxford University Press; 1993.

Brooks-Gunn J, Warren MP. The psychological significance of secondary sexual characteristics in 9-to-11-year-old girls. *Child Dev* 1989;59(4):1061–1069.

Brown B. Peer groups. In Feldman S, Elliot G (eds.). *At the Threshold: The Developing Adolescent*. Cambridge, Massachusetts: Harvard University Press; 1990.

Brown HN, Saunders RB, Dick MJ. Preventing secondary pregnancy in adolescents: a model program. *Health Care Women Int* 1999;20(1):5–15.

Brown JD, Cantor J. An agenda for research on youth and the media. *J Adolesc Health* 2000(27S):2–7.

Buchanan CM, Eccles JS, Becker JB. Are adolescents the victims of raging hormones? Evidence for activational effects of hormones on moods and behaviors at adolescence. *Psychol Bull* 1992;111(1):62–107.

Buchanan DR. *An Ethic for Health Promotion. Rethinking the Sources of Human Well-Being.* New York: Oxford University Press; 2000.

Burg MM, Seeman TE. Families and health: the negative side of social ties. *Ann Behav Med* 1994;16:109–115.

Burnett PC, Fanshawe JP. Measuring school-related stressors in adolescents. *J Youth Adolesc* 1997;26:415–429.

Burt M. *Why Should We Invest in Adolescents?* Washington, DC: Pan American Health Organization/W. K. Kellogg Foundation; 1998.

Bush PJ. Developmental issues in prevention. *The Prevention Researcher* 1996;3(1).

Buston K, Wight D, Hart G, Scott S. Implementation of a teacher-delivered sex education programme: obstacles and facilitating factors. *Health Educ Res* 2002;17(1):59–72.

Butterfoss FD, Goodman R, Wandersman A. Community coalitions for prevention and health promotion. *Health Educ Res* 1993;8(3):315–330.

Butterfoss FD, Kegler MC. Toward a comprehensive understanding of community coalitions. Moving from practice to theory. In DiClemente RJ, Crosby RA, Kegler MC (eds.). *Emerging Theories in Health Promotion Practice and Research*. San Francisco: Jossey-Bass; 2002.

Cáceres CF, Vanoss, MB, Sid Hudes E. Sexual coercion among youth and young adults in Lima, Peru. *J Adolesc Health* 2000;27(5):361–367.

Calderón V. Foro Nacional de Prevención y Atención de Embarazos en Adolescentes (Presentation). Juan Dolio, República Dominicana, October 2002.

Camacho-Hubner AV. *Perfil en salud sexual y reproductiva de los y las adolescentes de América Latina y el Caribe. Revisión bibliográfica, 1988-1998*. Washington, DC: OPS; 2000. (Serie OPS/FNUAP No.1).

Canada NewsWire. Assembly of First Nations National Chief Welcomes Report on Urban Youth by Standing Senate Committee on Aboriginal Peoples; Ottawa, 2003. (News release).

Cannon WB. *The Wisdom of the Body*. New York: WW Norton & Company Inc.; 1932.

Capella JN, Fishbein M, Hornik R, Kirkland Ahern R, Sayeed S. Using theory to select messages in antidrug media campaigns. Reasoned action and media priming. In Rice RE, Atkin CK (eds.). *Public Communication Campaigns*. 3rd ed. Newbury Park, California: Sage Publications; 2001.

Carey WB. Introduction-basic issues. In Carey WB, McDevitt SC (eds.). *Clinical and Educational Applications of Temperament Research*. Amsterdam/Lisse: Swets and Zeitlinger; 1989.

Caribbean Epidemiology Center. *Behavior Change Interventions for Sexual Health Promotion: A Manual*. Port of Spain, Trinidad and Tobago: CAREC; 2003.

Caribbean Food and Nutrition Institute. Obesity Prevention in the Caribbean: The Stages of Change Model. Diabetes and Obesity Conference, Ocho Rios, Jamaica, March 2002.

Carlini-Cotrim B. Country profile on alcohol in Brazil. In Riley L, Marshall M (eds.). *Alcohol and Public Health in 8 Developing Countries*. Geneva: World Health Organization; 1999.

Carlson C, Uppal S, Prosser EC. Ethnic differences in processes contributing to the self-esteem of early adolescent girls. *J Early Adolesc* 2000;20:44–67.

Carver CS, Pozo C, Harris SD, Noriega V, Scheier MF, Robinson DS, Ketcham AS, Moffat FL Jr, Clark KC. How coping mediates the effect of optimism on distress: a study of women with early stage breast cancer. *J Pers Soc Psychol* 1993;65(2):375–390.

Casey M, Nuttal R, Pezaris E, Benbow C. The influence of spatial ability on gender differences in mathematics college entrance test scores across diverse samples. *Dev Psychol* 1995;31:697–705.

Cassel J. The contribution of the social environment to host resistance: The Fourth Wade Hampton Frost Lecture. *Am J Epidemiol* 1976;104(2):107–123.

Chaloupka FJ, Grossman M, Saffer H. The effects of price on alcohol consumption and alcohol-related problems. *Alcohol Res Health* 2002;26(1):22–34.

Chaloupka FJ, Saffer H, Grossman M. Alcohol-control policies and motor-vehicle fatalities. *J Legal Stud* 1993;22(1):161–186.

Champion JD. Life histories of rural Mexican American adolescents experiencing abuse. *West J Nurs Res* 1999;21(5):699–717.

Chapman S, Wong WL. Smith W. Self-exempting beliefs about smoking and health: differences between smokers and ex-smokers. *Am J Public Health* 1993;83(2):215–219.

Chapple CL. Examining intergenerational violence: violent role modeling or weak parental controls? *Violence Vict* 2003;18(2):143–162.

Chavkin NF, González J. *Mexican Immigrant Youth and Resiliency: Research and Promising Programs*. Charleston, West Virginia: Eric Digest; 2000.

Chen X, Unger JB, Palmer P, Weiner MD, Johnson CA, Wong MM, Austin G. Prior cigarette smoking initiation predicting current alcohol use: evidence for a gateway drug effect among California adolescents from eleven ethnic groups. *Addict Behav* 2002;27(5):799–817.

Chess S, Thomas A. *Temperament. Theory and Practice*. New York: Brunner Mazel Publishers; 1996.

Child Trends. *Building a Better Teenager: A Summary of "What Works" in Adolescent Development*. Washington, DC: Child Trends; 2002. (Publication No. 2002–57).

Chile. Ministerio de Educación, Ministerio de Salud, Ministerio del Interior. Consejo Nacional para el Control de Estupefacientes. *Estudio del consumo de drogas en la población escolar de Chile*. Santiago de Chile: CONACE; 1999. www.conacedrogas.cl/inicio/obs_naci_encu_tema2.php

Chile. Ministerio del Interior. Consejo Nacional para el Control de Estupefacientes. *Estudio Nacional de Consumo de Drogas. Informe Final 1996*. Santiago de Chile: CONACE; 1996.

Chile. Ministerio del Interior. Consejo Nacional para el Control de Estupefacientes. *Estudio nacional de drogas en la población escolar de Chile*. Santiago de Chile: CONACE; 2001. www.conacedrogas.cl/inicio/obs_naci_encu_tema2.php

Chumlea WC, Schubert CM, Roche AF, Kulin HE, Lee PA, Himes JH, Sun SS. Age at menarche and racial comparisons in US girls. *Pediatrics* 2003;111(1):110–113.

Clubb RL. Promoting non-tobacco use in childhood. *Pediatr Nurs* 1991;17(6):566–570.

Coatsworth JD, Pantin H, Szapocznik J. Familias unidas: a family-centered ecodevelopmental intervention to reduce risk for problem behavior among Hispanic adolescents. *Clin Child Fam Psicol Rev* 2002;5(2):113–132.

Cobb RW, Elder CD. *Participation in American Politics: The Dynamics of Agenda Building*. Baltimore: Johns Hopkins University Press; 1983.

Cohen S, Wills TA. Stress, social support, and the buffering hypothesis. *Psychol Bull* 1985;98(2):310–357.

Comín Bertrán E, Torrubia Beltri R, Mor Sancho J. Relación entre personalidad, actitudes y consumo de alcohol, tabaco y ejercicio en escolares. *Gac Sanit* 1998;12(6):255–262.

Comisión Económica para América Latina y el Caribe (NU). *Panorama social de América Latina*. Santiago de Chile: CEPAL; 1997.

Comisión Económica para América Latina y el Caribe (NU). *Panorama social de América Latina*. Santiago de Chile: CEPAL; 2000.

Comisión Económica para América Latina y el Caribe (NU). *Anuario estadístico de América Latina y el Caribe, 2000*; Santiago de Chile: CEPAL; 2001.

Communication for Development Roundtable Report. New York: United Nations Population Fund; 2001.

Conger R, Conger K, Elder G, Lorenz F, Simons R. Economic stress, coercive family process and developmental problems of adolescents. *Child Dev* 1994;65:541–561.

Conger R, Conger K, Elder G, Lorenz F, Simons R, Whitbeck L. A family process model of economic hardship and adjustment of early adolescent boys. *Child Dev* 1992;63:526–541.

Conger R, Conger K, Elder G, Lorenz F, Simons R, Whitbeck L. Family economic stress and adjustment of early adolescent girls. *Dev Psychol* 1993;29:206–219.

Conger R, Neppl T, Kim KJ, Scaramella L. (2003). Angry and aggressive behavior across three generations: a prospective, longitudinal study of parents and children. *J Abnorm Child Psychol* 2003;31(2):143–160.

Conger R, Patterson G, Ge X. It takes two to replicate: a mediational model for the impact of parents' stress on adolescent adjustment. *Child Dev* 1995;66(1):80–97.

Connell RW. *Gender and Power*. Stanford, California: Stanford University Press; 1987.

Conway K, Tunks M, Henwood W, Casswell S. Te Whanau Cadillac—A waka for change. *Health Educ Behav* 2000;27(3):339–350.

Crawford AM, Pentz MA, Chou CP, Li C, Dwyer JH. Parallel developmental trajectories of sensation seeking and regular substance use in adolescents. *Psychol Addict Behav* 2003;17(3):179–192.

Crawford MA, Balch GI, Mermelstein R, and the Tobacco Control Network Writing Group. Responses to tobacco control policies among youth. *Tob Control* 2002;11:14–19.

Crosby RA, DiClemente RJ, Wingood GM, Cobb BK, Harrington K, Davies SL, Hook EW III, Oh MK. HIV/STD-protective benefits of living with mothers in perceived supportive families: a study of high-risk African American female teens. *Prev Med* 2001;33(3):175–178.

Crosby RA, DiClemente RJ, Wingood GM, Harrington K, Davies S, Hook EW III, Oh MK. Low parental monitoring predicts subsequent pregnancy among African-American adolescent females. *J Pediatr Adolesc Gynecol* 2002;15(1):43–46.

Crosby RA, DiClemente RJ, Wingood GM, Lang DL, Harrington K. Infrequent parental monitoring predicts sexually transmitted infections among low income African American female adolescents. *Arch Pediatr Adolesc Med* 2003;157(2):169–173.

Cullen KW, Baranowski T, Smith SP. Using goal setting as a strategy for dietary behavior change. *J Am Diet Assoc* 2001;101(5):562–566.

Cullen KW, Bartholomew LK, Parcel GS, Koehly L. Measuring stage of change for fruits and vegetable consumption in 9-to-12-year-old girls. *J Behav Med* 1998;21(3):241–254.

Cullen KW, Koehly LM, Anderson C, Baranowski T, Prokhorov A, Basen-Engquist K, Wetter D, Hergenroeder A. Gender differences in chronic disease risk behaviors through the transition out of high school. *Am J Prev Med* 1999;17(1):1–7.

Cunha, MM, Soares MJ, Novo SM, da Costa SP. Evaluation of an educative proposal on AIDS with teenagers of a public school in João Pessoa City, Paraiba, Brazil. *Rev Bras Cienc Saude* 1998;2(1/3): 27–32.

Damasio AR. *Descartes' Error: Emotion, Reason and the Human Brain*. New York: Putnam; 1994.

Damasio AR. On some functions of the human prefrontal cortex. In Grafma J, Holyoak KJ, Boller F (eds.). *Structure and Functions of the Human Prefrontal Cortex*. New York: New York Academy of Sciences; 1995.

Danaher A, Kato C. *Making a Difference in Your Community: A Guide for Policy Change*. Toronto: Ontario Public Health Association; 1995.

Davis M, Baranowski T, Resnicow K, Baranowski J, Doyle C, Smith M, Wang DT, Yaroch A, Herbert D. Gimme five fruit and vegetables for fun and health: process evaluation. *Health Educ Behav* 2000;27(2):167–176.

Derevensky JL, Gupta R, Della-Cioppa G. A developmental perspective of gambling behavior in children and adolescents. *J Gambl Stud* 1996;12(1):49–66.

DeVries H, Backbier E. Self-efficacy as an important determinant of quitting among pregnant women who smoke: the Phi-pattern. *Prev Med* 1994;23(2):167–174.

DeVries H, Weijts W, Dijkstra M, Kok G. The utilization of qualitative and quantitative data for health education program planning, implementation and evaluation: a spiral approach. *Health Educ Q* 1992;19(1): 101–115.

DiClemente CC, Crosby RA, Kegler MC (eds). *Emerging Theories in Health Promotion Practice and Research: Strategies for Improving Public Health*. San Francisco: Jossey-Bass; 2002.

DiClemente CC, Prochaska JO. Self change and therapy changes of smoking behavior: a comparison of processes of change in cessation and maintenance. *Addit Behav* 1982;192;7(2):133–142.

DiClemente RJ, Crosby RA, Wingood GM. Enhancing STD/HIV prevention among adolescents: the importance of parental monitoring. *Minerva Pediatr* 2001;54(3):171–177.

DiClemente RJ, Wingood GM. A randomized controlled trial of an HIV sexual risk-reduction intervention for young African-American women. *JAMA* 1995;274(16):1271–1276.

DiClemente RJ, Wingood GM, Crosby R, Sionean C, Cobb BK, Harrington K, Davies S, Hook EW III, Oh MK. Parental monitoring: association with adolescents' risk behaviors. *Pediatrics* 2001;107(6):1363–1368.

Dietz WH. Childhood weight affects adult morbidity and mortality. *J Nutr* 1998;128(2 Suppl.):411S–414S.

Dietz WH, Bland MG, Gortmaker SL, Molloy M, Schmidt TL. Policy tools for the childhood obesity epidemic. *J Law Med Ethics* 2002;30(3 Suppl.):83–87.

DiNardo J, Lemieux T. Alcohol, marijuana, and American youth: the unintended consequences of government regulation. *J Health Econ* 2001;20:991–1010.

Dinn WM, Aycicegi A, Harris CL. Cigarette smoking in a student sample: neurocognitive and clinical correlates. *Addict Behav* 2004;29(1):107–126.

Dishion TJ, McCord J, Poulin F. When interventions harm: peer groups and problem behavior. *Am Psychol* 1999;54(9):755–764.

Dishion TJ, Patterson G, Stoolmiller M, Skinner M. Family, school, and behavioral antecedents to early adolescent involvement with antisocial peers. *Dev Psychol* 1991;27:172–180.

Dryfoos JG. *Safe Passage, Making It through Adolescence in a Risky Society. What Parents, Schools, and Communities Can Do*. New York: Oxford University Press; 1998.

Dugan S, Lloyd B, Lucas K. Stress and coping as determinants of adolescent smoking behavior. *J Appl Soc Psychol* 1999;29:870–888.

Durant RH, Barkin S, Krowchuk DP. Evaluation of a peaceful conflict resolution and violence prevention curriculum for sixth-grade students. *J Adolesc Health* 2001;28(5):386–393.

Education Development Center. The science of healthy behavior: using research-based policies and strategies to promote health and safety. *Mosaic* 2001;3(2).

Eggleston E, Jackson J, Rountree W, Pan Z. Evaluation of a sexuality education program for young adolescents in Jamaica. *Rev Panam Salud Pública* 2000;7(2):102–112.

Emery S, White MM, Pierce JP. Does cigarette price influence adolescent experimentation? *J Health Econ* 2001;20:261–270.

Eng E, Parker E. Natural helper models to enhance a community's health and competence. In DiClemente CC, Crosby RA, Kegler MC (eds.). *Emerging Theories in Health Promotion Practice and Research: Strategies for Improving Public Health*. San Francisco: Jossey-Bass; 2002.

Eng E, Smith J. Natural helping functions of lay health advisers in breast cancer education. *Breast Cancer Res Treat* 1995;(35):23–29.

Ennett ST, Bauman KE. Peer group structure and adolescent cigarette smoking: a social network analysis. *J Health Soc Behav* 1993;34(3):226–236.

Ennett ST, Bauman KE. Adolescent social networks: school, demographic, and longitudinal considerations. *J Adolesc Res* 1996;11:194–215.

Ennett ST, Bauman KE, Koch GG. Variability in cigarette smoking within and between adolescent friendship cliques. *Addict Behav* 1994;19(3):295–305.

Ennett ST, Tobler NS, Ringwalt CL, Flewelling RL. How effective is drug abuse resistance education? A meta-analysis of Project DARE outcome evaluations. *Am J Public Health* 1994;84 (9):1394–1401.

Enright R, Levy V, Harris D, Lapsley D. Do economic conditions influence how theorists view adolescents? *J Youth Adolesc* 1987;16:541–560.

Ensminger M, Lamkin R, Jacobson N. School leaving: a longitudinal perspective including neighborhood effects. *Child Dev* 1996;67:2400–2416.

Epstein HT. Brain growth spurts. On the beam. *New Horizons for Learning* 1981;I(2).

Erickson EH. *Identity: Youth and Crisis*. New York: Norton; 1968.

Erickson EH. *The Life Cycle Completed*. New York: Norton; 1982.

Evans G, Newnham J. *The Dictionary of World Politics: A Reference Guide to Concepts, Ideas and Institutions*. New York: Harvester Wheatsheaf; 1992.

Everett S, Price J. Students' perceptions of violence in the public schools: The Metlife Survey. *J Adolesc Health Care* 1995;17:345–352.

Family Health International. *Behavior Change Communication Handbook Series*. Research Triangle Park, NC: FHI; 1996.

Farrely MC, Bray JW, Zarkin GA, Wendling BW. The joint demand for cigarettes and marijuana: evidence from the National Household Surveys on Drug Abuse. *J Health Econ* 2001;20(1):51–68.

Fasick F. On the "invention" of adolescence. *J Early Adolesc* 1994;14:6–23.

Feighery E, Ribisl KM, Scleicher N, Lee RE, Halvorson S. Cigarette advertising and promotional strategies in retail outlets: results of a statewide survey in California. *Tob Control* 2001;10:184–188.

Feighery E, Rogers T. *Building and Maintaining Effective Coalitions*. Palo Alto, California: Stanford Center for Research in Disease Prevention; 1990.

Feudo R, Vining-Bethea S, Shulman LC, Shedlin MG, Burleson JA. Bridgeport's Teen Outreach and Primary Services (TOPS) project: a model for raising community awareness about adolescent HIV risk. *J Adolesc Health* 1998;23(2 Suppl.):49–58.

Fichtenberg CM, Glantz SA. Youth access interventions do not affect youth smoking. *Pediatrics* 2002;109(6):1088–1092.

Figueroa ME, Kincaid DL, Rani M, Lewis G. *Communication for Social Change. An Integrated Model for Measuring the Process and Its Outcomes*. Baltimore: Johns Hopkins University Center for Communication Programs; 2002. (The Communication for Social Change Working Paper Series No. 1).

Filgueira C, Filgueira F, Fuentes A. *Critical Choices at a Critical Age: Youth Emancipation Paths and School Attainment in Latin America*. Washington, DC: Inter-American Development Bank; 2001. (Research Network Working Paper #R–432).

Fishbein M. AIDS and behavior change: an analysis based on the theory of reasoned action. *Int J Psychol* 1990;24:37–56.

Fishbein M, Ajzen I. *Belief, Attitude, Intention, and Behavior: An Introduction to Theory and Research*. Reading, Massachusetts: Addison-Wesley; 1975.

Flanagan D, Williams C, Mahler H. *Peer Education in Projects Supported by AIDSCAP: A Study of Twenty-one Projects in Africa, Asia and Latin America*. Arlington, Virginia: AIDSCAP/FHI; 1996.

Fleishman JA, Sherbourne CD, Crystal S, Collins RL, Marshall GN, Kelly M, Bozzette SA, Shapiro MF, Hays RD. Coping, conflictual social interactions, social support, and mood among HIV-infected persons. HCSUS Consortium. *Am J Community Psychol* 2000;28(4):421–453.

Folkman S. Positive psychological states and coping with severe stress. *Soc Sci Med* 1997;45(8):1207–1221.

Folkman S, Lazarus RS. An analysis of coping in a middle-aged community sample. *J Health Soc Behav* 1980;21(3):219–239.

Folkman S, Moskowotz J. Positive affect and the other side of coping. *Am Psychol* 2000;55(6):647–654.

Ford ME. *Motivating Humans: Goals, Emotions and Personal Agency Beliefs*. Newbury Park, California: Sage Publications; 1992.

Forehand R, Biggar H, Kotchic BA. Cumulative risk across family stressors: short- and long-term effects for adolescents. *J Abnorm Child Psychol* 1998;26(2):119–129.

Forster LM, Tannhauser M, Barros HM. Drug use among street children in southern Brazil. *Drug Alcohol Depend* 1996;43(1–2):57–62.

Foshee VA, Bauman KE, Arriaga, XB, Helms RW, Koch GG, Fletcher LG. An evaluation of safe dates, an adolescent dating violence prevention program. *Am J Public Health* 1998;88(1):45–50.

Foxcroft D, Lister-Sharp D, Lowe G, Breen R, Ireland, D. Preventive Programmes for Youth: What Works? Invited paper. World Health Organization European Ministerial Conference on Young People and Alcohol. Stockholm, February 19 to 22, 2001.

Frankish CJ, Green LW, Ratner PA, Chomik T, Larsen C. Health Impact Assessment as a Tool for Population Health Promotion and Public Policy. A report submitted to the Health Promotion Development Division of Health Canada. Vancouver: University of British Columbia; 1996.

Freedman DS, Khan LK, Serdula MK, Dietz WH, Srinivasan SR, Berenson GS. Relation of age at menarche to race, time period, and anthropometric dimensions: the Bogalusa Heart Study. *Pediatrics* 2002;110(4):e43.

Freeman R, Sheiham A. Understanding decision-making processes for sugar consumption in adolescence. *Community Dent Oral Epidemiol* 1997;25(3):228–232.

Freire P. *Pedagogy of the Oppressed*. New York: Seabury Press; 1970.

Frenk J. Dimensions of health system reform. *Health Policy* 1994;27(1):19–34.

Frijda NH. Emotions are functional, most of the time. In Ekman P, Davidson RJ (eds.). *The Nature of Emotion: Fundamental Questions.* (Series in Affective Science). New York: Oxford University Press; 1994.

Fuhrman T, Holmbeck GN. A contextual-moderator analysis of emotional autonomy and adjustment in adolescence. *Child Dev* 1995;66(3):793–811.

Fukuyama F. *Our Posthuman Future. Consequences of the Biotechnology Revolution*. New York: Farrar, Straus and Giroux; 2002.

Fulk J, Boyd B. Emerging theories of communication in organizations. *J Management* 1991;17(2):407–446.

Furano K, Roaf PA, Styles MB, Branch AY. *Big Brothers/Big Sisters: A Study of Program Practices*. Philadelphia: Public/Private Ventures; 1993.

Fuster JM. *The Prefrontal Cortex*. New York: Raven Press; 1989.

Fuster JM. Memory and planning: Two temporal perspectives of frontal lobe function. In Jasper HH, Riggio S, Goldman-Rakic PS (eds.). *Epilepsy and the Functional Anatomy of the Prefrontal Lobe*. New York: Raven Press; 1995.

Galduróz JCF, Noto AR, Carlini EA. Tendencies do uso de drogas no Brasil. São Paulo: Centro Brasileiro de Informacões Sobre Drogas Psicotrópicas (CEBRID); 1997.

Gans J. *America's Adolescents: How Healthy Are They?* Chicago: American Medical Association; 1990.

Gardner J. *Building Community*. Washington, DC: Independent Sector Studies Program; 1991.

Gaughan M. Predisposition and pressure: mutual influence and adolescent drunkenness. *Connections* 2003;25(2):17–31.

Gazzaniga MS, Heatherton TF. *Psychological Science. Mind, Brain, and Behavior*. New York: WW Norton and Company; 2003.

Gebhardt WA. *Health Behavior Goal Model: Towards a Theoretical Framework for Health Behavior Change*. Leiden, the Netherlands: Leiden University; 1997. (Health Psychology Series No.2).

Gebhardt WA, Maes S. Integrating social-psychological frameworks for health behavior research. *Am J Health Behav* 2001;25(6):528–536.

Gerrard M, Gibbons FX, Benthin A, Hessling RM. A longitudinal study of the reciprocal nature of risk behaviors and cognitions in adolescents: what you do shapes what you think, and vice versa. *Health Psychol* 1996;155:344–354.

Gerrard M, Gibbons FX, Warner TD. Perceived vulnerability to AIDS and AIDS preventive behavior: a critical review of the evidence. In Pryor JB, Reeder G (eds.). *The Social Psychology of HIV Infection*. Hillsdale, New Jersey: Erlbaum; 1993.

Gilligan C. *In a Different Voice: Psychological Theory and Women's Development*. Cambridge, Massachusetts: Harvard University Press; 1982.

Gilligan C, Taylor JM, Tolamn D, Sullivan A, Pleasants P, Dorney J. *The Relational World of Adolescent Girls Considered to Be at Risk*. Monograph. Cambridge, Massachusetts: Harvard Graduate School of Education; 1992.

Gillis AJ. Determinants of a health-promoting lifestyle: an integrative review. *J Adv Nurs* 1993;18(3):345–353.

Glanz K, Lewis F, Rimer B. *Health Behavior and Health Education: Theory, Research, and Practice*. 2nd ed. San Francisco: Jossey-Bass; 1997.

Glanz K, Rimer B. *Theory at a Glance: A Guide for Health Promotion Practice*. Washington, DC: National Institutes of Health; 1995.

Glanz K, Rimer B, Lewis FM. *Health Behavior and Health Education: Theory, Research, and Practice*. 3rd ed. San Francisco: Jossey-Bass; 2002.

Glantz SA, Jamieson P. Attitudes toward secondhand smoke, smoking and quitting among young people. *Pediatrics* 2000;106(6):E82.

Glied S. Is smoking delayed smoking averted? *Am J Public Health*;2003;93(3):412–416.

Godin G. Le non-usage du tabac. Une application des théories sociales cognitives à l'étude des comportements lies a la santé. *Alcoologie* 1996;18(3):237–242.

Golding JF, Harpur T, Brent-Smith H. Personality, drinking and drug-taking correlates of cigarette smoking. *Pers Individ Dif* 1983;4:703–706.

Goldman LK, Glantz SA. Evaluation of antismoking advertising campaigns. *JAMA* 1998;279:772–777.

Goldman-Rakic PS. Anatomical and functional circuits in prefrontal cortex of nonhuman primates: relevance to epilepsy. In Jasper HH, Riggio S, Goldman-Rakic PS (eds.). *Epilepsy and the Functional Anatomy of the Frontal Lobe*. New York: Raven Press; 1995a.

Goldman-Rakic PS. Architecture of the prefrontal cortex and the central executive. In Grafman J, Holyoak KJ, Boller F (eds.). *Structure and Functions of the Human Prefrontal Cortex*. New York: New York Academy of Sciences; 1995b.

Goodman RM, Steckler A, Kegler MC. Mobilizing organizations for health enhancement. Theories of organizational change. In Glanz K, Lewis F, Rimer B (eds.). *Health Behavior and Health Education: Theory, Research and Practice*. 2nd ed. San Francisco: Jossey-Bass; 1997.

Gotthoffer AR. Localization of relevant consequences in anti-drinking and driving PSAs (public service announcements): a new approach to targeting underage college students? *Health Mark Q* 1999;6(2):17–37.

Graber JA, Lewisohn PM, Seeley JR, Brooks-Gunn J. Is psychopathology associated with the timing of pubertal development? *J Am Acad Child Adolesc Psychiatry* 1997;36:1768–1776.

Green LW, Gottlieb N, Parcel G. Diffusion theory extended and applied. In Ward WB (ed.). *Advances in Health Education and Promotion*. Greenwich, Connecticut: JAI Press; 1987.

Green LW, Kreuter MW. *Health Promotion Planning: An Educational and Ecological Approach*. 3rd ed. Mountain View, California: Mayfield Publishing; 1999.

Green LW, Kreuter MW. Fighting back or fighting themselves? Community coalitions against substance abuse and their use of best practices. *Am J Prev Med* 2002;23(4):303–306.

Greenspan SI. *Infancy and Early Childhood: The Practice of Clinical Assessment and Intervention with Emotional and Developmental Challenges*. Madison, Connecticut: International Universities Press; 1992.

Greenspan SI. *Playground Politics: The Emotional Development of Your School-aged Child*. Reading, Massachusetts: Addison Wesley Publishers; 1993.

Greenspan SI. *The Challenging Child: Understanding, Raising, and Enjoying the Five "Difficult" Types of Children*. Reading, Massachusetts: Addison Wesley Publishers; 1995.

Greenspan SI. *The Growth of the Mind and the Endangered Origins of Intelligence*. Reading, Massachusetts: Addison Wesley Publishers; 1997a.

Greenspan SI. *Developmentally-Based Psychotherapy*. New York: International Universities Press; 1997b.

Greenspan SI. *The Secure Child*. Cambridge, Massachusetts: Perseus Books; 2002.

Greenspan SI, Shanker S. *Toward a Psychology of Global Interdependency: A Framework for International Collaboration. Council on Human Development*. Monographs. Bethesda, Maryland: Interdisciplinary Council on Learning and Developmental Disabilities; 2002.

Greenspan SI, Shanker S. *The Evolution of Intelligence: How Language, Consciousness, and Social Groups Come About*. Cambridge, Massachusetts: Perseus Books; 2003.

Greydanus D, Farrel E, Sladkin K, Rypma C. The gang phenomenon and the American teenager. *Adolesc Med State Art Review* 1990;1:55–70.

Griffin KW, Botvin GJ, Epstein JA, Doyle MM, Diaz T. Psychosocial and behavioral factors in early adolescence as predictors of heavy drinking among high school seniors. *J Stud Alcohol* 2000a;61(4):603–606.

Griffin KW, Botvin GJ, Scheier LM, Diaz T, Miller NL. Parenting practices as predictors of substance use, delinquency, and aggression among urban minority youth: moderating effects of family structure and gender. *Psychol Addict Behav* 2000b;14(2):174–184.

Groebel J. Media access and media use among 12-year-olds in the world. In von Feilitzen C, Carlsson U (eds). *Children and Media: Image, Education, Participation*. Gotenborg, Sweden: UNESCO International Clearinghouse on Children and Violence on the Screen; 1999.

Grossman M, Markowitz S. Alcohol regulation and violence on college campuses. In Grossman M, Hsieh CR (eds.). *Economic Analysis of Substance Use and Abuse: The Experience of Developed Countries and Lessons for Developing Countries*. Cheltenham, United Kingdom: Edward Elgar; 2001.

Grothberg E. *A Guide to Promoting Resilience in Children. Strengthening the Human Spirit. The International Resilience Project from the Early Childhood Development: Practice and Reflections*. The Hague, Netherlands: Bernard van Leer Foundation; 1995.

Guizar-Vázquez JJ, Rosales-López A, Ortiz-Jalomo R, Nava-Delgado SE, Salamanca-Gómez F. Edad de aparición de la espermaturia (espermaquia) en 669 niños mexicanos y su relación con caracteres sexuales secundarios y talla. *Bol Med Hosp Infant Mex* 1992;49(1):12–17.

Gullone E. The development of normal fear: a century of research. *Clin Psychol Rev* 2000;20(4):429–451.

Gupta R, Derevensky JL. Adolescent gambling behavior: a prevalence study and examination of the correlates associated with excessive gambling. *J Gambl Stud* 1998;14:319–345.

Gupta R, Derevensky JL, Hardoon K. Youth gambling attitudes and perceptions. Paper presented at the annual meeting of the Canadian Foundation on Compulsive Gambling. Ontario, Canada, April 2001.

Gur RC, Mozley LH, Mozley PD, Resnick SM, Karp JS, Alavi A, Arnold SE, Gur RE. (1995). Sex differences in regional cerebral glucose metabolism during a resting state. *Science* 1995;267:528–531.

Gurian M. *Boys and Girls Learn Differently!* 1st ed. San Francisco: Jossey-Bass; 2001.

Guzman BL, Schlehofer-Sutton MM, Villanueva CM, Dello Stritto ME, Casad BJ, Feria A. Let's talk about sex: how comfortable discussions about sex impact teen sexual behavior. *J Health Commun* 2003;8:583–598.

Hale S. A global developmental trend in cognitive processing speed. *Child Dev* 1990;61(3):653–663.

Hall P, Land H, Parker R, Webb A. *Change, Choice and Conflict in Social Policy*. London: Heinemann; 1975.

Hallfors D, Cho H, Livert D, Kadushin C. Fighting back against substance abuse: are community coalitions winning? *Am J Prev Med* 2002;23(4):237–245.

Hallfors D, Godette D. Will the 'principles of effectiveness' improve prevention practice? Early findings from a diffusion study. *Health Educ Res* 2002;17(4):461–470.

Hanson MJ. Cross-cultural study of beliefs about smoking among teenaged females. *West J Nurs Res* 1999;21(5):635–651.

Hardoon K, Derevensky J, Gupta R. *An Examination of the Influence of Familial, Emotional, Conduct, and Cognitive Problems, and Hyperactivity upon Youth Risk-Taking and Adolescent Gambling Problems*. Report to the Ontario Problem Gambling Research Centre. R & J Child Development Consultants, Inc. Montreal, Quebec; 2002. www.education.mcgill.ca/gambling/en/researchreports.htm

Hatcher JL, Scarpa J. Encouraging Teens to Adopt a Safe, Healthy Lifestyle: A Foundation for Improving Future Adult Behaviors. Research Brief. Washington, DC: Child Trends; 2002.

Hauser S, Powers S, Noam G. *Adolescents and Their Families*. New York: Free Press; 1991.

Hawkins K, Hane AC. Adolescents' perceptions of print cigarette advertising: a case for counteradvertising. *J Health Commun* 2000;5(1):83–96.

Hayward C, Sanborn K. Puberty and the emergence of gender differences in psychopathology. *J Adolesc Health* 2002;30S:49–58.

Health Canada; 2003. http://www.hc-sc.gc.ca/hppb/phdd/determinants/index.html#determinants

Heaney CA, Israel A. Social networks and social support. In Glanz K, Lewis F, Rimer B (eds.). *Health Behavior and Health Education: Theory, Research and Practice*. 2nd ed. San Francisco: Jossey-Bass; 1997.

Heaney CA, Israel A. Social networks and social support. In Glanz K, Lewis F, Rimer B (eds.). *Health Behavior and Health Education: Theory, Research and Practice*. 3rd ed. San Francisco: Jossey-Bass; 2002.

Heath EM, Coleman KJ. Adoption and institutionalization of the Child and Adolescent Trial for Cardiovascular Health (CATCH) in El Paso, Texas. *Health Promot Pract* 2003;4:157–164.

Henderson M, Wight D, Raab G, Abraham C, Buston K, Hart G, Scott S. Heterosexual risk behavior among young teenagers in Scotland. *J Adolesc* 2002;25(5):483–494.

Herman-Giddens ME, Slora EJ, Wasserman RC, Bourdony CJ, Bhapkar MV, Koch GG, Hasemeier CM. Secondary sexual characteristics and menses in young girls seen in office practice: a study from the Pediatric Research in Office Settings Network. *Pediatrics* 1997;99(4):505–512.

Herman-Stahl M, Petersen AC. The protective role of coping and social resources for depressive symptoms among young adolescents. *J Youth Adolesc* 1996;25:733–754.

Hernández JT, DiClemente RJ. Self-control and ego identity development as predictors of unprotected sex in late adolescent males. *J Adolesc* 1992;15(4):437–447.

Hill J. Early adolescence: a framework. *J Early Adolesc* 1983;3:1–21.

Hilton JF, Walsh MM, Massouredis CM, Drues JC, Grady DG, Ernster VL. Planning a spit tobacco cessation intervention: identification of beliefs associated with addiction. *Addict Behav* 1994;19(4):381–391.

Hochbaum GM. *Public Participation in Medical Screening Programs: A Sociopsychological Study*. Washington, DC: Government Printing Office; 1958. (PHS Publication No. 572).

Hoelscher DM, Kelder SH, Murray N, Cribb PW, Conroy J, Parcel GS. Dissemination and adoption of the Child and Adolescent Trial for Cardiovascular Health (CATCH): a case study in Texas. *J Public Health Manag Pract* 2001;7(2):90–100.

Holden D, Pendergast K, Austin D. *Literature Review for American Legacy Foundation's Statewide Youth Movement against Tobacco Use*. Research Triangle Park, North Carolina: Center for Economics Research; 2000.

Holmes TH, Rahe RH. The social readjustment rating scale. *J Psychosom Res* 1967;11:213–218.

Holtgrave DR, Tinsley BJ, Kay LS. Encouraging risk reduction: a decision-making approach to message design. In Meibach E, Parrot RL (eds.). *Designing Health Messages: Approaches from Communication Theory and Public Health Practice*. Newbury Park, California: Sage Publications; 1995.

Holzmann R, Jorgensen S. Social risk management: a new conceptual framework for social protection and beyond. Washington, DC: World Bank; 2000. (Social Protection Discussion Paper No. 006).

Hopenhayn M, Bello A. *Discriminación étnico-racial y xenofobia en América Latina y el Caribe*. Santiago de Chile: CEPAL; 2001. (Serie Políticas Sociales No. 47).

Howard D, Qiu Y, Boekeloo B. Personal and social contextual correlates of adolescent dating violence. *J Adolesc Health* 2003;33(1):9–17.

Huebner AJ, Howell LW. Examining the relationship between adolescent sexual risk-taking and perceptions of monitoring, communication, and parenting styles. *J Adolesc Health* 2003;33(2):71–78.

Huston AC, Donnerstein E, Fairchild H, Feshbach ND, Katz PA, Murria JP, Rubinstein EA, Wilcox BL, Zuckerman D. *Big World, Small Screen: The Role of Television in American Society*. Lincoln, Nebraska: University of Nebraska Press; 1992.

Inciardi JA, Surrat HL. Children in the streets of Brazil: drug use, crime, violence and HIV risks. *Subst Use Misuse* 1998;33(7):1461–1480.

Infante F. *Five Open Questions to Resilience: A Review of Recent Literature*. The Hague, Netherlands: Bernard van Leer Foundation; 2001.

Infante F. Resilience and biculturalism: the Latino experience in the U.S. In Grothberg E (ed). *Resilience for Today: Gaining Strength from Adversity*. Westport, Connecticut: Greenwood Publishing Group; 2003.

Instituto Promundo. Project H. *Manual Series Working with Young Men*. Rio de Janeiro: Instituto Promundo; 2001.

Inter-American Observatory on Drugs; 2002. http://www.cicad.oas.org/oid/

International Centre for Youth Gambling Problems and High Risk Behaviors. *General Facts about Youth Gambling*. Montreal, Quebec: McGill University; 2003.

International Labor Organization. Convention Concerning Minimum Age for Admission to Employment (C138). Geneva: ILO; 1973. http://www.ilo.org/public/english/employment/skills/recomm/instr/c_138.htm

International Resilience Research Project. Birmingham, Alabama: Civitan International Research Center, University of Alabama; 2004. http://www.circ.uab.edu/cpages/resbg1.htm

Iowa State University. *Strengthening Families Program: For Parents and Youth 10–14*; 1997. http://www.extension.iastate.edu/sfp/

Israel BA. Social networks and health status: linking theory, research and practice. *Patient Couns Health Educ* 1982;4(2):65–79.

Jacinto C, Lasida J, Ruetalo J, Berruti E. Formación para el trabajo de jóvenes de sectores de pobreza en América Latina. Qué desafios y qué estrategias. In *Por una segunda oportunidad. La formación para el trabajo de jóvenes vulnerables*. Montevideo, Cinterfor/OIT; 1998.

Jackson C, Henriksen L, Dickinson D. Alcohol-specific socialization, parenting behaviors and alcohol use by children. *J Stud Alcohol* 1999;60(3):362–367.

Jackson C, Henriksen L, Fosheen VA. The authoritative parenting index: predicting health risk behaviors among children and adolescents. *Health Educ Behav* 1998;25(3):319–337.

Jacobs, DF. Juvenile gambling in North America: an analysis of long term trends and future prospects. *J Gambl Stud* 2000;16(2–3):119–152.

Jemmott JB III, Jemmott LS. Abstinence and safer sex HIV risk-reduction interventions for African American adolescents: a randomized controlled trial. *JAMA* 1998;279(19):1529–1536.

Jemmott JB III, Jemmott LS. HIV behavioral interventions for adolescents in community settings. In Peterson JL, DiClemente RJ (eds). *Handbook of HIV Prevention*. New York: Kluwer Academic/Plenum Publishers; 2000.

Jernigan D. Effective Policies to Control Alcohol Consumption and Problems in the Region of the Americas: A Review of the Evidence. Washington, DC: Pan American Health Organization; 2002. (Internal Document SDE/RA).

Jessor R. Reply-risk behavior in adolescence: a psychosocial framework for understanding and action. *Dev Rev* 1992;12:374–390.

Jessor R. Successful adolescent development among youth in high-risk settings. *Am Psychol* 1993;48(2):117–126.

Johns Hopkins University Center for Communications Program. Evaluated Programmes-JHU/CCP. *The Drum Beat* 1999;28. www.comminit.com

Joint United Nations Programme on HIV/AIDS. *Epidemic Update*. Geneva: UNAIDS; 1998.

Joint United Nations Programme on HIV/AIDS. *Summary Booklet of Best Practices*. Geneva: UNAIDS; 1999a.

Joint United Nations Programme on HIV/AIDS. *Peer Education and HIV/AIDS: Concepts, Uses and Challenges*. UNAIDS Best Practice Collection. Geneva: UNAIDS; 1999b.

Joint United Nations Programme on HIV/AIDS/World Health Organization/Pan American Health Organization. *HIV and AIDS in the Americas: An Epidemic with Many Faces*. UNAIDS, WHO, PAHO; 2001.

Jomphe Hill A, Boudreau F, Amyot E, Dery D, Godin G. Predicting the stages of smoking acquisition according to the theory of planned behavior. *J Adolesc Health* 1997;21:107–115.

Joyce T, Kaestner R. State reproductive policies and adolescent pregnancy resolution: the case of parental involvement laws. *J Health Econ* 1996;15:579–607.

Jucovy L. *Building Relationships: A Guide for New Mentors*. Portland, Oregon: Northwest Regional Educational Laboratory; 2001.

Juszczak L, Sadler L. Adolescent development: setting the stage for influencing health behaviors. *Adolesc Med* 1999;10(1):7–17.

Kaldmae P, Priimagi L, Raudsepp A, Grintchak M, Valjaots E. Promotion of safer sexual behavior and HIV/STD prevention among adolescent students and army recruits. *AIDS Care* 2000;12(6):783–788.

Kaplan PS, The State University of New York at Stony Brook, and Suffolk County Community College. *Adolescence*. Boston: Houghton Mifflin Company; 2004.

Kazis R. *Improving the Transition from School to Work in the United States*. Cambridge, Massachusetts: Jobs for the Future; 1993.

Kegler MC, Wyatt VH. A multiple case study of neighborhood partnerships for positive youth development. *Am J Health Behavior* 2003;27(2):156–169.

Kelly JA. Behavior changes and disease prevention: Medical College of Wisconsin research shows effectiveness of HIV/AIDS risk reduction interventions. *WMJ* 2000;99(1):41–43, 47.

Kennedy MG, Mizuno Y, Seals BF, Myllyluoma J, Weeks-Norton K. Increasing condom use among adolescents with coalition-based social marketing. *AIDS* 2000;14(12):1809–1818.

Kenney JW, Reinholtz C, Angelini PJ. Ethnic differences in childhood and adolescent sexual abuse and teenage pregnancy. *J Adolesc Health* 1997;21(1):3–10.

Kerr M, Stattin H, Trost K. To know you is to trust you: parents' trust is rooted in child disclosure of information. *J Adolesc* 1999;22(6):737–752.

Killgore WDS, Oki M, Yurgelun-Todd DA. Sex-specific developmental changes in amygdala responses to affective faces. *Neuroreport* 2001;12(2):427–433.

Kim KJ, Conger RD, Lorenz FO, Elder GH Jr. Parent-adolescent reciprocity in negative affect and its relation to early adult social development. *Dev Psychol* 2001;37(6):775–790.

Kim SC, Crutchfield C, Williams C, Hepler N. Toward a new paradigm in substance abuse and other problem behavior prevention for youth: youth development and empowerment approach. *J Drug Educ* 1998;28(1):1–17.

Kingdon JW. *Agendas, Alternatives, and Public Policies*, 2nd ed. New York: Harper Collins; 1995.

Kipnis D. Accounting for the use of behavior technologies in social psychology. *Am Psychol* 1994;49(3):165–172.

Kirby D. *Emerging Answers: Research Findings on Programs to Reduce Teen Pregnancy.* Summary. Washington, DC: National Campaign to Prevent Teen Pregnancy; 2001.

Kirby D, Korpi M, Adivi C, Weismann J. An impact evaluation of project SNAPP: an AIDS and pregnancy prevention middle school program. *AIDS Educ Prev* 1997;9(1 Suppl.):44–61.

Klepp KI, Ndeki SS, Thuen F, Leshabari M, Seha AM. Predictors of intention to be sexually active among Tanzanian school children. *East Afr Med J* 1996;73(4):218–24.

Kobasa SC. Stressful life events, personality, and health: an inquiry into hardiness. *J Pers Soc Psychol* 1979;37(1):1–11.

Kohlberg L. Moral stages and moralization: the cognitive-development approach. In Lickona T (ed.). *Moral Development and Behavior*. New York: Holt, Rinehart & Winston; 1976.

Kohnstamm GA, Bates JE, Rothbart MK. *Temperament in Childhood*. New York: John Wiley & Sons; 1989.

Kok G, Schaalma H, De Vries H, Parcel G, Paulussen T. Social psychology and health education. *Eur J Soc Psychol* 1996;7:241–282.

Komro KA, Perry CL, Williams CL, Stigler MH, Farbakhsh K, Veblen-Mortenson S. How did Project Northland reduce alcohol use among young adolescents? Analysis of mediating variables. *Health Educ Res* 2001;16(1):59–70.

Kopp CB. Antecedents of self-regulation: a developmental perspective. *Dev Psychol* 1982;18:199–214.

Kotler P, Roberto EL. *Social Marketing Strategies for Changing Public Health Behavior*. New York: Free Press; 1989.

Kremers SP, Brug J, de Vries H, Engels RC. Parenting style and adolescent fruit consumption. *Appetite* 2003;41(1):43–50.

Kwan CM, Love GD, Ryff CD, Essex MJ. The role of self-enhancing evaluations in a successful life transition. *Psychol Aging* 2003;18(1):3–12.

Laflin MT, Moore-Hirschl S, Weis DL, Hayes BE. Use of the theory of reasoned action to predict drug and alcohol use. *Int J Addict* 1994;29(7):927–940.

Langlois MA, Petosa R, Hallam JS. Why do effective smoking prevention programs work? Student changes in social cognitive theory constructs. *J Sch Health* 1999;69(8):326–331.

Laniado-Laborin R, Molgaard CA, Elder JP. Efectividad de un programa de prevención de tabaquismo en escolares mexicanos. *Salud Pública Mex* 1993;35(4):403–408.

Lantz PM, Jacobson PD, Warner KE, Wasserman J, Pollack HA, Berson J, Ahlstrom A. Investing in youth tobacco control: a review of smoking prevention and control strategies. *Tob Control* 2000;9(1):47–63.

Lapsley D, Enright R, Serlin R. Toward a theoretical perspective on the legislation of adolescence. *J Early Adolesc* 1985;5:441–466.

Larraque D, McLean DE, Brown-Peterside P, Ashton D, Diamond B. Predictors of reported condom use in Central Harlem youth as conceptualized by the Health Belief Model. *J Adolesc Health* 1997;21(5):318–327.

Laufer A, Harel Y. The role of family, peers, and school perceptions in predicting involvement in youth violence. *Int J Adolesc Med Health* 2003;15(3):235–244.

Lavoie F, Herbert M, Tremblay R, Vitaro F, Vezina L, McDuff P. History of family dysfunction and perpetration of dating violence by adolescent boys: a longitudinal study. *J Adolesc Health* 2002;30(5):375–383.

Lawson EJ. The role of smoking in the lives of low-income pregnant adolescents: a field study. *Adolescence* 1994;29(113):61–79.

Lazarus RS. Coping theory and research: past, present, and future. *Psychosom Med* 1993;55:234–247.

Lazarus RS, Cohen JB. Environmental stress. In Altman I, Wohlwill JF (eds.). *Human Behavior and Environment*. New York: Plenum; 1977.

Lazarus RS, Folkman S. *Stress, Appraisal and Coping*. New York: Springer; 1984.

Lee V, Croninger R, Linn E, Chen X. The culture of sexual harassment in secondary schools. *Am Educ Res J* 1996;33:383–417.

Lerman, C, Glanz, K. Stress, coping and health behavior. In Glanz K, Lewis F, Rimer B (eds.). *Health Behavior and Health Education: Theory, Research and Practice*. 2nd ed. San Francisco: Jossey-Bass; 1997.

Leung SF, Phelps CE. My kingdom for a drink…? A review of estimates of the price sensitivity of demand for alcoholic beverages. In Hilton ME, Bloss G (eds.). *Economics and the Prevention of Alcohol-related Problems*. Bethesda, MD: National Institute on Alcohol Abuse and Alcoholism; 1993. (NIAAA Research Monograph No. 25).

Levin HS, Culhane KA, Hartmann J, Evankovich K, Mattson AJ, Harwood H, Ringholz G, Ewing-Cobbs L, Fletcher JM. Developmental changes in performance on tests of purported frontal lobe functions. *Dev Neuropsychol* 1991;7:377–396.

Levine PB. Parental involvement laws and fertility behavior. *J Health Econom* 2003;22(5):861–878.

Levy DT, Cummings KM, Hyland A. A simulation of the effects of youth initiation policies on overall cigarette use. *Am J Public Health* 2000;90(8):1311–1314.

Levy DT, Friend KB. A simulation model of tobacco youth access policies. *Journal Health Polit Policy Law* 2000;25(6):1023–1050.

Lewis JM. *Textbook of Child & Adolescent Psychiatry*. 2nd ed. Washington, DC: American Psychiatric Press; 1997.

Leyva GF, Salas RM, Salas SS, Velasco RJ. Conocimiento de las medidas para prevenir el VIH por parte de los adolescentes. *Rev Med IMSS* 1995;33(6):577–580.

Limber SP, Nation MA. Violence within the neighborhood and community. In Trickett PK, Schellenbach CJ (eds.). *Violence Against Children in the Family and the Community*. Washington, DC: American Psychological Association; 1998.

Lloyd B, Lucas K. *Smoking in Adolescence*. London: Routledge; 1998.

Locke EA, Latham GP. *A Theory of Goal Setting and Task Performance*. Englewood Cliffs, New Jersey: Prentice Hall; 1991.

Loewenstein GF, Weber EU, Hsee CK, Welch N. Risk as feelings. *Psychol Bull* 2001;127:267–286.

loveLife. *Behavior Change: the Cornerstone of HIV Prevention*; 2002. http://www.lovelife.org.za

Luepker RV, Perry CL, McKinlay SM, Nader PR, Parcel GS, Stone EJ, Webber LS, Elder JP, Feldman HA, Johnson CC. Outcomes of a field trial to improve children's dietary patterns and physical activity: the Child and Adolescent Trial for Cardiovascular Health. CATCH Collaborative Group. *JAMA* 1996; 275(10):768–776.

Maccoby E. *The Two Sexes: Growing up Apart, Coming Together*. Cambridge, Massachusetts: Belknap/Harvard; 1998.

Maccoby E, Martin J. Socialization in the context of the family: parent-child interaction. In Mussen PH, Hetherington EM (eds.). *Handbook of Child Psychology: Vol. 4: Socialization, Personality and Social Development*. 4th ed. New York: Wiley; 1983.

MacDonald MA, Green LW. Reconciling concept and context: the dilemma of implementation in school-based health promotion. *Health Educ Behav* 2001;28(6):749–768.

MacKellar DA, Valleroy LA, Hoffmann JP, Glebatis D, Lalota M, McFarland W, Westerholm J, Janssen, RS. Gender differences in sexual behaviors and factors associated with nonuse of condoms among homeless and runaway youths. *AIDS Educ Prev* 2000;12(6):477–491.

Maes S, Gebhardt WA. Self-regulation and health behavior: the health behavior goal model. In Boekaerts M, Pintrich PR, Zeidner M (eds.). *Handbook of Self-regulation: Theory, Research and Applications*. San Diego, California: Academic Press; 2000.

Mahoney CA, Thombs DL, Ford OJ. Health belief and self-efficacy models: their utility in explaining college student condom use. *AIDS Educ Prev* 1995;7(1):32–49.

Maibach EW, Cotton D. Moving people to behavior change: a staged social cognitive approach to message design. In Maibach EW, Parrot RL (eds.). *Designing Health Messages: Approaches from Communication Theory and Public Health Practice*. Thousand Oaks: Sage; 1995.

Maibach EW, Rothschild M, Novelli W. Social marketing. In Glanz K, Rimer B, Lewis FM (eds.). *Health Behavior and Health Education: Theory, Research and Practice*. 3rd ed. San Francisco: Jossey-Bass; 2002.

Mandu ENT, Correa AC, Vieira MA. Adolescents' knowledge, values and practices regarding sexually transmitted diseases and AIDS. *Rev Bras Cresc Desenv Hum* 2000;10(1).

Markowitz S, Chatterji P, Kaestner R. Estimating the impact of alcohol policies on youth suicides. *J Ment Health Policy Econ* 2003;6(1):37–46.

Markowitz S, Grossman M. Alcohol regulation and domestic violence towards children. *Contemp Econ Policy* 1998;16(3):309–320.

Martin JD, Ribisi KM, Jefferson D, Houston A. Teen empowerment movement to prevent tobacco use by North Carolina's youth. *N C Med J* 2001;62(5):260–265.

Masten AS. Children who overcome adversity to succeed in life. Minnesota: University of Minnesota, Extension Service; 2000. Available at http://www.extension.umn.edu/distribution/familydevelopment/components/7565_06.html

Masten AS. Ordinary magic: resilient processes in development. *Am Psychol* 2001;56(3):227–238.

Mayhew KP, Flay BR, Mott JA. Stages in the development of adolescent smoking. *Drug Alcohol Depend* 2000;59(1 Suppl.):S61–81.

McAdoo M. Project GRAD's strength is the sum of its parts. *Ford Foundation Report*; spring/summer, 1998.

McAlister A, Perry C, Killen J, Slinkard LA, Maccoby N. Pilot study of smoking, alcohol and drug abuse prevention. *Am J Public Health* 1980;70(7):719–721.

McArthur L, Peña M, Holbert D. Effects of socioeconomic status on the obesity knowledge of adolescents from six Latin American cities. *Int J Obes Relat Metab Disord* 2001;25(8):1262–1268.

McLeroy KR, Bibeau D, Steckler A, Glanz K. An ecological perspective on health promotion programs. *Health Educ Q* 1988;15(4):351–377.

McLoyd V. The impact of hardship on black families and children: psychological distress, parenting and socioemotional development. *Child Dev* 1990;61(2):311–346.

McNeely CA, Nonnemaker JM, Blum R.W. Promoting school connectedness: evidence from the National Longitudinal Study of Adolescent Health. *J School Health* 2002;72(4):138–146.

Medina-Mora ME. Country profile on alcohol in Mexico. In Riley L, Marshall M (eds.). *Alcohol and Public Health in 8 Developing Countries*. Geneva: World Health Organization; 1999.

Mehan HI, Villanueva LH, Lintz A. *Constructing School Success: The Consequences of Untracking Low-achieving Students*. New York: Cambridge University Press; 1996.

Mellin AE, Neumark-Sztainer D, Story M, Ireland M, Resnick MD. Unhealthy behaviors and psychosocial difficulties among overweight adolescents: the potential impact of familial factors. *J Adolesc Health* 2002;31(2):145–153.

Mercer University Students Together Against Negative Decisions (STAND); 1998. http://www.mercer.edu/publications/discoveries/riskybus.htm

Merson MH, Dayton JM, O'Reilly K. Effectiveness of HIV prevention interventions in developing countries. *AIDS* 2000;14(2 Suppl.):S68–S84.

Mesters I, Oostveen T. Why do adolescents eat low nutrient snacks between meals? An analysis of behavioral determinants with the Fishbein and Ajzen model. *Nutr Health* 1994;10(1):33–47.

Michael JL, Colditz GA, Coakley E, Kawachi I. Health behaviors, social networks, and healthy aging: cross-sectional evidence from the nurses' health study. *Qual Life Res* 1999;8:711–722.

Migneault JP, Pallonen UE, Velicer WF. Decisional balance and stage of change for adolescent drinking. *Addict Behav* 1997;22(3):339–351.

Miller JM, DiIorio C, Dudley W. Parenting style and adolescents' reaction to conflict: is there a relationship? *J Adolesc Health* 2002;31(6):463–468.

Minkler M, Wallerstein, N. Improving health through community organization and community building. In Glanz K, Lewis F, Rimer B (eds.). *Health Behavior and Health Education: Theory, Research and Practice.* 2nd ed. San Francisco: Jossey-Bass; 1997.

Minkler M, Wallerstein N. Improving health through community organization and community building. In Glanz K, Rimer B, Lewis F (eds.). *Health Behavior and Health Education: Theory, Research and Practice*. 3rd ed. San Francisco: Jossey-Bass; 2002.

Modell J, Goodman M. Historical perspectives. In Feldman, S, Elliot G (eds.). *At the Threshold: The Developing Adolescent*. Cambridge, Massachusetts: Harvard University Press; 1990.

Molnar BE, Buka SL, Brennan RT, Holton JK, Earls F. A multilevel study of neighborhoods and parent-to-child physical aggression: results from the project on human development in Chicago neighborhoods. *Child Maltreat* 2003;8(2):84–97.

Monitoring the Future. Teen smoking declines sharply in 2002, more than offsetting large increases in the early 1990s. (Press release). Ann Arbor, MI: The University of Michigan News and Information Services; 2002. www.monitoringthefuture.org/press.html

Montgomery KS. Planned adolescent pregnancy: what they needed. *Issues Compr Pediatr Nurs* 2001;24(1):19–29.

Moos RH. *Coping Response Inventory-Youth Form: Professional Manual*. Odessa, Florida: Psychological Assessment Resources Inc; 1993.

Moraes CL, Reichenheim ME. Domestic violence during pregnancy in Rio de Janeiro, Brazil. *Int J Gynaecol Obstet* 2002;79(3):269–277.

Morral AR, McCaffrey DF, Paddock SM. Reassessing the marijuana gateway effect. *Addiction* 2002;97(12):1493–1504.

Mummery WK, Spence JC, Hudec JC. Understanding physical activity intention in Canadian school children and youth: an application of the theory of planned behavior. *Res Q Exerc Sport* 2000;71(2):116–124.

Muss RE. *Theories of Adolescence*. 6th ed. New York: McGraw-Hill; 1996.

Nader PR, Stone EJ, Lytle LA, Perry CL, Osganian SK, Kelder S, Webber LS. Three-year maintenance of improved diet and physical activity: the CATCH cohort. Child and Adolescent Trial for Cardiovascular Health. *Arch Pediatr Adolesc Med* 1999;153(7):695–704.

National Research Council. *Losing Generations*. Washington, DC: National Academy Press; 1993.

Neinstein L. *Adolescent Health Care: A Practical Guide*. 4th ed. Philadelphia: Lippincott, Williams and Wilkins; 2002.

Neumark-Sztainer D. The social environment of adolescents: associations between socioenvironmental factors and health behaviors during adolescence. *Adolesc Med* 1999;10(1):41–55.

NIZW International Centre. Youth & Policy in the Netherlands; 2001. http://www.nizw.nl/

Nolen-Hoeksema S. The role of rumination in depressive disorders and mixed anxiety/depressive symptoms. *J Abnorm Psychol* 2000;109:504–511.

Nolen-Hoeksema S, Girgus JS. The emergence of gender differences in depression during adolescence. *Psychol Bull* 1994;115:424–443.

Nolen-Hoeksema S, Larson J, Grayson C. Explaining the gender difference in depressive symptoms. *J Pers Soc Psychol* 1999;77:1061–1072.

Norris R, Carrol D, Cochrane R. The effects of physical activity and exercise training on psychological stress and well-being in an adolescent population. *J Psychosom Res* 1992;36(1):55–65.

Norton BL, McLeroy KR, Burdine JN, Felix MRJ, Dorsey AM. Community capacity. Concept, theory, and methods. In DiClemente RJ, Crosby RA, Kegler MC (eds.). *Emerging Theories in Health Promotion Practice and Research*. San Francisco: Jossey-Bass; 2002.

Novak SP, Clayton RR. The influence of school environment and self-regulation on transitions between stages of cigarette smoking: a multilevel analysis. *Health Psychol* 2001;20(3):196–207.

Nyswander DB. Education for health: some principles and their applications. *Health Educ Monogr* 1956;14:65–70.

Observatorio Brasileño de Información Sobre Drogas (OBID); 2002. www.obid.senad.gov.br/OBID/Portal

O'Callaghan FV, Callan VJ, Baglioni A. Cigarette use by adolescents: attitude-behavior relationships. *Subst Use Misuse* 1999;34(3):455–468.

O'Callaghan FV, Chang DC, Callan VJ, Baglioni A. Models of alcohol use by young adults: an examination of various attitude-behavior theories. *J Stud Alcohol* 1997;58(5):502–507.

Ollendick T. Violence in youth: where do we go from here? Behavior therapy's response. *Behav Ther* 1996;27(4):485–514.

Ontario Heart Health and Nutrition Resource Centres. *Policies in Action*. Toronto, Ontario; 2002. http://www.hhrc.net/pdfs/toc.pdf

Organización Panamericana de la Salud. *Medios y salud: la voz de los adolescentes. Informe Regional*. Washington, DC: OPS; 2003a. (OPS/FCH/CA No. 1).

Organización Panamericana de la Salud. Visita oficial de la Dra. Mirta Roses Periago, Directora de la OPS, a la República Dominicana, del 14 al 16 de octubre de 2003b.

Orlandi MA, Landers C, Weston R, Haley N. Diffusion of health promotion innovations. In Glanz, K, Lewis FM, Rimer BK (eds.). *Health Behavior and Health Education: Theory, Research and Practice*. San Francisco: Jossey Bass; 1990.

Orpinas P, Kelder S, Frankowski R, Murray N, Zhang Q, McAlister A. Outcome evaluation of a multi-component violence-prevention program for middle schools: the Students for Peace project. *Health Educ Res* 2000;15(1):45–58.

Orpinas P, Murray N, Kelder S. Parental influences on students' aggressive behaviors and weapon carrying. *Health Educ Behav* 1999;26(6):774–787.

Padgett DI, Selwyn BJ, Kelder SH. Ecuadorian adolescents and cigarette smoking: a cross-sectional survey. *Rev Panam Salud Pública* 1998;4(2):87–93.

Pallonen UE, Prochaska JO, Velicer WF, Prokhorov AV, Smith NF. Stages of acquisition and cessation for adolescent smoking: an empirical integration. *Addict Behav* 1998;23(3):303–324.

Palmgreen P, Donohew L, Lorch EP, Hoyle RH, Stephenson MT. Television campaigns and adolescent marijuana use: tests of sensation seeking targeting. *Am J Public Health* 2001;91(2):292–296.

Palmgreen P, Lorch E, Donohew L, Harrington NG, Dsilva M, Helm D. Reaching at-risk populations in a mass media drug abuse prevention campaign: sensation seeking as a target variable. *Drugs Soc* 1995;8(3–4):27–45.

Pan American Health Organization. *Plan of Action for Health and Development of Adolescents and Youth in the Americas 1998–2001*. Washington, DC: PAHO; 1998.

Pan American Health Organization, WHO Collaborating Center on Adolescent Health, University of Minnesota. *A Portrait of Adolescent Health in the Caribbean*; 2000a.

Pan American Health Organization. *Why Should We Invest in Adolescents?* Washington, DC: PAHO; 2000b.

Pan American Health Organization. *Developing Legislation for Tobacco Control: Template and Guidelines*. Washington, DC: PAHO; 2002a.

Pan American Health Organization. *Health in the Americas*. Vol. I. Washington, DC: PAHO; 2002b.

Pan American Health Organization. *Health in the Americas*. Vol. II. Washington, DC: PAHO; 2002c.

Pan American Health Organization. *Quadrennial Report*. Washington, DC: PAHO; 2002d.

Pan American Health Organization/Belize. *Situational Analysis of Adolescent Health in Belize*. Washington, DC: PAHO; 2002e.

Parcel GS, Edmundson E, Perry CL, Feldman HA, O'Hara-Tompkins N, Nader PR, Johnson CC, Stone EJ. Measurement of self-efficacy for diet-related behaviors among elementary school children. *J Sch Health* 1995a;65(1):23–27.

Parcel GS, Erikson MP, Lovato CY, Gottlieb NH, Brink SG, Green LW. The diffusion of school-based tobacco-use prevention programs; project description and baseline data. *Health Educ Res* 1989;4:111–124.

Parcel GS, O'Hara-Tompkins N, Harrist RB, Basen-Engquist K, McCornick LK, Gottlieb NH, Eriksen MP. Diffusion of an effective tobacco prevention program. Part II. Evaluation of the adoption phase. *Health Educ Res* 1995;10(3):297–307.

Parkerson GR Jr, Connis RT, Broadhead WE, Patrick DL, Taylor TR, Tse CK. Disease-specific versus generic measurement of health-related quality of life in insulin-dependent diabetic patients. *Med Care* 1993;31(7):629–637.

Parrot AC. Does cigarette smoking cause stress? *Am Psychol* 1999;54:817–820.

Parson JT, Siegel AW, Cousins JH. Late adolescent risk-taking: effect of perceived benefits and perceived risks on behavioral intentions and behavioral change. *J Adolesc* 1997;20:381–392.

Partnership for a Drug-Free America. Partnership Attitude Tracking Study (PATS). *Transitions: From 5th grade to 8th grade, Tweens and Illegal Drugs*. New York: PDFA; 1999.

Patrick K, Sallis JF, Prochaska JJ, Lydston DD, Calfas KJ, Zabinski M, Wilfley DE, Saelens BE, Brown DR. A multi-component program for nutrition and physical activity change in primary care: PACE + for Adolescents. *Arch Pediatr Adolesc Med* 2001;155:940–946.

Paulussen Th. GW. *Adoption and Implementation of AIDS Education in Dutch Secondary Schools*. Utrecht: National Center for Health Promotion and Health Education; 1994.

Paulussen Th. GW, Kok G, Schaalma HP. Antecedents to adoption of classroom-based AIDS education in secondary schools. *Health Educ Res* 1994;9:485–496.

Paulussen Th. GW, Kok G, Schaalma HP, Parcel GS. Diffusion of AIDS curricula among Dutch secondary school teachers. *Health Educ Q* 1995;22:227–243.

Pearlman DN, Camberg L, Wallace LJ, Symons P, Finison L. Tapping youth as agents for change: evaluation of a peer leadership HIV/AIDS intervention. *J Adolesc Health* 2002;31(1):31–39.

Pechansky F, Barros FC. Problems related to alcohol consumption by adolescents living in the city of Porto Alegre, Brazil. *J Drug Issues* 1995;25(4):735–750.

Pederson W, Clausen SE, Lavik NJ. Patterns of drug use and sensation seeking among adolescents in Norway. *Acta Psychiatr Scand* 1989;79:386–390.

Pender NJ. Motivation for physical activity among children and adolescents. *Annu Rev Res* 1998;16:139–172.

Penfold S, Kirkman R. Social marketing of condoms—an unconventional approach. *J Fam Plann Reprod Health Care* 2002;28(4):218–219.

Perrin KM, Dindial K, Eaton D, Harrison V, Matthews T, Henry T. Responses of seventh grade students to 'do you have a partner with whom you would like to have a baby?' *Psychol Rep* 2000;86(1):109–118.

Perry CL, Komro KA, Veblen-Mortenson S, Bosma L, Munson K, Stigler M, Lytle LA, Forster JL, Welles SL. The Minnesota DARE PLUS Project: creating community partnerships to prevent drug use and violence. *J Sch Health* 2000;70(3):84–88.

Perry CL, Williams CL, Komro KA, Veblen-Mortenson S, Stigler MH, Munson KA, Farbakhsh K, Jones RM, Forster JL. Project Northland: Long-term outcomes of community action to reduce adolescent alcohol use. *Health Educ Res* 2002;17(1):117–132.

Peterson AV, Kealey KA, Mann SL, Marek PM, Sarason IG. Hutchinson Smoking Prevention Project: long-term randomized trial in school-based tobacco use prevention—results on smoking. *J Natl Cancer Inst* 2000;92(24):1979–1991.

Petosa R, Jackson K. Using the health belief model to predict safer sex intentions among adolescents. *Health Educ Q* 1991;18(4):463–476.

Pettit GS, Laird RD, Dodge KA, Bates JE, Criss MM. Antecedents and behavior-problem outcomes of parental monitoring and psychological control in early adolescence. *Child Dev* 2001;72(2):583–598.

Pierce JP, Choi WS, Gilpin EA, Farkas AJ, Berry CC. Tobacco industry promotion of cigarettes and adolescent smoking. *JAMA* 1998;279(7):511–515.

Pierce JP, Distefan JM, Kackson C, White MM, Gilpin EA. Does tobacco marketing undermine the influence of recommended parenting in discouraging adolescents from smoking? *Am J Prev Med* 2002;23(2):73–81.

Pierce JP, Lee L, Gilpin EA. Smoking initiation by adolescent girls, 1944 through 1988: an association with targeted advertising. *JAMA* 1994;23:608–611.

Pipher M. *Reviving Ophelia. Saving the Selves of Adolescent Girls*. New York: Ballantine Books; 1994.

Pleck JH, O'Donnell LN. Gender attitudes and health risk behaviors in urban African American and Latino early adolescents. *Matern Child Health J* 2001;5(4):265–272.

Prochaska JO. *Systems of Psychotherapy: A Transtheoretical Analysis*. Pacific Grove, California: Brooks-Cole; 1979.

Prochaska JO, DiClemente CC. *The Transtheoretical Approach: Crossing Traditional Boundaries of Change*. Homewood, Illinois: Dorsey Press; 1984.

Prochaska JO, DiClemente CC, Norcross JC. In search of how people change: applications to addictive behaviors. *Am Psychol* 1992;47:1102–1114.

Prochaska JO, Velicer WF, Rossi JS, Goldstein MG, Marcus BH, Rakowski W, Fiore C, Harlow LL, Redding CA, Rosenbloom D, Rossi SR. Stages of change and decisional balance for twelve problem behaviors. *Health Psychol* 1994;13:39–46.

Project Northland. University of Minnesota, School of Public Health. Minneapolis, Minnesota; 2003. http://www.epi.umn.edu/projectnorthland/

Prokhorov AV, Hudmon KS, de Moor CA, Kelder SH, Conroy JL, Ordway N. Nicotine dependence, withdrawal symptoms and adolescents' readiness to quit smoking. *Nicotine Tob Res* 2001;3(2):151–155.

Pruitt D, American Academy of Child and Adolescent Psychiatry. *Your Adolescent. Emotional, Behavioral, and Cognitive Development from Early Adolescence through the Teen Years.* New York; Harper Collins; 1999.

Puskar KR, Lamb JM, Bartolovic M. Examining the common stressors and coping methods of rural adolescents. *Nurse Pract* 1993;18(11):50–53.

Raboteg-Saric Z, Rijavec M, Brajsa-Zganec A. The relation of parental practices and self-conceptions to young adolescent problem behaviors and substance use. *Nord J Psychiatry* 2001;55(3):203–209.

Reich RB. *The Work of Nations: Preparing Ourselves for 21st Century Capitalism*. New York: Alfred A. Knopf; 1991.

Resnick MD, Bearman PS, Blum RW, Bauman KE, Harris KM, Jones J, Tabor J, Beuhring T, Sieving RE, Shew M et al. Protecting adolescents from harm. Findings from the National Longitudinal Study on Adolescent Health. *JAMA* 1997;278(10):823–832.

Richard R, Van der Plight J, DeVries N. Anticipated affective reactions and prevention of AIDS. *Br J Soc Psychol* 1995;34:9–21.

Rimal RN. Closing the knowledge-behavior gap in health promotion: the mediating role of self-efficacy. *Health Commun* 2000;12(3):219–237.

Ringbäck Weitoft G, Hjern A, Haglund B, Rosen M. Mortality, severe morbidity and injury in children living with single parents in Sweden: A population-based study. *The Lancet* 2002;361(9354).

Risor H. Reducing abortion: the Danish experience. *Plan Parent Eur* 1989;18(1):17–19.

Rivers K, Aggleton P. Adolescent sexuality, gender and the HIV epidemic. *BETA* 2001;14(2):35–40.

Roberts D. Media and youth: access, exposure and privatization. *J Adolesc Health* 2000;(2 Suppl.):8–14.

Rodríguez-García R, Russell J, Maddaleno M, Kastrinakis M. *The Legislative and Policy Environment for Adolescent Health in Latin America and the Caribbean*. Washington, DC: Pan American Health Organization; 1999.

Rogers EM. *Diffusion of Innovations*. 3rd and 4th eds. New York: Free-Press; 1983, 1995.

Rogers EM, Vaughan PW, Swalehe RM, Rao N, Svenkerud P, Sood S. Effects of an entertainment-education radio soap opera on family planning behavior in Tanzania. *Stud Fam Planning* 1999;30(3):193–211.

Rosen JE. *Formulating and Implementing National Youth Policy: Lessons from Bolivia and the Dominican Republic*. Washington, DC: FOCUS on Young Adults; 2001. http://www.pathfind.org/focus.htm

Rosenstock IM, Stretcher VJ, Becker MH. Social learning theory and the health belief model. *Health Educ Q* 1988;15(2):175–183.

Rothman J. Approaches to Community Intervention. In Rothman J, Erlich JL, Tropman JE (eds.). *Strategies of Community Intervention*. Itasca, Illinois: Peacock Publishers; 2001.

Rothshild ML. Carrots, sticks and promises: a conceptual framework for the management of public health and social issue behaviors. *J Mark* 1999;63:24–37.

Rudd RA, Goldberg J, Dietz W. A five-stage model for sustaining a community campaign. *J Health Commun* 1999;4(1):37–48.

Rudolph K. Gender differences in emotional responses to interpersonal stress during adolescence. *J Adoles Health* 2002;30S:3–13.

Rueter MA, Conger RD. Interaction style, problem-solving behavior and family problem-solving effectiveness. *Child Dev* 1995;66(1):98–115.

Russo MF, Lahey BB, Christ MAG, Frick PJ, McBurnett K, Walker JL, Loeber R, Stouthhamer-Loeber M, Green S. Preliminary development of a sensation seeking scale for children. *Pers Individ Dif* 1991; 12:399–405.

Russo MF, Stoke GS, Lahey BB, Christ MAG, McBurnett K, Loeber R, Stouthhamer-Loeber M, Green SM. A sensation seeking scale in children: further refinement and psychometric development. *J Psychopathol Behav Assess* 1993;15:69–86.

Ryff CD, Keyes CL. The structure of psychological well-being revisited. *J Pers Soc Psychol* 1995;69(4):719–727.

Ryff CD, Lee YH, Essex MJ, Schmutte PS. My children and me: midlife evaluations of grown children and of self. *Psychol Aging* 1994;9(2):195–205.

Sabido M. *El tono: Andanzas teóricas, aventuras prácticas, el entretenimiento con beneficio social*. 1ra. ed. México, DF: Universidad Nacional Autónoma de México; 2002.

Saffer H, Chaloupka F. The effect of tobacco advertising bans on tobacco consumption. *J Health Econ* 2000;19(6):1117–1137.

Saffer H, Grossman M. Beer taxes, the legal drinking age, and youth motor vehicle fatalities. *J Legal Stud* 1987;16(2):351–374.

Sallis JF, Simons-Morton BG, Stone EJ, Corbin CB, Epstein LH, Faucette N, Iannotti RJ, Killen JD, Klesges RC, Petray CK et al. Determinants of physical activity and interventions in youth. *Med Sci Sports Exerc* 1992;24(6 Suppl.):S248–S257.

Salovey P, Rothman AJ, Rodin J. Health behavior. In Gilbert DT, Fiske ST, Lindzey G (eds.). *The Handbook of Social Psychology*. 4th ed. New York: McGraw-Hill; 1998.

Sanderson CA, Cantor N. Social dating goals in late adolescence: implications for safer sexual activity. *J Pers Soc Psychol* 1995;68(6):1121–1134.

Santacruz Giralt ML, Concha-Eastman A. *Barrio adentro. La solidaridad violenta de las pandillas*. San Salvador, El Salvador: Universidad Centroamericana José Simeon Canas; 2001.

Santrock JW. *Adolescence*. 7th ed. New York: McGraw Hill; 1997.

Sargent JD, Dalton MA, Beach ML, Mott LA, Tickle JJ, Ahrens MB, Heatherton TF. Viewing tobacco use in movies. Does it shape attitudes that mediate adolescent smoking? *Am J Prev Med* 2002;22(3):137–145.

Scales P. *A Portrait of Young Adolescents in the 1990s: Implications for Promoting Healthy Growth and Development*. Chapel Hill, North Carolina: Center for Early Adolescence; 1991.

Scales P, Leffert N. *Developmental Assets: A Synthesis of the Scientific Research on Adolescent Development*. Minneapolis, Minnesota: Search Institute; 1999.

Scaramella LV, Conger RD, Spoth R, Simons RL. Evaluation of a social contextual model of delinquency: a cross-study replication. *Child Dev* 2002;73(1):175–195.

Schaalma H, Kok G, Peters L. Determinants of consistent condom use by adolescents: the impact of experience of sexual intercourse. *Health Educ Res* 1993;8:255–269.

Schmitz KH, Lytle LA, Phillips GA, Murray DM, Birnbaum AS, Kubik MY. Psychosocial correlates of physical and sedentary leisure habits in young adolescents: the Teens Eating for Energy and Nutrition at School study. *Prev Med* 2002;34(2):266–278.

Schnoll R, Zimmerman BJ. Self-regulation training enhances dietary self-efficacy and dietary fiber consumption. *J Am Diet Assoc* 2001;101(9):1006–1011.

Schunk DE. Teaching elementary students to self-regulate practice of mathematical skills with modeling. In Schunk DH, Zimmerman BJ (eds.). *Self-regulated Learning: From Teaching to Self-reflective Practice*. New York: Guilford Press; 1998.

Schutt-Aine J, Maddaleno M. *Sexual Health and Development of Adolescents and Youth in the Americas: Program and Policy Implications*. Washington, DC: Pan American Health Organization; 2003.

Search Institute 2004. [Internet site]. Available at: www.search-institute.org. Search Institute. http://www.search-institute.org/research/assets/assetpower/html

Selman RL. A structural-developmental model of social cognition. *Couns Psychol* 1977;6:3–6.

Selvan MS, Ross MW, Kapadia AS, Mathai R, Hira S. Study of perceived norms, beliefs and intended sexual behavior among higher secondary school students in India. *AIDS Care* 2001;13(6):779–788.

Senderowitz J. *Making Reproductive Health Services Youth Friendly*. Washington, DC: FOCUS on Young Adults; 1999. (Research Program and Policy Series).

Sheeber L, Allen N, Davis B, Sorensen E. Regulation of negative affect during mother-child problem solving interactions: adolescent depressive status and family processes. *J Abnorm Child Psychol* 2000;28(5):467–479.

Shimai S, Kawabata T, Nishioka N, Haruki T. Snacking behavior among elementary and junior high school students and its relationship to stress-coping. *Nippon Koshu Eisei Zasshi* 2000;47(1):8–19.

Shoemaker K, Gordon L, Hutchins V, Rom M. Educating Others with Peers: Others Do—Should You? Background Briefing Report. Washington, DC: Georgetown Public Policy Institute/Georgetown University; 1998.

Short MB, Succop PA, Mills L, Stanberry LR, Biro FM, Rosenthal SL. Non-exclusivity in adolescent girls' romantic relationships. *Sex Transm Dis* 2003;30(10):752–755.

SIECUS. *Innovative Approaches to Increase Parent-Child Communication about Sexuality: Their Impact and Examples from the Field*; 2002. www.siecus.org

Siegel M, Albers AB, Cheng DM, Biener L, Rigotti NA. Effect of local restaurant smoking regulations on environmental tobacco smoke exposure among youths. *Am J Public Health* 2004;94(2):321–325.

Sieving RE, Oliphant JA, Blum RW. Adolescent sexual behavior and sexual health. *Pediatr Rev* 2002;23(12).

Simons-Morton B, Hartos J. Application of the authoritative parenting model to adolescent health behavior. In DiClemente CC, Crosby RA, Kegler MC (eds.). *Emerging Theories in Health Promotion Practice and Research: Strategies for Improving Public Health*. San Francisco: Jossey-Bass; 2002.

Singhal A, Rogers E. *Entertainment-Education: A Communication Strategy for Social Change*. Mahwah, New Jersey: Lawrence Erlbaum Associates; 1999.

Siqueira LM, Rolnitzky LM, Rickert VI. Smoking cessation in adolescents: the role of nicotine dependence, stress and coping methods. *Arch Pediatr Adolesc Med* 2001;155(4):489–495.

Slater MD. Sensation-seeking as a moderator of the effects of peer influences, consistency with personal aspirations, and perceived harm on marijuana and cigarette use among younger adolescents. *Subst Use Misuse* 2003;38(7):865–880.

Slovic P, Finucane M, Peters E, MacGregor DG. The affect heuristic. In Gilovich T, Griffin D, Kahneman D (eds.). *Heuristic and Biases*. New York: Cambridge University Press; 2002.

Smith C, Carlson BE. Stress, coping, and resilience in children and youth. *Soc Serv Rev* 1997;71:231–257.

Smith CA, Haynes KN, Lazarus RS, Pope LK. In search of the "hot" cognitions: attributions, appraisals, and their relation to emotion. *J Pers Soc Psychol* 1993;65(5):916–929.

Smith CA, Lazarus RS. Appraisal components, core relational themes, and the emotions. *Cognition and Emotion* 1993;7(3–4):233–269.

Smith KW, McGraw SA, Costa LA, McKinlay JB. A self-efficacy scale for HIV risk behaviors: development and evaluation. *AIDS Educ Prev* 1996;8(2):97–105.

Sonenstein F. *Young Men's Sexual and Reproductive Health: Toward a National Strategy. Framework and Recommendations*. Washington, DC: Urban Institute; 2000. http://www.urban.org

Sowell ER, Thompson PM, Tessner KD, Toga AW. Mapping continued brain growth and gray matter density reduction in dorsal frontal cortex: inverse relationships during postadolescent brain maturation. *J Neurosci* 2001;21(22):8819–8829.

Sports Illustrated for Kids. Omnibus Study. New York: Sports Illustrated for Kids; 1998.

Stanton B, Li X, Cottrell L, Kaljee L. (2001). Early initiation of sex, drug-related risk behaviors, and sensation-seeking among urban, low-income African-American adolescents. *J Natl Med Assoc* 2001;93(4):129–138.

Stanton B, Li X, Pack R, Cottrell L, Harris C, Burns JM. Longitudinal influence of perceptions of peer and parental factors on African American adolescent risk involvement. *J Urban Health* 2002;79(4):536–548.

Statistics Canada. *How Healthy Are Canadians? Annual Report 2003.* Health Reports 2003;14(Suppl.).

Stattin H. Candid, not monitored children run less risk of becoming delinquent. *Lakartidningen* 2001;20;98(25):3009–3013.

Steinberg L. *Adolescence.* 5th ed. New York: McGraw-Hill; 1999.

Steinberg L, Morris AS. Adolescent development. *Annu Rev Psychol* 2001;52:83–110.

Steiner H, Erickson S, Hernández N, Pavelski R. Coping styles as correlates of health in high school students. *J Adolesc Health* 2002;30:326–335.

Stevenson J. The treatment of the long-term sequelae of child abuse. *J Child Psychol Psychiatry* 1999;40(1):89–111.

Stokols D. Translating social ecological theory into guidelines for community health promotion. *Am J Health Promot* 1996;10(4):282–298.

Strasburger VC, Wilson BJ. *Children, Adolescents and the Media.* Newbury Park, California: Sage Publications, Inc.; 2002.

Strauss RS, Rodzilsky D, Burack G, Colin M. Psychosocial correlates of physical activity in healthy children. *Arch Pediatr Adolesc Med* 2001;155:897–902.

Strecher VJ. Seijts GH, Kok GJ, Latham GP, Glasgow R, DeVellis B, Meertens RM, Bulger DW. Goal setting as a strategy for health behavior change. *Health Educ Q* 1995;22(2):190–200.

Stronski SM, Ireland M, Michaud P, Narring F, Resnick MD. Protective correlates of stages in adolescent substance use: a Swiss National Study. *J Adolesc Health* 2000;26(6):420–427.

Sturges JW, Rogers RW. Preventive health psychology from a developmental perspective: an extension of protection motivation theory. *Health Psychol* 1996;15(3):158–166.

Sullivan HS. *The Interpersonal Theory of Psychiatry.* New York: Norton; 1953.

Sussman S, Brannon, BR, Dent CW, Hansen WB, Johnson CA, Flay BR. Relations of coping effort, perceived stress and cigarette smoking among adolescents. *Int J Addict* 1993;28(7):599–612.

Sussman S, Dent CW. One year prospective prediction of drug use from stress-related variables. *Subst Use Misuse* 2000;35:717–735.

Sussman S, Lichtman K, Ritt A, Pallonen UE. Effects of thirty-four adolescent tobacco use cessation and prevention trials on regular users of tobacco products. *Subst Use Misuse* 1999;34(11):1469–1503.

Sussman S, Sussman AN. Praxis in health behavior program development. In Sussman S (ed.). *Handbook of Program Development for Health Behavior Research and Practice.* Newbury Park, California: Sage Publications; 2001.

Takanishi R, Hamburg DA (eds.). *Preparing Adolescents for the 21st Century: Challenges Facing Europe and the United States*. New York: Cambridge University Press; 1996.

Tarter RE, Blackson T, Brigham J, Moss H, Caprara GV. The association between childhood irritability and liability to substance use in early adolescence: a 2-year follow-up study of boys at risk for substance abuse. *Drug Alcohol Depend* 1995;39(3):253–261.

Tavares CH, Haeffner LS, Barbieri MA, Bettiol H, Barbieri MR, Souza L. Idade da menarca em escolares de uma comunidade rural do Sudeste do Brasil. [Age at menarche among schoolgirls from a rural community in southeast Brazil]. *Cad Saude Publica* 2000;16(3):709–715.

Taylor R. Adolescents' perceptions of kinship support and family management practices: association with adolescent adjustment in African American families. *Dev Psychol* 1996;32:687–695.

Taylor SE, Klein LC, Lewis BP, Gruenewald TL, Gurung RA, Updegraff JA. Biobehavioral responses to stress in females: tend-and-befriend, not fight-or-flight. *Psychol Rev* 2000;107:411–429.

Taylor WC, Yancey AK, Leslie J, Murray NG, Cummings SS, Sharkey SA, Wert C, James J, Miles O, McCarthy WJ. Physical activity among African American and Latino middle school girls: consistent beliefs, expectations and experiences across two sites. *Women Health* 1999;30(2).

Teichman M, Barnea Z, Rahav G. Sensation seeking, state and trait anxiety and depressive mood in adolescent substance users. *Int J Addict* 1989;24:87–89.

The Communication Initiative. *Soul Buddyz—South Africa*. Victoria, British Columbia; 2003. Available at http://www.comminit.com/pds12-99/sld-945.html

The Global Youth Tobacco Survey Collaborative Group. Tobacco use among youth: a cross country comparison. *Tob Control* 2002;11:252–270.

The Henry J. Kaiser Family Foundation. Sex on TV; www.kff.org

The National Center on Addiction and Substance Abuse at Columbia University. *The Formative Years: Pathways to Substance Abuse among Girls and Young Women Ages 8–22*. New York: CASA; 2003. www.casacolumbia.org

Thoits PA. Stress, coping, and social support processes: where are we? What next? *J Health Soc Behav* 1995 (1 Suppl.):53–79.

Thomas A, Chess S, Birch HG. *Temperament and Behavior Disorders in Childhood*. New York: Brunner/Mazel; 1968.

Tomeo CA, Field AE, Berkey CS, Colditz GA, Frazier AL. Weight concerns, weight control behaviors and smoking initiation. *Pediatrics* 1999;104:918–924.

Unger JB, Chen X. The role of social networks and media receptivity in predicting age of smoking initiation: a proportional hazards model of risk and protective factors. *Addict Behav* 1999;24(3):371–381.

Unger JB, Rohrbach LA, Howard-Pitney B, Ritt-Olson A, Mouttapa M. Peer influences and susceptibility to smoking among California adolescents. *Subst Use Misuse* 2001;36(5):551–571.

Unger JB, Molina GB, Teran L. Perceived consequences of teenage childbearing among adolescent girls in an urban sample. *J Adolesc Health* 2000;26(3):205–212.

United Nations. Convention on the Rights of the Child. New York: UN; 1989. http://www.unhchr.ch/html/menu3/b/k2crc.htm

United Nations Children's Fund. *Young Health—For a Change*. New York: UNICEF; 1997.

United Nations Children's Fund. *The State of Eastern Caribbean Children*. Bridgetown, Barbados: UNICEF Caribbean Area Office; 1998.

United Nations Children's Fund. *The Progress of Nations*. New York: UNICEF; 2000.

United Nations Population Fund. UNFPA and Adolescents. New York: UNFPA; 1997.

United States. National Youth Anti-Drug Media Campaign. Tween Behavior Brief, Ages 11–13; 1999. http://www.mediacampaign.org/publications/index.html

United States. Department of Health and Human Services. Centers for Disease Control and Prevention. *Reducing Tobacco Use: A Report of the Surgeon General—Executive Summary*. Atlanta, Georgia: CDC; 2000.

United States. Department of Health and Human Services. Center for Substance Abuse Prevention. *Principles of Substance Abuse Prevention. Guide to Science-Based Practices 3*; Washington, DC: CSAP; 2001a.

United States. National Campaign to Prevent Teen Pregnancy with One Voice: America's Adults and Teens Sound Off about Teen Pregnancy. Washington, DC; 2001b.

United States. Department of Health and Human Services. *Youth Violence: A Report of the Surgeon General*. Washington, DC: DHHS; 2001c.

United States. Department of Health and Human Services. Center for Substance Abuse Prevention. *Science-Based Substance Abuse Prevention: A Guide*. Bethesda, Maryland: SAMHSA/CSAP; 2001d.

United States. Department of Health and Human Services. Centers for Disease Control and Prevention. Technical Strategies. National Center for HIV, STD and TB Prevention; 2001e. www.cdc.gov/nchstp/od/gap/text/strategies/default.htm

United States. Department of Health and Human Services. Center for Substance Abuse Prevention. *The Three Keys to Success in Prevention*. Bethesda, Maryland: SAMHSA/CSAP; 2002a.

United States. Office of National Drug Control Policy. National Youth Anti-Drug Media Campaign. Scientific and Situational Bases for the Strategy; 2002b. http://www.mediacampaign.org/publications/strat_statement/basis.html

United States. Office of National Drug Control Policy. National Youth Anti-Drug Media Campaign. Communication Strategy Statement: Target Audiences; 2002c. http://www.mediacampaign.com/publications/strat_statement/contents.html

United States. Department of Health and Human Services. Centers for Disease Control and Prevention. Physical activity levels among children aged 9–13 years–United States, 2002. *Morb Mortal Wkly Rep* 2003a;52(33):785–788.

United States. Department of Health and Human Services. *Results from the 2002 National Survey on Drug Use and Health: National Findings*. Rockville, Maryland: Office of Applied Studies; 2003b. (NHSDA Series H–22, DHHS Publication No. SMA 03–3836).

United States. Department of Health and Human Services. Centers for Disease Control and Prevention. Youth Media Campaign. Resources and Reports; 2004. http://www.cdc.gov/youthcampaign/research/resources.htm

University of California. EatFit Health Promotion Program for Adolescents. UC Davis Nutrition Department; 2004. http://www.eatfit.net/

Urzúa RF. Risk factors and youth: the role of family and community. *J Adolesc Health* 1993;14:619–625.

Valente T. Social network influences on adolescent substance use: an introduction. *Connections* 2003;25(2): 11–16. http://www.sfu.ca/~insna/Connections-Web/Volume25-2/Cover 25-2.htm

Valente TW, Davis RL. Accelerating the diffusion of innovations using opinion leaders. *Ann Am Acad Pol Soc Sci* 1999;566:55–67.

Vaughan PW, Rogers EM, Singhal A, Swalehe RM. Entertainment-education and HIV/AIDS prevention: a field experiment in Tanzania. *J Health Communication* 2000(5 Suppl.):81–100.

Veblen-Mortenson S, Rissel C, Perry CL, Wolfson M, Finnegan JR, Forster J, Wolfson M. Lessons learned from Project Northland: community organization in rural communities. In Bracht N (ed.). *Health Promotion at the Community Level*. Thousand Oaks, California: Sage Publications; 1999.

Vik PW, Culbertson KA, Sellers K. Readiness to change drinking among heavy-drinking college students. *J Stud Alcohol* 2000;61(5):674–680.

Vittes KA, Sorenson SB, Gilbert D. High school students' attitudes about firearms policies. *J Adolesc Health* 2003;33:471–478.

Vygotsky LS. *Thought and Language*. Cambridge, Massachusetts: MIT Press; 1962.

Vygotsky LS. *Mind in Society*. Cambridge, Massachusetts: Harvard University Press; 1978.

Vygotsky LS. Thinking and speech. In *The Collected Works of L.S. Vygotsky*: Vol. 1: *Problems in General Psychology*. New York: Plenum Press; 1987.

Wagenaar AC, Murray DM, Gehan JP, Wolfson M, Forster JL, Toomey TL, Perry CL, Jones-Webb R. Communities Mobilizing for Change on Alcohol: outcomes from a randomized community trial. *J Stud Alcohol* 2000;61(1):85–94.

Wagenaar AC, Murray DM, Toomey TL. Communities Mobilizing for Change on Alcohol (CMCA): effects of a randomized trial on arrest and traffic crashes. *Addiction* 2000;95(2):209–217.

Wagner FA, Anthony JC. Into the world of illegal drug use: exposure opportunity and other mechanisms linking the use of alcohol, tobacco, marijuana and cocaine. *Am J Epidemiol* 2002;155(10):918–925.

Wakefield M, Chaloupka F. Effectiveness of comprehensive tobacco control programs in reducing teenage smoking in the USA. *Tob Control* 2000;9:177–186.

Wakefield M, Flay B, Nichter M, Giovino G. Role of the media in influencing trajectories of youth smoking. *Addiction* 2003;98(1 Suppl.):79–103.

Wall AM, Hinson RE, McKee SA. Alcohol outcome expectancies, attitudes towards drinking and the theory of planned behavior. *J Stud Alcohol* 1998;59(4):409–419.

Wallace LS, Buckworth J, Kirby TE, Sherman WM. Characteristics of exercise behavior among college students: application of social cognitive theory to predicting stage of change. *Prev Med* 2000;31(5):494–505.

Wallach L, Dorfman L, Jernigan D, Themba M. *Media Advocacy and Public Health*. Newbury Park, California: Sage Publications; 1993.

Wallerstein N. Powerlessness, empowerment and health: implications for health promotion programs. *Am J Health Promot* 1992;6(3):197–205.

Walsh SM, Corbett RW. Helping postpartum rural adolescents visualize future goals. *MCN Am J Matern Child Nurs* 1995;20(5):276–279.

Walt G. *Health Policy: An Introduction to Process and Power*. London: Witwatersrand University Press, Johannesburg & Zed Books; 1994.

Walter C. Community building practice. In Minkler M (ed.) *Community Organizing and Community Building to Improve Health*. New Brunswick, New Jersey: Rutgers University Press; 1997.

Wasserman J, Manning W, Newhouse J, Winkler J. The effects of excise taxes and regulations on cigarette smoking. *J Health Econ* 1991;10(1):43–64.

Webber J. Comprehending youth violence: a practical perspective. *Remedial and Special Education* 1997;18(2):94–104.

Weist MD, Cooley-Quille M. Advancing efforts to address youth violence involvement. *J Clin Child Psychol* 2001;30(1):147–151.

Weitoft GR, Hjern A, Haglund B, Rosen M. Mortality, severe morbidity and injury in children living with single parents in Sweden: a population-based study. *Lancet* 2003;361(9354):289–295.

Wenzel L, Glanz K, Lerman C. Stress, coping and health behavior. In Glanz K, Rimer B, Lewis FM (eds.). *Health Behavior and Health Education: Theory, Research and Practice*. 3rd ed. San Francisco: Jossey-Bass; 2002.

Werch CE, DiClemente CC. A multi-component stage model for matching drug prevention strategies and messages to youth stage of use. *Health Educ Res* 1995;9(1):37–46.

Werner E, Smith R. *Overcoming the Odds: High-risk Children from Birth to Adulthood*. Ithaca, New York: Cornell University Press; 1992.

Westera DA, Bennet LR. Population-focused research: a broad-based survey of teens' attitudes, beliefs and behaviors. *Int J Nurs Stud* 1994;31(6):521–531.

Westoff C, Bankole A. *Mass Media and Reproductive Behavior in Africa. Demographic and Health Surveys Analytical Reports No. 2*. Calverton, Maryland: Macro International; 1997.

Whitt M. *Fighting Tobacco: A Coalition Approach to Improving Your Community's Health*. Lansing, Michigan: Department of Public Health; 1993.

Wills TA, Cleary SD. How are social support effects mediated? A test with parental support and adolescent substance use. *J Pers Soc Psychol* 1996;7(5):937–952.

Wills TA, Cleary SD, Filer M, Shinar O, Mariani J, Spera K. Temperament related to early-onset substance use: test of a developmental model. *Prev Sci* 2001a;2(3):145–163.

Wills TA, Sandy JM, Yaeger AM. Moderators of the relationship between substance use level and problems: test of a self-regulation model in middle adolescence. *J Abnorm Psychol* 2002a;111(1):3–21.

Wills TA, Sandy JM, Yaeger AM. Stress and smoking in adolescence: a test of directional hypotheses. *Health Psychol* 2002b;21(2):122–130.

Wills TA, Sandy JM, Yaeger AM, Cleary SD, Shinar O. Coping dimensions, life stress and adolescent substance use: a latent growth analysis. *J Abnorm Psychol* 2001b;110(2):309–323.

Wilson WJ. *The Truly Disadvantaged: The Inner City, the Underclass and Public Policy*. Chicago: University of Chicago Press; 1987.

Wingood GM, DiClemente RJ. The theory of gender and power. A social structural theory for guiding public health interventions. In DiClemente RJ, Crosby RA, Kegler MC (eds.). *Emerging Theories in Health Promotion Practice and Research. Strategies for Improving Public Health*. San Francisco: Jossey-Bass; 2002.

World Bank. *Youth-Strategic Directions for the World Bank*. Washington, DC: World Bank; 2002.

World Health Organization. *Tobacco or Health*. Geneva: WHO; 1989. (WHA42/19).

World Health Organization. *Ottawa Charter for Health Promotion*. Geneva: WHO; 1996.

World Health Organization. *What in the World Works?* International Consultation on Tobacco and Youth. Singapore, 28–30 September 1999. Final Conference Report.

World Health Organization. *Global Status Report: Alcohol and Young People*. Geneva: WHO; 2001.

World Health Organization. Briefing Note 1 on Adolescent Health: Sexual Abstinence. Department of Child and Adolescent Health and Development. Geneva: WHO; 2002a.

World Health Organization. Briefing Note 2 on Adolescent Health: Confidentiality and Parental Consent. Geneva: WHO; 2002b.

World Health Organization. Briefing Note 4 on Adolescent Health: Provision of Information on Sexuality. Geneva: WHO; 2002c.

World Health Organization. *World Report on Violence and Health*. Geneva: WHO; 2002d. http://www5.who.int/violence_injury_prevention/main.cfm?p=0000000682

World Health Organization. Strategy for Child and Adolescent Health and Development. Report by the Secretariat. Fifty-sixth World Health Assembly, 27 March, 2003.

World Health Organization, UNAIDS. Very Young Adolescents: The Hidden Young People. Technical Meeting on 10–14 years old. WHO, Geneva, 29 April–2 May 2003. http://www.who.int/child-adolescent-health/New_Publications/NEWS/NEWS_20/Participants_background.pdf

World Health Organization. HIV/AIDS and Young People: WHO Takes Action. Brief, March 2004. Geneva: WHO; 2004a.

World Health Organization. Noncommunicable Disease Prevention and Health Promotion Web site; 2004b. http://www.who.int/hpr/physactiv/population.groups.shtml

Wu T, Mendola P, Buck GM. Ethnic differences in the presence of secondary sex characteristics and menarche among US girls: the Third National Health and Nutrition Examination Survey, 1988–1994. *Pediatrics* 2001;110(4):752–757.

Yep GA. HIV prevention among Asian-American college students: does the health belief model work? *J Am Coll Health* 1993;41(5):199–205.

Zamboni BD, Crawford I, Williams P. Examining communication and assertiveness as predictors of condom use: implications for HIV prevention. *AIDS Educ Prev* 2002;12(6):492–504.

Zimmerman MA, Bingenheimer JB, Notaro PC. Natural mentors and adolescent resiliency: a study with urban youth. *Am J Community Psychol* 2002;30(2):221–243.

Zucker D, Hopkins RS, Sly DF, Urich J, Kershaw JM, Solari S. Florida's "truth" campaign: a counter-marketing, anti-tobacco media campaign. *J Public Health Manag Pract* 2000;6(3):1–6.

Zuckerman M. Sensation seeking, risk taking, and health. In Janisse MP (ed.). *Individual Differences, Stress and Health*. New York: Springer-Verlag; 1988.

Zuckerman M. *Behavioral Expressions and Biosocial Bases of Sensation Seeking*. Cambridge University Press; 1994.

Zuckerman M, Kolin I, Price L, Zoob I. Development of a sensation seeking scale. *J Consult Psychol* 1964;28:477–482.

Selected List of Web Resources on Adolescence and Health Behaviors

Communication and Media
- Centers for Disease Control and Prevention. Youth Media Campaign Resources and Reports. http://www.cdc.gov/youthcampaign/research/resources.htm
- The Communication Initiative. http://www.comminit.com/adolescents
- Henry J. Kaiser Family Foundation. Study of Entertainment Media. http://www.kff.org/entmedia/index.cfm
- Population Media Center. http://www.populationmedia.org/index.html

Education
- Educational Resources Information Center. Topics related to ethnic minority, rural, small school, and migrant education. http://www.ael.org/page.htm?&index=752&pd=1&pv=x
- Latin American Youth Center. http://www.layc-dc.org/

Latin American and Caribbean Bibliographic Databases Search
- Adolescent Virtual Health Library. (Spanish only). http://www.adolec.org/
- Pan American Health Organization. Family and Community Health Area, Child and Adolescent Health Unit. http://www.paho.org/adolescence
- Virtual Health Library. (English, Portuguese, Spanish). http://bases.bvs.br/public/scripts/php/page_show_main.php?lang=en&form=simple

Mental Health
- American Academy of Child and Adolescent Psychiatry. Facts for Families. http://www.aacap.org/publications/factsfam/index.htm
- National Institute of Mental Health. Child and Adolescent Mental Health. http://www.nimh.nih.gov/healthinformation/childmenu.cfm
- Substance Abuse and Mental Health Services Administration. National Mental Health Information Center. http://www.mentalhealth.org/topics

Physical Activity and Nutrition
- University of California, UC-Davis Nutrition Department. EatFit Health Promotion Program for Adolescents. http://groups.ucanr.org/nutrition/Eatfit%5FHealth%5FPromotion%5Fprogram%5Ffor%5FAdolescents/
- World Health Organization. Child and Adolescent Health and Development. http://www.who.int/child-adolescent-health/OVERVIEW/AHD/adh_over.htm
- World Health Organization. Noncommunicable Disease Prevention and Health Promotion. http://www.who.int/hpr/physactiv/children.youth.shtml

Policy
- Education Development Center. "The Science of Healthy Behavior: Using Research-Based Policies and Strategies to Promote Health and Safety." *Mosaic*, Fall 2001, Vol. 3, No. 2. http://main.edc.org/mosaic/Mosaic5/toc5.asp

- FOCUS on Young Adults. Pathfinder International. "Formulating and Implementing National Youth Policy: Lessons from Bolivia and the Dominican Republic," by J.E. Rosen (2001).
  http://www.pathfind.org/pf/pubs/focus/pubs/bolivia.pdf
- Health Canada. What Determines Health?
  http://www.hc-sc.gc.ca/hppb/phdd/determinants/index.html
- The Health Communication Unit. Policy Development Resources.
  http://www.thcu.ca/infoandresources/policy_resources.htm#tp
- NIZW International Centre. Youth Policy in the Netherlands. (English and Dutch).
  http://www.youthpolicy.nl/smartsite.htm?id=3298
- Ontario Heart Health and Nutrition Resource Centres. *Policies in Action*.
  http://action.web.ca/home/nutritio/readingroom_details.shtml?x=18889
- Ontario Public Health Association. *Making a Difference in Your Community: A Guide for Policy Change*, by A. Danaher and C. Kato (1995).
  http://www.thcu.ca/infoandresources/policy_resources.htm#tp
- U.N. Convention on the Rights of the Child. http://www.unhchr.ch/html/menu3/b/k2crc.htm
- The World Bank. Children and Youth.
  http://wbln0018.worldbank.org/HDNet/hddocs.nsf/ChildrenandYouth/566328FF4C7BDDCB85256AED0066F4FA?OpenDocument

Sexual and Reproductive Health

- Centers for Disease Control and Prevention Global AIDS Program. National Center for HIV, STD, and TB Prevention. Technical Strategies.
  http://www.cdc.gov/nchstp/od/gap/text/strategies/default.htm
- Family Health International. Focus on Youth. http://www.fhi.org/en/Youth/index.htm
- loveLife Initiative. http://www.lovelife.org.za
- National Campaign to Prevent Teen Pregnancy. http://www.teenpregnancy.org/Default.asp?bhcp=1
- Pathfinder International. Adolescents.
  http://www.pathfind.org/site/PageServer?pagename=Priorities_Adolescents
- National Center for Health Statistics. *Sexual Activity and Contraceptive Practices among Teenagers in the United States, 1988 and 1995*, by J.C. Abma and F.L. Sonenstein (2002).
  http://www.cdc.gov/nchs/data/series/sr_23/sr23_021.pdf
- Sexuality Information and Education Council. "Innovative Approaches to Increase Parent-Child Communication about Sexuality: Their Impact and Examples from the Field" (2002).
  http://www.siecus.org/pubs/pubs0004.html#REPORT
- Urban Institute. *Young Men's Sexual and Reproductive Health: Toward a National Strategy. Framework and Recommendations*, by F. Sonenstein (2000). http://www.urban.org
- Youth and HIV. (English, French, Italian, Spanish). http://www.youthandhiv.org
- YouthNet. Family Health International. http://www.fhi.org/en/youth/youthnet/ynetindex.html

Tobacco, Alcohol, and Drug Use Prevention

- American Legacy Foundation. http://www.americanlegacy.org
- Campaign for Tobacco-Free Kids Research Center.
  http://tobaccofreekids.org/research/factsheets/index23.shtml
- Center for Substance Abuse Prevention. The Three Keys to Success in Prevention.
  http://www.northeastcapt.org/science/default.asp
- Inter-American Observatory on Drugs. (English and Spanish).
  http://www.cicad.oas.org/oid/default.htm
- Monitoring the Future. Studies on teen substance use. http://www.monitoringthefuture.org
- National Council on Addiction and Substance Abuse. *The Formative Years: Pathways to Substance Abuse among Girls and Young Women Ages 8–22* (2003).
  http://www.casacolumbia.org/pdshopprov/shop/category.asp?catid=2
- National Council for Drug Control. Ministry of the Interior, Chile. Results of a national study of drug use among schoolchildren conducted in 2003. (Spanish only).
  http://www.conacedrogas.cl/inicio/obs_naci_encu_tema2.php

- National Institute on Alcohol Abuse and Alcoholism, National Institute of Health. *Haga la diferencia. Hable con sus hijos sobre el uso del alcohol*. (Publication in Spanish for parents to discuss alcohol use with their children).
  http://www.niaaa.nih.gov/publications/SpanParents.pdf
- Office of National Drug Control Policy. National Youth Anti-Drug Media Campaign.
  http://www.mediacampaign.org
- Project Northland. University of Minnesota School of Public Health.
  http://www.epi.umn.edu/projectnorthland/Default.Html
- Tobacco Control Network. http://www.tobaccocontrol.com

Violence
- Children and Youth in Organized Armed Violence. (English, Portuguese, Spanish).
  http://www.coav.org.br
- Department of Health and Human Services. *Youth Violence: A Report of the Surgeon General* (2001).
  http://www.surgeongeneral.gov/library/youthviolence/
- International Center for the Prevention of Crime.
  http://www.crime-prevention-intl.org/publications.php?type=REPORT
- National Center for Injury Prevention and Control. Youth Violence.
  http://www.cdc.gov/ncipc/factsheets/yvfacts.htm
- Public Safety and Emergency Preparedness Canada. National Crime Prevention Strategy. (English and French). http://www.prevention.gc.ca/en/index.asp
- World Health Organization. *World Report on Violence and Health* (2002). (English, French, Russian).
  http://www.who.int/violence_injury_prevention/violence/world_report/wrvh1/en/

Other related resources:
- ConflictWeb. Resource on conflict prevention, mitigation, and management; conflict resolution, recovery, and post-conflict reconstruction. http://www.usaid.gov/regions/afr/conflictweb/
- University of Virginia. Virginia Youth Violence Project. Effective Methods for Youth Violence Prevention and School Safety. http://youthviolence.edschool.virginia.edu/
- The World Bank Group. Policy Research on the Causes and Consequences of Conflict in Developing Countries. http://www.worldbank.org/research/conflict/crime.htm

Youth Development
- Child Trends. "Building a Better Teenager: A Summary of 'What Works' in Adolescent Development," by K.A. Moore and J. Zaff. Publication # 2002-57, November 2002.
  http://www.childtrends.org
- International Resilience Research Project (2004). Civitan International Research Center, University of Alabama. http://www.circ.uab.edu/cpages/resbg1.htm
- Iowa State University. Strengthening Families Program: For Parents and Youth 10–14.
  http://www.extension.iastate.edu/sfp/sfpback.html
- Search Institute. Youth Developmental Assets.
  http://www.search-institute.org/research/assets/assetpower.html
- Society for Adolescent Medicine. http://www.adolescenthealth.org
- University of Minnesota. "Children Who Overcome Adversity to Succeed in Life," by A.S. Masten (2002).
  http://www.extension.umn.edu/distribution/familydevelopment/components/7565_06.html

Youth Employment
- Inter-American Development Bank. "Latin American Youth in Transition: A Policy Paper on Youth Unemployment in Latin America and the Caribbean," by C. Fawcett (2002).
  http://www.eldis.org/static/DOC11803.htm
- International Labor Organization. Convention Concerning Minimum Age for Admission to Employment (C138). http://www.ilo.org/ilolex/english/convdisp2.htm

- International Labor Organization. Inter-American Research and Documentation Centre on Vocational Training. Youth, Training, and Employment (English and Spanish). http://www.cinterfor.org.uy/public/english/region/ampro/cinterfor/index.htmhttp:/

Youth Participation

- Adolescentes por la vida. Web site developed in Argentina by adolescents for adolescents featuring health news and related topics of interest. (Spanish only).
http://www.adolescentesxlavida.com.ar/index2.htm
- Ecoclubes. International youth movement promoting citizen participation in improving community environmental health. (English, French, Portuguese, Spanish).
http://www.ecoclubes.org/index_ing.html
- Mercer University (1998). Students Together against Negative Decisions (STAND).
http://www.mercer.edu/publications/discoveries/riskybus.htm